Arthritis: Diagnosis and Treatment

Arthritis: Diagnosis and Treatment

Edited by **Sharlton Pierce**

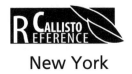

New York

Published by Callisto Reference,
106 Park Avenue, Suite 200,
New York, NY 10016, USA
www.callistoreference.com

Arthritis: Diagnosis and Treatment
Edited by Sharlton Pierce

International Standard Book Number: 978-1-63239-772-0 (Hardback)

Printed in the United States of America.

Contents

Preface

Arthritis is a disorder related to joints. The symptoms of this disease are characterized by severe pain, weight loss, tenderness, stiffness, etc. Osteoarthritis, lupus, gout, and rheumatoid arthritis are some common forms of this disease. The aim of this book is to present researches that have transformed this discipline and aided its advancement. It is a valuable compilation of topics, ranging from the basic to the most complex advancements made in development of new medications and diagnostic treatments. Orthopedics, professionals and students actively engaged in this field will find this book full of crucial and unexplored concepts.

Significant researches are present in this book. Intensive efforts have been employed by authors to make this book an outstanding discourse. This book contains the enlightening chapters which have been written on the basis of significant researches done by the experts.

Finally, I would also like to thank all the members involved in this book for being a team and meeting all the deadlines for the submission of their respective works. I would also like to thank my friends and family for being supportive in my efforts.

Editor

Multifaceted role of TNF-α during the pathogenesis of rheumatoid arthritis

Ramanjaneya V. R. Mula, Rangaiah Shashidharamurthy[*]

Department of Pharmaceutical Sciences, Philadelphia College of Osteopathic Medicine, School of Pharmacy, Suwanee, USA
Email: [*]rangaiahsh@pcom.edu

ABSTRACT

Tumor necrosis factor alpha (TNF-α) a cytokine has been shown to be the key player during the pathogenesis of several autoimmune inflammatory disorders (presumably sterile inflammation) including rheumatoid arthritis (RA). Several studies have shown that TNF-α is mainly involved in the proinflammatory responses. However recent studies have reported multifunctional role of TNF-α during the development of RA. Therefore, in this article we have highlighted the distinct functions of TNF-α during pathogenesis of RA.

Keywords: Cytokines; Tumor Necrosis Factor-α; Rheumatoid Arthritis; Inflammation

1. TNF-α AS CHEMO-ATTRACTANT AT SYNOVIAL JOINTS FOR CD4+ T CELLS

The organization of infiltrated cells in the arthritic microenvironment resembles the secondary lymphoid organ including the presence of CD4+ T cells [1]. Typically, in secondary lymphoid organs the presence of chemokine gradient is necessary for the localization of T cells, especially to interact maximally with antigen presenting cells [2]. The cytokine TNF-α plays a crucial role during the pathogenesis of RA [3]. The focal immunological function of TNF-α is thought to be the induction of several proinflammatory cytokines and stimulate the effector immune cells through interaction with TNF-α receptors. In addition TNF-α is also known to act as chemoattractant for various cells including T cells [4,5]. However, the additional role of TNF-α in early phase of T cell migration to arthritic microenvironment, especially adhesion

and transmigration through endothelium is not clear. Therefore, Rossol et al. [6] observed that the interactions of TNF-α and TNFRI are necessary for T-cell migration into synovium using in vitro and ex vivo experiments.

"The results of Rossol et al. [6] study show that the interaction of TNF-α with receptor type1 (TNFR1) is indeed a migratory stimulus for CD4+ T cells in RA patients which is a TNF-α gradient dependent".

In this article, the authors used horizontally oscillating microtome for synovial sections and confocal as well as fluorescent microscopic methods to follow the T lymphocyte migration. They also collected the migrated T lymphocytes for phenotyping. The in vitro transwell experiment was performed to ascertain that TNF-α is indeed required for T cell migration. In support of this, they also carried out the ex vivo T cell migration assay using synovial tissue section from RA patients by coincubating with autologous peripheral CD4+ T cells. The migrated CD4+ T cells in the tissue sections were visualized by Fluorescent microscopy. The results showed that only the CD4+ T cells form RA patients migrated into synovial tissue but not from the healthy controls. In continuation with this observation, they found that the expression of TNFR1 and ICAM-1 is necessary for activated CD4+ T cells to migrate into synovium. Subsequent flow cytometry results of cells isolated from synovial tissue show that expression of TNFR1 is specific in transmigrated activated CD4+ T cells but not in control healthy volunteer CD4+ T cells. Taken together, these results suggest that the TNF-α is necessary for CD4+ T cell migration in arthritic joints. At the conclusive point the goal of the investigation on the role of TNF-α in synovium which was proven concretely as a potential chemoattractnat may possibly pave way to develop therapy of TNF-α inhibitors as well as new approaches that can be more focused towards targeting T-cells that express TNFR1 in excess.

---

[*]Corresponding author.

2. DISTINCT EFFECT OF TNF-α ON MACROPHAGES AND FIBROBLAST-LIKE SYNOVIOCYTES DURING RA

A step-by-step manifestation of synovial inflammation in RA quietly transforms into chronic inflammation through elevated levels of many inflammatory mediators [7] of which TNF-α plays a key role during synovial inflammation. Both macrophages and fibroblast-like synovial cells (FLS) are most prominent among multiple cell types for prolonged synovial inflammation [8,9] in RA. In addition, TNF-α secreted at the arthritic microenvironment is known to influence these two cells differently. Activation of macrophages through TNF-α is transient, while the FLS are responsible for prolonged synovial inflammation [10]. The distinct role of TNF-α in activating the macrophages and FLS is not clearly understood. However, it can be postulated that the main function of macrophages is to promote the inflammation and later dampen the inflammation by triggering the tissue repair mechanism as protective role to avoid the local and systemic toxicity caused by high levels of inflammatory mediators [11]. Therefore, they may transiently respond to the TNF-α to initiate the inflammation in the early phase. Whereas, since FLS normal function is to create a mechanical platform of synovium [12] and usually never exposes to foreign antigens, therefore they may lack the haemostatic mechanism to control their activation during RA. However, the molecular mechanism of FLS activation leading to prolonged synovial inflammation is not clearly understood. An attempt to investigate the possible mechanism was carried out by Lee *et al.* [13] have shown that TNF-α induced FLS activation leads to uncontrolled NF-κB signaling in FLS resulting in secretion of cytokines, chemokines and metalloproteinases for longer period of time leading to persistent synovial inflammation.

"*TNF-α induces prolonged canonical NF-κB signaling resulting in uncontrolled production of inflammatory mediators contributing to the persistent synovial inflammation during RA through FLS but not macrophages. In other words FLS may be the contributing cell type for chronic inflammation during RA*".

The authors studied the distinct functional role of TNF-α using macrophages and FLS. The signaling mechanisms of NF-κB were elucidated by western blot analyses and the protein involvement in transcriptional regulation was analyzed by histone acetylation, chromatin accessibility, and NF-κB, p65 and RNA polymerase II (Pol II) occupancy at the interleukin-6 (IL-6) promoter using chromatin immunoprecipitation and restriction enzyme accessibility assays. Lee *et al.* have shown macrophage and FLS stimulation by TNF-α is transient and

sustained respectively during the inflammatory RA condition. The feedback inhibition of inflammatory responses mediated by ABIN-3, IRAK-M, SOCS-3, ATF-3 and STAT-3 are expressed at high level in macrophages while at a low level in FLS. This may be a contributing factor for persistence of synovial inflammation in RA through FLS. Further, TNF-α facilitated histone modification and increased accessibility for RNA polymerase II at IL-6 promoter site resulting in secretion of proinflammatory cytokine IL-6 in FLS. Taken together this investigation has shown that sustained inflammatory response by FLS through TNF-α mediated inflammatory gene transcriptions and protein expressions prolong the synovial inflammation. This may pave a way to make FLS as an additional target in countering the unresolved synovitis.

3. DIFFERENTIAL FUNCTION OF TNF-α DURING INFLAMMATION AND OSTEOCLASTOGENESIS IN RA

TNF-α, a proinflammatory cytokine initiates the inflammatory response leading to edematic joint and subsequent bone destruction during the development of rheumatoid arthritis [3]. The bone destruction is mainly mediated by osteoclast, a cell of myeloid origin (OC). OC differentiation, maturation and activation are primarily mediated by RANKL and its receptor RANK. Recent studies have shown that TNF-α can magnify the process of osteoclastogenesis in the presence of RANKL [14-16] as an additional role apart from its proinflammatory response. It has been shown that monoclonal antibody therapy (infliximab, etanercept and adalimumab) against TNF-α, though inhibited/reduced the bone erosion after the treatment, the clinical symptoms of inflammation were not affected [17]. Nonetheless, the mechanism of the biphasic effect of biological TNF-α inhibitors was not yet fully understood. Therefore, Binder *et al.* [18] investigated the fundamental mechanism of TNF-α during RA by *in vitro* studies and human TNF-α (hTNF) transgenic destructive arthritis mouse model. Binder *et al.* have shown the differential effects of TNF-α on osteoclastogenesis and bone erosion activity using above mentioned mouse model of experimental arthritis.

"*High level of TNF-α is required for osteoclastogenesis than to initiate the inflammation at the synovial joints. Hence, low doses of TNF-α inhibitor used in present investigation lead to expression of low levels of TNF-α, which impede osteoclastogenesis but do not inhibit synovial inflammation. Therefore, high levels of TNF-α inhibitors are required to inhibit both inflammation and bone resorption*".

The authors have chosen monocytes derived from spleen cells and tested the osteoclastogenesis *in vitro* using different concentrations of TNF-α inhibitor adalimumab and activator RANKL. An hTNF-transgenic destructive arthritis mouse model was employed for *in vivo* studies of inhibition of osteoclast precursors by the therapeutic. The dose dependent differential effect of TNF-α on osteoclastogenesis though countered with low doses of immunotherapeutic inhibitor adalimumab even in the absence of RANKL, the inflammation of synovium was not affected. These data suggested that TNF-α alone can activate the osteoclasts. The mRNA levels of proinflammatory mediators such as IL-1, matrix metalloproteinase (MMP) 3, and MMP13 are significantly upregulated in untreated hTNF-transgenic mice compared to hTNF-transgenic mice treated with high concentration (10 mg/kg body weight) of adalimumab. Whereas low dose (0.1 mg/kg) did not have any affect. Osteoclast associated genes such as NF-ATc1, cathepsin K, c-Fms, and M-CSF were also upregulated at higher dose but, interestingly not at lower dose. These data suggest that antiresorptive activity of TNF-α was not affected at lower concentration but not synovial inflammation. Taken together Binder *et al.* [18] exemplified the need of controlling both cartilage destruction as well as inflammation mediated by TNF-α during the treatment of rheumatoid arthritis.

4. ACKNOWLEDGEMENTS

This work was supported by American Heart Association award (11SDG5710004) to R.S. The authors declare no competing financial interests.

REFERENCES

[1] Lundy, S.K., Sarkar, S., Tesmer, L.A. and Fox, D.A. (2007) Cells of the synovium in rheumatoid arthritis. T lymphocytes. *Arthritis Research & Therapy*, 9, 202. http://dx.doi.org/10.1186/ar2107

[2] Crotty, S. (2011) Follicular helper CD4 T cells (TFH). *Annual Review of Immunology*, 29, 621-663. http://dx.doi.org/10.1146/annurev-immunol-031210-101400

[3] Feldmann, M. and Maini, R.N. (2001) Anti-TNF alpha therapy of rheumatoid arthritis: What have we learned? *Annual Review of Immunology*, 19, 163-196. http://dx.doi.org/10.1146/annurev.immunol.19.1.163

[4] de Jong, A.L., Green, D.M., Trial, J.A. and Birdsall, H.H. (1996) Focal effects of mononuclear leukocyte transendothelial migration: TNF-alpha production by migrating monocytes promotes subsequent migration of lymphocytes. *Journal of Leukocyte Biology*, 60, 129-136.

[5] Green, D.M., Trial, J. and Birdsall, H.H. (1998) TNF-alpha released by comigrating monocytes promotes transendothelial migration of activated lymphocytes. *The Journal of Immunology*, 161, 2481-2489.

[6] Rossol, M., Schubert, K., Meusch, U., Schulz, A., Biedermann, B., Grosche, J., Pierer, M., Scholz, R., Baerwald, C., Thiel, A., Hagen, S. and Wagner, U. (2013) Tumor necrosis factor receptor type I expression of CD4+ T cells in rheumatoid arthritis enables them to follow tumor necrosis factor gradients into the rheumatoid synovium. *Arthritis & Rheumatism*, 65, 1468-1476. http://dx.doi.org/10.1002/art.37927

[7] Riegsecker, S., Wiczynski, D., Kaplan, M.J. and Ahmed, S. (2013) Potential benefits of green tea polyphenol EGCG in the prevention and treatment of vascular inflammation in rheumatoid arthritis. *Life Sciences*, 93, 307-312. http://dx.doi.org/10.1016/j.lfs.2013.07.006

[8] McInnes, I.B. and Schett, G. (2011) The pathogenesis of rheumatoid arthritis. *The New England Journal of Medicine*, 365, 2205-2219. http://dx.doi.org/10.1056/NEJMra1004965

[9] Fox, D.A. (1997) The role of T cells in the immunopathogenesis of rheumatoid arthritis: New perspectives. *Arthritis & Rheumatism*, 40, 598-609. http://dx.doi.org/10.1002/art.1780400403

[10] Firestein, G.S. (2003) Evolving concepts of rheumatoid arthritis. *Nature*, 423, 356-361. http://dx.doi.org/10.1038/nature01661

[11] Ivashkiv, L.B. (2011) Inflammatory signaling in macrophages: transitions from acute to tolerant and alternative activation states. *European Journal of Immunology*, 41, 2477-2481. http://dx.doi.org/10.1002/eji.201141783

[12] Noss, E.H. and Brenner, M.B. (2008) The role and therapeutic implications of fibroblast-like synoviocytes in inflammation and cartilage erosion in rheumatoid arthritis. *Immunological Reviews*, 223, 252-270. http://dx.doi.org/10.1111/j.1600-065X.2008.00648.x

[13] Lee, A., Qiao, Y., Grigoriev, G., Chen, J., Park-Min, K.H., Park, S.H., Ivashkiv, L.B. and Kalliolias, G.D. (2013) Tumor necrosis factor alpha induces sustained signaling and a prolonged and unremitting inflammatory response in rheumatoid arthritis synovial fibroblasts. *Arthritis & Rheumatism*, 65, 928-938. http://dx.doi.org/10.1002/art.37853

[14] Lam, J., Takeshita, S., Barker, J.E., Kanagawa, O., Ross, F.P. and Teitelbaum, S.L. (2000) TNF-alpha induces osteoclastogenesis by direct stimulation of macrophages exposed to permissive levels of RANK ligand. *Journal of Clinical Investigation*, 106, 1481-1488. http://dx.doi.org/10.1172/JCI11176

[15] Abu-Amer, Y., Ross, F.P., Edwards, J. and Teitelbaum, S.L. (1997) Lipopolysaccharide-stimulated osteoclastogenesis is mediated by tumor necrosis factor via its P55 receptor. *The Journal of Clinical Investigation*, 100, 1557-1565. http://dx.doi.org/10.1172/JCI119679

[16] Kobayashi, K., Takahashi, N., Jimi, E., Udagawa, N., Takami, M., Kotake, S., Nakagawa, N., Kinosaki, M., Yamaguchi, K., Shima, N., Yasuda, H., Morinaga, T., Higashio, K., Martin, T.J. and Suda, T. (2000) Tumor necrosis factor alpha stimulates osteoclast differentiation by a mechanism independent of the ODF/RANKL-RANK interaction. *The Journal of Experimental Medicine*, 191, 275-286. http://dx.doi.org/10.1084/jem.191.2.275

[17] Smolen, J.S., Han, C., Bala, M., Maini, R.N., Kalden,

J.R., van der Heijde, D., Breedveld, F.C., Furst, D.E., Lipsky, P.E. and Group, A.S. (2005) Evidence of radiographic benefit of treatment with infliximab plus methotrexate in rheumatoid arthritis patients who had no clinical improvement: A detailed subanalysis of data from the anti-tumor necrosis factor trial in rheumatoid arthritis with concomitant therapy study. *Arthritis & Rheumatism*, **52**, 1020-1030. http://dx.doi.org/10.1002/art.20982

[18] Binder, N.B., Puchner, A., Niederreiter, B., Hayer, S., Leiss, H., Bluml, S., Kreindl, R., Smolen, J.S. and Redlich, K. (2013) Tumor necrosis factor-inhibiting therapy preferentially targets bone destruction but not synovial inflammation in a tumor necrosis factor-driven model of rheumatoid arthritis. *Arthritis & Rheumatism*, **65**, 608-617. http://dx.doi.org/10.1002/art.37797

Reactive Arthritis: From Clinical Features to Pathogenesis

Ethelina Cargnelutti[1,2], María Silvia Di Genaro[1,2*]

[1]Division of Immunology, Faculty of Chemistry, Biochemistry and Pharmacy, National University of San Luis, San Luis, Argentina;
[2]Laboratory of Immunopathology, Multidisciplinary Institute of Biological Investigations-San Luis (IMIBIO-SL), National Council of Scientific and Technical Investigations (CONICET), San Luis, Argentina.
Email: [*]sdigena@unsl.edu.ar

ABSTRACT

Reactive arthritis (ReA) is a sterile synovitis which occurs after a gastrointestinal or urogenital infection. ReA belongs to Spondyloarthritis (SpA), a group of diseases that share several clinical and radiological features including familiar clustering, absence of rheumatoid factor and association with HLA-B27. Clinically, ReA is characterized by an asymmetric arthritis predominantly affecting the lower limbs, often associated with urethritis, conjunctivitis and other extra-articular symptoms. The ReA prevalence depends on the incidence of causative pathogens. The ReA diagnosis is based on clinical features and serological tests to evidence previous infection. Different treatment including antibiotics, disease modifying antirheumatic drugs (DMARs) and biologic agents has been recommended. Even though knowing that infections trigger the joint inflammation, the ReA pathogenesis remains to be poorly understood. Several animal models and *in vitro* studies have been used to elucidate the mechanisms involved in ReA development. In this sense, HLA-B27 transgenic rat or mice have been used to explain the role of this molecule in SpA aetiopathogenesis. Moreover, the infectious model of *Yersinia*-induced ReA in rodents has shed some lights on the relationship between host genetic susceptibility to infection and abnormal immune response in ReA development. Understanding the immune mediators triggering ReA will contribute to find a specific treatment for this arthritis. In this review, we focus on clinical features, epidemiology, treatment, and the different attempts to understand the pathogenesis of ReA.

Keywords: Reactive Arthritis; HLA-B27; Spondyloarthritis; *Yersinia*-Induced ReA; Therapy

1. Introduction

Reactive arthritis (ReA) is arthritis that arises following a gastrointestinal or urogenital infection. It is a form of Spondyloarthritis (SpA), a group of diseases with common features including inflammatory arthritis (generally an asymmetrical oligoarthritis), absence of rheumatoid factor and genetic association with the human leukocyte antigen (HLA)-B27. In addition to ReA, SpA also includes ankylosing spondylitis (AS), psoriatic arthritis (PsA), arthritis related to inflammatory bowel disease (IBD-SpA) and undifferentiated SpA (U-SpA) [1]. Nevertheless, at present it exist a discussion whether this classification represent alternative presentations of one entity with heterogeneous phenotype [2]. Currently, according to the Assessment of Spondylo Arthritis International Society

(ASAS) classification criteria (2009-2011), the SpA is classified as axial and peripheral arthritis [3].

The term "ReA" was introduced by Avohen *et al.* in 1969 to describe arthritis induced by *Yersinia enterocolitica* [4]. Moreover, the clinical features of this disease were characterized and the diagnosis of the preceding infection through serological methods was established [5]. The name ReA involves the immunological origin of this arthritis in which microorganisms do not enter in the joint cavity and antibiotic treatment has no effect on its development or outcome [6]. Even though none cultivable microorganism has been isolated from the joints of patients with ReA, bacterial antigens have been demonstrated in synovial fluid or tissue using different techniques, indicating deficient clearance of the inducer bacteria [7-10]. In addition, *Chlamydia trachomatis* mRNA has been detected in the joints of patients with post-ve-

[*]Corresponding author.

nereal ReA, raising the possibility that viable forms of this microorganism may be present [11,12].

A controversy exists in relation to the clinical findings to diagnose ReA [13]. According to the 4th International Workshop on Reactive Arthritis (Berlin, 1999), the term ReA must apply to a patient with typical clinical features of this disease and in those whose preceding infection was caused by the classic microorganisms involved in their development. The minimum time interval between the gastrointestinal/genitourinary infection symptoms and arthritis should be of 1 - 7 days, maximum 4 weeks. It is advisable for the investigation of microorganisms inducers of ReA by culturing urine/feces or through serological methods [14]. The current diagnosis of ReA is performed considering clinical features, radiologic examination and laboratory tests. However, for diagnosis of ReA, there is not a single laboratory test, and the radiological images do not help much in diagnosing an acute episode. The investigations performed to ReA diagnosis, and also to make a differential diagnosis are based on hematologic, microbiologic, serologic and radiologic findings, and on synovial fluid studies (**Table 1**).

2. Epidemiology

The incidence and prevalence of ReA depends of geographic region and the prevalence of causative pathogens. The ReA incidence is estimated to be 5 - 14/100,000 patients aged 18 - 60 years [15,16]. Most patients are aged 20 - 40 and it is more common in Caucasians affecting equally men and women [16]. A population-based study in Oregon and Minnesota (US) reported a ReA incidence following documented enteric bacterial infections ranged from 0.6 to 3.1 cases per 100,000, depending upon the

organism [17]. Two registry-based studies from Spain reported that 1.2% to 1.4% of all patients with SpA was diagnosed with ReA [18]. A recent epidemiological study in Argentina informed that from 402 patients with SpA aged 38.3 - 58 years, 25 (6.2%) had ReA [19]. In outbreaks triggered by a single source of infection, 0% - 22% of infected subjects developed subsequent ReA [20].

The HLA-B27 antigen is found in 30% - 70% of patients with ReA, which is a lower frequency compare to others SpA, such as AS with 90% of patients positive for this antigen [21]. Patients with this molecule manifest a more severe arthritis with a tendency to progress to a chronic stage and also they have greater chance of developing extra-articular symptoms [22]. At present, there are descript more than 100 isoforms of the HLA-B27 molecule (http://www.ebi.ac.uk/ipd/imgt/hla) that differ in the aminoacidic sequence. Most HLA-B27 molecules seem to be associated with SpA; however, there would be a hierarchy of association between the different subtypes of these molecules. Thus, HLA-B*2704 shows higher association with SpA, followed by HLA-B*2705, HLA-B*2702 and HLA-B*2707, while HLA-B*2706 and HLA-B*2709 are less associated to these diseases [23]. Furthermore, there is a geographical distribution of these isoforms, with a prevalence of HLA-B*2704 and HLA-B*2707 for Asians, and HLA-B*2705 and HLA-B*2702 for Caucasians [24]. In regional studies in South America, the most frequent HLA-B27 isoforms are HLA-B*2705 and HLA-B*2702 [25-27]. In Argentina, it is estimated a prevalence of 4% of HLA-B27 in the general population [28]. A study in 11 Rheumatology Centers in Argentina reported in 405 patients with SpA that 50% of patients with ReA were positive for HLA-B27 [29].

Table 1. Methods and expected results for ReA diagnosis.

Hematology	Erythrocyte sedimentation rate (ESR): usually elevated.
	C-reactive protein level (CRP): usually elevated.
	Complete blood cell count: in the acute phase may show leukocytosis.
	Rheumatoid factor: negative.
	Antinuclear antibody: negative.
	HLA-B27 testing: not diagnosis, but has prognostic value as positive results may indicate more serious disease.
Microbiology	Urine culture: may be positive for *Chlamydia* at the beginning of the infection.
	Stool culture: positive for *Salmonella*, *Shigella* or *Yersinia* whether obtained early.
Synovial fluid studies	Cell count: at early time of ReA is high and dominated by polymorphonuclears.
	Microscopy under polarized light: negative for urate crystals.
	Synovial fluid culture: negative.
Serology	Antibodies against *Yersinia*, *Salmonella*, *Campylobacter*, *Chlamydia*, *Neisseria gonorrhoeae*, *Borrelia burgdorferi*, and also against β-hemolytic streptococci should be determined and followed: positive for *Salmonella*, *Shigella*, *Yersinia* or *Chalmydia*.
Radiological images	Early disease: soft tissue swelling around affected joints that can represent large effusions; tendon swelling as in the calcaneal region.
	Chronic disease: bone and cartilage erosions with adjacent bone proliferation specially in the lower extremities; paravertebral ossification.

3. Clinical Features

The classic clinical characteristics of ReA involve an axial joint arthritis, enthesitis and peripheral oligoarthritis (less than 5 joint affected) usually asymmetrically accompanied by extra-articular symptoms [30]. The musculoskeletal symptoms are commonly acute and at beginning associated with systemic features such as malaise, fever, fatigue and weight loss [31].

Urogenital infection precedes 1 - 6 weeks the musculoskeletal symptoms. Their presentation varies from mild to severe with prostatitis or cervicitis. However, it can be asymptomatic in both sex. It is often accompanied by other signs such as penis discharge in males, pain with urination, or hematuria [32]. On the other hand, acute diarrhea appears approximately one month before articular manifestations in post-dysenteric ReA. Gastrointestinal symptoms are absent or mild in ReA triggered by *Yersinia*, unlike in patients with *Salmonella* and *Campylobacter* infections where symptoms are more severe and of longer duration [33].

Joint inflammation could be axial, involving the lumbar spine or sacroiliac joints, alternatively it is peripheral, commonly affecting the large joints of lower extremities, being knees, foot joints and ankles the most frequently involved. However, affectation of upper extremities (elbow, shoulder) and polyarticular forms have been reported in which the subtalar, metatarsophalangeal and toe interphalangeal joints tend to be affected [34,35]. Some patients suffer from dactylitis which is a diffuse swelling of entire finger or toe, sometimes referred as "sauce digit". This feature is common in ReA, but also in PsA and it is used to make a diagnosis of axial SpA using the ASAS criteria [36] or PsA using the ClASsification criteria for Psoriatic ARthritis (CASPAR) [37].

Enthesitis is an inflammation of the transitional zone where tendons and ligaments insert into the bone and sometimes it is the unique manifestation of this arthritis. Achilles tendonitis and plantar fasciitis are the most common types of enthesitis in ReA, but another enthesis can be involved [38].

Extra-articular symptoms are frequently observed in ReA and include mucocutaneous, ocular and occasionally cardiac manifestations. Mucocutaneous lesions are very specific of ReA and more frequent in HLA-B27 positive patients. Circinate balanitis is the most common skin manifestation of this arthritis following by keratoderma blennorrhagicum, occurring in almost 50% and 10% of the patients, respectively [39]. A well recognized complication of *Yersinia*-infection is erythema nodosum which is a painful rash predominantly on the extensor surfaces of the arms and legs [40]. Nails changes (nail dystrophy, subungual debris, and periungual pustules), hyperkeratosis and oral lesions also may occur [38]. One-third of patients with ReA suffer of conjunctivitis

once it is established, being more common after a genitourinary infection or enteric infection by *Shigella*, *Salmonella* and *Campylobacter*. The conjunctivitis is unilateral or bilateral with a mucopurulent discharge and its course is often mild and transient [41]. Acute anterior uveitis (AAU) may be observed in about a 5% patients with acute ReA and more than 50% patients with AAU are HLA-B27 positive. This manifestation is very painful and is characterized by sudden-onset, mostly unilateral [42-44]. Others less frequent ocular symptoms are keratitis [45], corneal ulceration, retrobulbar neutritis, scleritis and hypema which appear in persistent or chronic ReA [28]. The persistence of ocular inflammation may result in complications such as posterior synechiae, glaucoma, cystoids macular edema and cataract formation [46].

Cardiovascular manifestations in ReA and in other members of the SpA family have long been recognized and related to HLA-B27 positivity. Disturbances of the cardiac conduction system are found early [47,48] and cases with severe aortic insufficiency are found in late disease [49].

4. Triggering Microbes

Different bacteria species are associated with ReA development [15]. The classical enteric pathogens capable of triggering this arthritis belong to the genders *Salmonella*, *Yersinia*, *Shigella* and *Campylobacter*. On the other hand, *C. trachomatis* is the most common urogenital pathogen related to ReA [11,12]. *Salmonella*, *Yersinia*, *Shigella* and *Campylobacter* are Gram-negative bacteria with lipopolysaccharide (LPS) in their outer membrane. Furthermore, they are facultative or obligate intracellular, aerobic or microaerophilic bacteria. These characteristics probably account for their relation with ReA [31]. Epidemiological studies support the high association between infection with these bacteria and ReA development. Thus, in a study performed in different Rheumatology clinics in Berlin, Germany, from 52 patients with ReA a causative pathogen was identified in 29/52 (56%) [50]. In 17 (52%) of the patients with enteric ReA one of the enteric bacteria was identified: *Salmonella* in 11/33 (33%) and *Yersinia* in 6/33 (18%). *C. trachomatis* was the causative pathogen in 12/19 (63%) of the patients with urogenic ReA [50]. In 74 patients with the clinical picture of U-SpA, a specific triggering bacterium was also identified in 35/74 (47%) patients: *Yersinia* in 14/74 (19%), *Salmonella* in 9/74 (12%), and *C. trachomatis* in 12/74 (16%) [50]. Moreover, a 2-year epidemiological study on ReA and possible ReA in Oslo (Norway) reported an annual minimum incidence of *Chlamydia*-induced ReA (n = 25) of 4.6/100,000, and of enteric ReA (n = 27) of 5/100,000 individuals between 18 and 60 years [16]. In addition, a population-based cohort study (n = 71) in Southern Sweden showed in patients with a new-onset arthritis that 45% had had a prior infection, 27 (38%) had ReA and *Campylobacter*-induced ReA dominated the ReA group [51]. In addition, in a study performed in our laboratory in patients with musculoskeletal symptoms, we found immunoglobulin (Ig) A to *Yersinia* LPS in 13/124 (6%) sera and in 3/47 synovial fluids (6%). By Western blot, IgA to *Yersinia* outer proteins (Yops) was found in 14/124 sera (11%) and 2/47 synovial fluids (4%) [52].

Among the less common triggering microorganisms *Clostridium difficile* and pathogens strains of *Escherichia coli* have been described cause ReA [17,53,54]. Other microorganisms have been implicated as potential causes of ReA, these include *Chlamydia pneumoniae* [55,56], *Ureaplasma urealyticum* [57], *Helicobacter pylori* [58] and multiple intestinal parasites [59-61]. Nevertheless, most descriptions involving these microorganisms are isolated cases and even in discussion [38].

5. Pathogenesis

Despite knowing the initial event (gastrointestinal or urogenital infection), the pathogenesis of ReA is not completely understood. Environmental and genetic factors are involved and different aspects should be considered in the development of ReA including impaired elimination of causative microbes, persistence of their antigens in the joints, host immune response and genetics factors like the presence of the molecule HLA-B27 (**Figure 1**).

The classical bacteria triggering this arthritis are invasive and cause primary infection in the gastrointestinal (enteric pathogens) or genitourinary mucosa (*C. thrachomatis*), from there they disseminate to other organs such as lymphoid tissue, spleen and liver [28]. As mentioned above, mRNA of *C. thrachomatis* and DNA from other enteric pathogens or their products have been de-

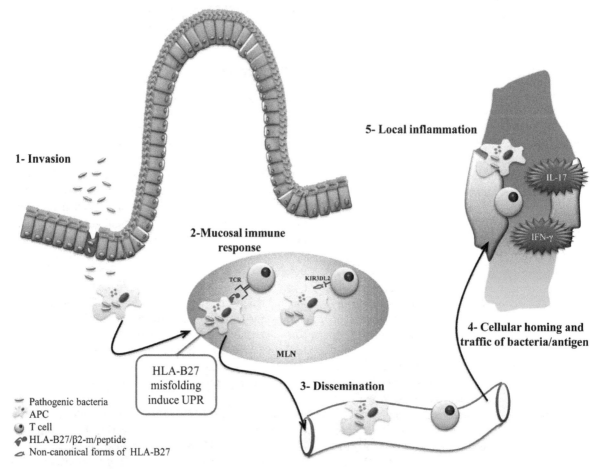

Figure 1. Model of ReA pathogenesis. (1) Pathogenic bacteria attach and invade the intestinal epithelium. HLA-B27 in antigen presenting cell (APC) such as macrophages may be responsible for bacterial persistence; (2) In mesenteric lymph node (MLN), APC could present arthritogenic peptides through HLA-B27 to CD8+ T cells, or HLA-B27 itself could be recognized through killer immunoglobulin receptor (KIR)3DL2 on CD4+ T cells. Moreover, HLA-B27 misfolding induces an unfolded protein response (UPR); (3-4) APC with non-active bacteria or with bacterial antigens, and T cells disseminate within peripheral blood and eventually reach the joint; (5) In the target joint, gut derived APC and T cells induce immune response with IFN-γ and IL-17 production, recruitment of other cells and induction of mesenchymal cells activation, which enhance and sustain inflammation.

tected in the synovial fluid or tissue of patients with ReA. These facts demonstrate that the entire bacteria or their products traffic from the initial site of infection to the joint. On the other hand, persistence of *Y. enterocolitica* has been informed in peripheral blood up to 4 year after initial infection in patients with ReA [62], as well in different organs in ReA rat models [63]. Furthermore, persistence of *Salmonella enteritidis* has been demonstrated in human epithelial cells after 14 days of *in vitro* infection [64]. The impaired elimination of causative microbes plus the traffic of their antigens to the joint could be responsible of pathological immune response in the joint [28]. However, the detailed mechanisms by which those antigens reach the joint and induce inflammation remain to be fully elucidated.

An imbalance in the cytokine levels may be responsible for persistence of causative microbes and also reflect the pathological immune response in the joint. In this way, diminished levels of TNF produced by peripheral blood mononuclear cells (PBMC) of patients with ReA [65] and elevated amounts of IL-10 have been demonstrated at the beginning of the disease [66]. However, in patients at chronic stage of arthritis, elevated amounts of TNF produced by PBMC and $CD3^+IFN\text{-}\gamma^+$ cells from blood and synovial fluid have been reported [66]. Another authors observed in patients with ReA enriched amounts of $CD4^+IL\text{-}17^+$ cells within synovial fluid supporting the hypothesis that IL-17 could contribute to pathogenesis of ReA [67]. In line with these results, we detected higher IL-17 and IFN-γ levels in regional lymph nodes of $TNFRp55^{-/-}$ mice with *Y. enterocolitica*-induced ReA and significantly increased number of $CD4^+IL\text{-}17^+$ cells in these mice compared to their counterpart wild-type [68]. In addition, in this animal model we observed decreased amounts of IL-10 and Treg cells at arthritis onset (day 14 after infection) in contrast with chronic stage of arthritis [69]. These works and others advocate the idea that in ReA, a specific cellular immune response take place in the joint and chronic stimuli allows to the cells maintain the inflammatory process for long periods [70].

The first genetic factor described to be related to ReA and SpA in general, is the molecule HLA-B27. The role of HLA-B27 in SpA is not completely known and several hypotheses try to explain it. Since HLA-B27 is a class I histocompatibility molecule, it has been postulated that it presents arthritogenic bacterial peptides to $CD8^+T$ cells, thus stimulating an autoimmune response (molecular mimicry) [71-73]. However, in HLA-B27/human β2-microglobulin (hβ2-m) transgenic rats, two different approaches demonstrated that $CD8^+T$ cells are not necessary for development of SpA-like phenotype. Furthermore, the depletion of $CD8^+T$ cells through antibodies [74] or the elimination of CD8α protein expression by chemical mutation of *CD8α* gene [75] does not prevent disease in this SpA rodent model.

It was found that heavy chains of HLA-B27 have a tendency to misfold forming homodimers and heterodimers due to aberrant disulfide bound formation by unpaired Cys residues at position 67 [76]. HLA-B27 misfolding causes a stress response in the endoplasmic reticulum and the cell activates multiple signaling pathways that orchestrate what is known as the unfolded protein response (UPR). One consequence of UPR activation is the polarization of cell to responding to patter recognition receptors (PRR) agonists (TLR 4, 2 and 3) toward the production of greater amount of IL-23 over IL-12, which in turns provide a stimulus for Th17 survival and activation in individual with permissive IL-23R polymorphism [77]. Additionally, the non-canonical forms of HLA-B27 antigen expressed on cell surface are plausible to be recognized by killer immunoglobulin receptors (KIR) such as KIR3DL2 on $CD4^+$ T cells, and then, trigger inflammation [1,21,78].

Other genetic factors (e.g. *IL-23R*, *IL-1R2*, *TNFRS1*, *TRADD*, etc.) has been associated with AS, PsA and IBD-SpA [79]; therefore, it is possible that these factors may also have significance in ReA since even individuals negative for HLA-B27 also develop ReA following mucosal infection.

6. Treatment

Since infections trigger ReA, the use of antibiotic therapy in this arthropathy has been proposed and it is possible when the trigger bacterium has been isolated. However, the use of antibiotics is controversial probably because several studies have been conducted enrolling patients with ReA caused by heterogeneous pathogens. Moreover, other studies have often employed antibiotic monotherapy that may be not effective in the aberrant forms of bacteria causing ReA. In contrast, a clinical trial in 2010 enrolled only patients with blood or synovial tissue positive for *Chlamydia* detected by PCR [80]. In this study, the patients were randomized to receive doxycycline + rifampin, azithromycin + rifampin or placebo. After six months, 63% of the patients with combination antibiotic therapy versus 20% of placebo group had clinical improvement as measured by swollen joint count [80]. Therefore, this was the first trial that provide evidence supporting antibiotic therapy efficacy in *Chlamydia*-induced ReA.

The current treatment of ReA is based on rest, nonsteroidal anti-inflammatory drugs (NSAIDs) [81]. In case of NSAID-resistance or active disease for more than 4 weeks, intra-articular injection of corticosteroids is recommended in patients with mono or oligoarthritis [82,83]. Topical corticosteroids are useful for ReA extra-articular symptoms such as uveitis, circinate balanitis and keratoderma blennorrhagicum [84].

In chronic and severe ReA, disease-modifying antirheumatic drugs (DMARDs) are recommended and the most used is sulfasalazine (SSZ) [81] which shows limited effectiveness in patients with ReA acute episodes [85]. Another DMARD is methotrexate, which may be used as an alternative to SSZ in patients who are allergic or intolerant to SSZ or who do not respond to this drug [84]. The DMARDs treatment is an alternative to anti-TNF therapy and may delay the switch to biologic agents.

The TNF antagonists such as infliximab, etanercept and adalimumab showed impressive short-term improvements in AS [86], however, data on the use of this anti-TNF therapy in ReA are limited [87-92]. A largest recent experience with TNF antagonists in ReA supported the safety and efficacy of these agents in refractory ReA [89]. In this study, 10 patients with ReA previously refractory to NSAIDs and DMARDs received anti-TNF therapy within a median of 6 months (range 2 - 12 months) between the onset of ReA and the initiation of the treatment. After a follow-up of 20.6 months, no severe adverse events, including severe infection, were observed. Anti-TNF therapy was rapidly effective in 9 patients (90%), as shown by the rapid effect on a visual analog scale pain score, tender joint count, swollen joint count, and extra-articular manifestations. Only mild infections were documented, none of which were associated with the triggering infection [89].

Our findings in *Yersinia*-induced ReA in *TNFRp55$^{-/-}$* mice demonstrated that, in the absence of TNF signaling, redundant pathways, particularly Th17 and Th1 effector cells, may act in concert to sustain inflammation in bacterial induced ReA [68]. Recently, we reported that TNFRp55 modulates macrophage functions in response to *Yersinia* LPS stimulation suggesting an essential regulatory role of TNF via TNFRp55 signaling [93]. Furthermore, we have reported that this pathway controlled the induction and function of Treg cells through differential regulation of cytokine production [69]. Our data support the concept that TNFRp55 signaling may participate in the modulation of immune response in ReA, suggesting caution in the use of TNF blockers in cases of chronic ReA.

Treatment switch to a second anti-TNF agent can be an effective strategy in AS. There is a need for more long-term studies to examine the longitudinal efficacy in SpA of the newer biological therapies such as golimumab, a fully human antibody anti-TNF, and rituximab, an antibody that induces B cell depletion [86]. Ustekinumab, an anti-p40 antibody blocking both IL-23 and IL-12 has demonstrated clinical efficacy in PsA [94]. Secukinumab, an anti-IL-17A antibody, has been used in a randomized controlled trial with short duration of follow-up for AS treatment showing good efficacy [86]. A trend towards improvement was also demonstrated for secukinumab in PsA [95]. Until now, these newer biological agents have not been used in patients with ReA.

7. ReA Prognosis

ReA usually has a self-limiting course since the most patients recover fully in 2 to 6 months. However, 15% - 30% of patients may develop chronic disease (>6 months with clinical symptoms) [15]. The prognosis of enteric ReA is best known being frequent recurrent acute attacks in patients with ReA triggered by *Salmonella*, *Shigella* and *Yersinia* [1,15]. In a Finnish study at mean of 11 years after *Salmonella*-induced ReA, 8/50 (16%) developed chronic SpA and 5 (12%) of these patients fulfilled the criteria of AS [96]. In a similar study in 85 patients with acute *Yersinia*-induced ReA, half to the patients showed peripheral joint symptoms and one-third of them had radiologic evidence of sacroiliitis [97]. A 20-year follow up study found that 32/100 of patients with *Shigella*-induced ReA had AS [98]. Only HLA-B27 positive patients ReA developed recurrent or chronic symptoms [96]. Therefore, the prognosis is less favorable in patients who are HLA-B27 positive [28].

8. Conclusion

A gastrointestinal or urogenital infection may trigger ReA and genetic factors such as HLA-B27 which are associated with chronic and more severe arthritis. However, the pathogenesis of this arthropathy is not completely known. Therefore, there are no specific treatment for this disease. Anti-TNF therapy in ReA has been recommended for refractory ReA suggesting an association with cytokine response and ReA development. Our experimental evidence indicates caution in the use of TNF blockers in bacterial-triggered chronic arthritis. We believe that further investigation in animal models should delineate the immunopathogenic mechanisms involved in ReA and contribute to more specific therapeutic intervention.

9. Sources of Funding

This work was supported by grants from Agencia Nacional de Promoción Científica y Tecnológica (PICT 2008-763; PICT 2011-0732), Universidad Nacional de San Luis (Project 0401), M.S.D.G. is member of the Scientific Career of National Council of Scientific and Technical Investigations; E. C. is National Council of Scientific and Technical Investigations fellow.

REFERENCES

[1]   M. Dougados and D. Baeten, "Spondyloarthritis," *Lancet*, Vol. 377, No. 9783, 2011, pp. 2127-2137.

http://dx.doi.org/10.1016/S0140-6736(11)60071-8

[2]   D. Baeten, M. Breban, R. Lories, G. Schett and J. Sieper, "Are Spondylarthritides Related but Distinct Conditions or a Single Disease with a Heterogeneous Phenotype?" *Arthritis & Rheumatism*, Vol. 65, No. 1, 2013, pp. 12-20. http://dx.doi.org/10.1002/art.37829

[3]   A. Van Tubergen and U. Weber, "Diagnosis and Classification in Spondyloarthritis: Identifying a Chameleon," *Nature Reviews Rheumatology*, Vol. 8, No. 5, 2012, pp. 253-261. http://dx.doi.org/10.1038/nrrheum.2012.33

[4]   P. Ahvonen, K. Sievers and K. Aho, "Arthritis Associated with *Yersinia enterocolitica* Infection," *Acta Rheumatologica Scandinavica*, Vol. 15, No. 3, 1969, pp. 232-253.

[5]   O. Laitenen, J. Tuuhea and P. Ahvonen, "Polyarthritis Associated with *Yersinia enterocolitica* Infection. Clinical Features and Laboratory Findings in Nine Cases with Severe Joint Symptoms," *Annals of the Rheumatic Diseases*, Vol. 31, No. 1, 1972, pp. 34-39. http://dx.doi.org/10.1136/ard.31.1.34

[6]   K. Aho, P. Ahvonen, T. Juvakoski, M. Kousa, M. Leirisalo and O. Laitinen, "Immune Responses in *Yersinia*-Associated Reactive Arthritis," *Annals of the Rheumatic Diseases*, Vol. 38, Suppl. 1, 1979, pp. 123-126.

[7]   C. J. Cox, K. E. Kempsell and J. S. Gaston, "Investigation of Infectious Agents Associated with Arthritis by Reverse Transcription PCR of Bacterial rRNA," *Arthritis Research & Therapy*, Vol. 5, No. 1, 2003, pp. R1-R8. http://dx.doi.org/10.1186/ar602

[8]   K. Granfors, S. Jalkanen, A. A. Lindberg, O. Maki-Ikola, R. Von Essen, R. Lahesmaa-Rantala, H. Isomaki, R. Saario, W. J. Arnold and A. Toivanen, "*Salmonella* Lipopolysaccharide in Synovial Cells from Patients with Reactive Arthritis," *Lancet*, Vol. 335, No. 8691, 1990, pp. 685-688. http://dx.doi.org/10.1016/0140-6736(90)90804-E

[9]   J. S. Hill Gaston, C. Cox and K. Granfors, "Clinical and Experimental Evidence for Persistent *Yersinia* Infection in Reactive Arthritis," *Arthritis & Rheumatism*, Vol. 42, No. 10, 1999, pp. 2239-2242. http://dx.doi.org/10.1002/1529-0131(199910)42:10<2239::AID-ANR29>3.0.CO;2-L

[10] R. Merilahti-Palo, K. O. Soderstrom, R. Lahesmaa-Rantala, K. Granfors and A. Toivanen, "Bacterial Antigens in Synovial Biopsy Specimens in *Yersinia* Triggered Reactive Arthritis," *Annals of the Rheumatic Diseases*, Vol. 50, No. 2, 1991, pp. 87-90. http://dx.doi.org/10.1136/ard.50.2.87

[11] A. M. Beutler, J. A. Whittum-Hudson, R. Nanagara, H. R. Schumacher and A. P. Hudson, "Intracellular Location of Inapparently Infecting *Chlamydia* in Synovial Tissue from Patients with Reiter's Syndrome," *Immunologic Research*, Vol. 13, No. 2-3, 1994, pp. 163-171. http://dx.doi.org/10.1007/BF02918277

[12] H. C. Gerard, P. J. Branigan, H. R. Schumacher Jr. and A. P. Hudson, "Synovial *Chlamydia trachomatis* in Patients with Reactive Arthritis/Reiter's Syndrome Are Viable but Show Aberrant Gene Expression," *The Journal of Rheumatology*, Vol. 25, No. 4, 1998, pp. 734-742.

[13] J. M. Townes, "Reactive Arthritis after Enteric Infections in the United States: The Problem of Definition," *Clinical Infectious Diseases*, Vol. 50, No. 2, 2010, pp. 247-254. http://dx.doi.org/10.1086/649540

[14] J. Braun, G. Kingsley, D. Van Der Heijde and J. Sieper, "On the Difficulties of Establishing a Consensus on the Definition of and Diagnostic Investigations for Reactive Arthritis. Results and Discussion of a Questionnaire Prepared for the 4th International Workshop on Reactive Arthritis, Berlin, Germany, July 3-6, 1999," *The Journal of Rheumatology*, Vol. 27, No. 9, 2000, pp. 2185-2192.

[15] T. Hannu, "Reactive Arthritis," *Best Practice & Research Clinical Rheumatology*, Vol. 25, No. 3, 2011, pp. 347-357. http://dx.doi.org/10.1016/j.berh.2011.01.018

[16] T. K. Kvien, A. Glennas, K. Melby, K. Granfors, O. Andrup, B. Karstensen and J. E. Thoen, "Reactive Arthritis: Incidence, Triggering Agents and Clinical Presentation," *The Journal of Rheumatology*, Vol. 21, No. 1, 1994, pp. 115-122.

[17] J. M. Townes, A. A. Deodhar, E. S. Laine, K. Smith, H. E. Krug, A. Barkhuizen, M. E. Thompson, P. R. Cieslak and J. Sobel, "Reactive Arthritis Following Culture-Confirmed Infections with Bacterial Enteric Pathogens in Minnesota and Oregon: A Population-Based Study," *Annals of the Rheumatic Diseases*, Vol. 67, No. 12, 2008, pp. 1689-1696. http://dx.doi.org/10.1136/ard.2007.083451

[18] E. Collantes, P. Zarco, E. Munoz, X. Juanola, J. Mulero, J. L. Fernandez-Sueiro, J. C. Torre-Alonso, J. Gratacos, C. Gonzalez, E. Batlle, P. Fernandez, L. F. Linares, E. Brito and L. Carmona, "Disease Pattern of Spondyloarthropathies in Spain: Description of the First National Registry (REGISPONSER) Extended Report," *Rheumatology (Oxford)*, Vol. 46, No. 8, 2007, pp. 1309-1315. http://dx.doi.org/10.1093/rheumatology/kem084

[19] E. Buschiazzo, J. A. Maldonado-Cocco, P. Arturi, G. Citera, A. Berman, A. Nitsche and O. L. Rillo, "Epidemiology of Spondyloarthritis in Argentina," *The American Journal of the Medical Sciences*, Vol. 341, No. 4, 2011, pp. 289-292. http://dx.doi.org/10.1097/MAJ.0b013e31820f8cc3

[20] M. Vasala, S. Hallanvuo, P. Ruuska, R. Suokas, A. Siitonen and M. Hakala, "High Frequency of Reactive Arthritis in Adults after *Yersinia pseudotuberculosis* O:1 Outbreak Caused by Contaminated Grated Carrots," *Annals of the Rheumatic Diseases*, 2013. http://dx.doi.org/10.1136/annrheumdis-2013-203431

[21] A. Mcmichael and P. Bowness, "HLA-B27: Natural Function and Pathogenic Role in Spondyloarthritis," *Arthritis Research*, Vol. 4, Suppl. 3, 2002, pp. S153-158.

[22] A. Toivanen and P. Toivanen, "Reactive Arthritis," *Best Practice & Research Clinical Rheumatology*, Vol. 18, No. 5, 2004, pp. 689-703. http://dx.doi.org/10.1016/j.berh.2004.05.008

[23] A. Chatzikyriakidou, P. V. Voulgari and A. A. Drosos, "What Is the Role of HLA-B27 in Spondyloarthropathies?" *Autoimmunity Reviews*, Vol. 10, No. 8, 2011, pp. 464-468. http://dx.doi.org/10.1016/j.autrev.2011.01.011

[24] G. P. Thomas and M. A. Brown, "Genetics and Genomics of Ankylosing Spondylitis," *Immunological Reviews*, Vol. 233, No. 1, 2010, pp. 162-180.

http://dx.doi.org/10.1111/j.0105-2896.2009.00852.x

[25] R. Bonfiglioli, R. A. Conde, P. D. Sampaio-Barros, P. Louzada-Junior, E. A. Donadi and M. B. Bertolo, "Frequency of HLA-B27 Alleles in Brazilian Patients with Psoriatic Arthritis," *Clinical Rheumatology*, Vol. 27, No. 6, 2008, pp. 709-712.
http://dx.doi.org/10.1007/s10067-007-0770-3

[26] A. Cipriani, S. Rivera, M. Hassanhi, G. Marquez, R. Hernandez, C. Villalobos and M. Montiel, "HLA-B27 Subtypes Determination in Patients with Ankylosing Spondylitis from Zulia, Venezuela," *Human Immunology*, Vol. 64, No. 7, 2003, pp. 745-749.
http://dx.doi.org/10.1016/S0198-8859(03)00085-5

[27] B. Martinez, L. Caraballo, M. Hernandez, R. Valle, M. Avila and A. Iglesias Gamarra, "HLA-B27 Subtypes in Patients with Ankylosing Spondylitis (as) in Colombia," *Revista de Investigación Clínica*, Vol. 51, No. 4, 1999, pp. 221-226.

[28] J. S. Hill Gaston and M. S. Lillicrap, "Arthritis Associated with Enteric Infection," *Best Practice & Research Clinical Rheumatology*, Vol. 17, No. 2, 2003, pp. 219-239. http://dx.doi.org/10.1016/S1521-6942(02)00104-3

[29] V. Bellomio, A. Berman, R. Sueldo, M. J. Molina, A. Spindler, E. Lucero, H. Berman, A. Nitsche, C. Asnal, J. A. Maldonado Cocco, G. Citera, S. Paira, C. Sandoval, R. Wong, R. Gallo, O. Rillo, R. Chaparro, A. Alvarellos, J. A. Albiero, C. Graf, A. Zunino, C. G. Casado, C. B. Romeo, J. C. Barreira and E. Aroca Briones, "Respondia. Iberoamerican Spondyloarthritis Registry: Argentina," *Reumatología Clínica*, Vol. 4, Suppl. 4, 2008, pp. S23-29.

[30] S. Kobayashi and I. Kida, "Reactive Arthritis: Recent Advances and Clinical Manifestations," *Annals of Internal Medicine*, Vol. 44, No. 5, 2005, pp. 408-12.
http://dx.doi.org/10.2169/internalmedicine.44.408

[31] M. Leirisalo-Repo, "Reactive Arthritis," *Scandinavian Journal of Rheumatology*, Vol. 34, No. 4, 2005, pp. 251-259. http://dx.doi.org/10.1080/03009740500202540

[32] W. F. Barth and K. Segal, "Reactive Arthritis (Reiter's Syndrome)," *American Family Physician*, Vol. 60, No. 2, 1999, pp. 499-503, 507.

[33] B. Kwiatkowska and A. Filipowicz-Sosnowska, "Reactive Arthritis," *Polskie Archiwum Medycyny Wewnętrznej*, Vol. 119, No. 1-2, 2009, pp. 60-65.

[34] T. Hannu, L. Mattila, H. Rautelin, P. Pelkonen, P. Lahdenne, A. Siitonen and M. Leirisalo-Repo, "Campylobacter-Triggered Reactive Arthritis: A Population-Based Study," *Rheumatology (Oxford)*, Vol. 41, No. 3, 2002, pp. 312-318.
http://dx.doi.org/10.1093/rheumatology/41.3.312

[35] T. Rathod, A. Chandanwale, S. Chavan and M. Shah, "Polyarthritic, Symmetric Arthropathy in Reactive Arthritis," *Journal of Natural Science, Biology and Medicine*, Vol. 2, No. 2, 2011, pp. 216-218.
http://dx.doi.org/10.4103/0976-9668.92312

[36] M. Rudwaleit, D. Van Der Heijde, R. Landewe, J. Listing, N. Akkoc, J. Brandt, J. Braun, C. T. Chou, E. Collantes-Estevez, M. Dougados, F. Huang, J. Gu, M. A. Khan, Y. Kirazli, W. P. Maksymowych, H. Mielants, I. J. Sorensen, S. Ozgocmen, E. Roussou, R. Valle-Onate, U. Weber, J.

Wei and J. Sieper, "The Development of Assessment of Spondyloarthritis International Society Classification Criteria for Axial Spondyloarthritis (Part II): Validation and Final Selection," *Annals of the Rheumatic Diseases*, Vol. 68, No. 6, 2009, pp. 777-783.
http://dx.doi.org/10.1136/ard.2009.108233

[37] W. Taylor, D. Gladman, P. Helliwell, A. Marchesoni, P. Mease and H. Mielants, "Classification Criteria for Psoriatic Arthritis: Development of New Criteria from a Large International Study," *Arthritis & Rheumatism*, Vol. 54, No. 8, 2006, pp. 2665-2673.
http://dx.doi.org/10.1002/art.21972

[38] J. D. Carter and A. P. Hudson, "Reactive Arthritis: Clinical Aspects and Medical Management," *Rheumatic Disease Clinics of North America*, Vol. 35, No. 1, 2009, pp. 21-44.
http://dx.doi.org/10.1016/j.rdc.2009.03.010

[39] I. B. Wu and R. A. Schwartz, "Reiter's Syndrome: The Classic Triad and More," *Journal of the American Academy of Dermatology*, Vol. 59, No. 1, 2008, pp. 113-121.
http://dx.doi.org/10.1016/j.jaad.2008.02.047

[40] B. M. Rosner, D. Werber, M. Hohle and K. Stark, "Clinical Aspects and Self-Reported Symptoms of Sequelae of *Yersinia enterocolitica* Infections in a Population-Based Study, Germany 2009-2010," *BMC Infectious Diseases*, Vol. 13, 2013, p. 236.

[41] I. Colmegna, R. Cuchacovich and L. R. Espinoza, "HLA-B27-Associated Reactive Arthritis: Pathogenetic and Clinical Considerations," *Clinical Microbiology Reviews*, Vol. 17, No. 2, 2004, pp. 348-369.
http://dx.doi.org/10.1128/CMR.17.2.348-369.2004

[42] T. E. Feltkamp and J. H. Ringrose, "Acute Anterior Uveitis and Spondyloarthropathies," *Current Opinion in Rheumatology*, Vol. 10, No. 4, 1998, pp. 314-318.
http://dx.doi.org/10.1097/00002281-199807000-00006

[43] M. Huhtinen, K. Laasila, K. Granfors, M. Puolakkainen, I. Seppala, L. Laasonen, H. Repo, A. Karma and M. Leirisalo-Repo, "Infectious Background of Patients with a History of Acute Anterior Uveitis," *Annals of the Rheumatic Diseases*, Vol. 61, No. 11, 2002, pp. 1012-1016.
http://dx.doi.org/10.1136/ard.61.11.1012

[44] D. Monnet, M. Breban, C. Hudry, M. Dougados and A. P. Brezin, "Ophthalmic Findings and Frequency of Extraocular Manifestations in Patients with HLA-B27 Uveitis: A Study of 175 Cases," *Ophthalmology*, Vol. 111, No. 4, 2004, pp. 802-809.
http://dx.doi.org/10.1016/j.ophtha.2003.07.011

[45] N. Kozeis, M. Trachana and S. Tyradellis, "Keratitis in Reactive Arthritis (Reiter Syndrome) in Childhood," *Cornea*, Vol. 30, No. 8, 2011, pp. 924-925.
http://dx.doi.org/10.1097/ICO.0b013e3182000916

[46] S. Kiss, E. Letko, S. Qamruddin, S. Baltatzis and C. S. Foster, "Long-Term Progression, Prognosis, and Treatment of Patients with Recurrent Ocular Manifestations of Reiter's Syndrome," *Ophthalmology*, Vol. 110, No. 9, 2003, pp. 1764-1769.

[47] L. Bergfeldt, "HLA B27-Associated Rheumatic Diseases with Severe Cardiac Bradyarrhythmias. Clinical Features and Prevalence in 223 Men with Permanent Pacemakers,"

American Journal of Medicine, Vol. 75, No. 2, 1983, pp. 210-215.
http://dx.doi.org/10.1016/0002-9343(83)91193-2

[48] H. Nielsen, "Complete Heart Block in Reiter's Syndrome," *Acta Cardiologica*, Vol. 41, No. 6, 1986, pp. 451-455.

[49] L. E. Brown, P. Forfia and J. A. Flynn, "Aortic Insufficiency in a Patient with Reactive Arthritis: Case Report and Review of the Literature," *HSS Journal*, Vol. 7, No. 2, 2011, pp. 187-189.
http://dx.doi.org/10.1007/s11420-010-9184-x

[50] C. Fendler, S. Laitko, H. Sorensen, C. Gripenberg-Lerche, A. Groh, J. Uksila, K. Granfors, J. Braun and J. Sieper, "Frequency of Triggering Bacteria in Patients with Reactive Arthritis and Undifferentiated Oligoarthritis and the Relative Importance of the Tests Used for Diagnosis," *Annals of the Rheumatic Diseases*, Vol. 60, No. 4, 2001, pp. 337-343. http://dx.doi.org/10.1136/ard.60.4.337

[51] M. K. Söderlin, H. Kautiainen, M. Puolakkainen, K. Hedman, M. Söderlund-Venermo, T. Skogh and M. Leirisalo-Repo, "Infections Preceding Early Arthritis in Southern Sweden: A Prospective Population-Based Study," *Journal of Rheumatology*, Vol. 30, No. 3, 2003, pp. 459-464.

[52] M. G. Lacoste, H. Tamashiro, S. G. Correa, A. M. de Guzmán and M. S. Di Genaro, "Correlation between *Yersinia enterocolitica* and Type I Collagen Reactivity in Patients with Arthropathies," *Rheumatology International*, Vol. 27, No. 7, 2007, pp. 613-620.
http://dx.doi.org/10.1007/s00296-006-0274-5

[53] J. Birnbaum, J. G. Bartlett and A. C. Gelber, "*Clostridium difficile*: An under-Recognized Cause of Reactive Arthritis?" *Clinical Rheumatology*, Vol. 27, No. 2, 2008, pp. 253-255. http://dx.doi.org/10.1007/s10067-007-0710-2

[54] P. Schiellerup, K. A. Krogfelt and H. Locht, "A Comparison of Self-Reported Joint Symptoms Following Infection with Different Enteric Pathogens: Effect of HLA-B27," *Journal of Rheumatology*, Vol. 35, No. 3, 2008, pp. 480-487.

[55] T. Hannu, M. Puolakkainen and M. Leirisalo-Repo, "*Chlamydia pneumoniae* as a Triggering Infection in Reactive Arthritis," *Rheumatology*, Vol. 38, No. 5, 1999, pp. 411-414.

[56] A. Rizzo, M. D. Domenico, C. R. Carratelli and R. Paolillo, "The Role of *Chlamydia* and *Chlamydophila* Infections in Reactive Arthritis," *Internal Medicine*, Vol. 51, No. 1, 2012, pp. 113-117.
http://dx.doi.org/10.2169/internalmedicine.51.6228

[57] I. Galadari and H. Galadari, "Nonspecific Urethritis and Reactive Arthritis," *Clinics in Dermatology*, Vol. 22, No. 6, 2004, pp. 469-475.
http://dx.doi.org/10.1016/j.clindermatol.2004.07.010

[58] M. K. Soderlin, E. Alasaarela and M. Hakala, "Reactive Arthritis Induced by *Clostridium difficile* Enteritis as a Complication of *Helicobacter pylori* Eradication," *Clinical Rheumatology*, Vol. 18, No. 4, 1999, pp. 337-338.
http://dx.doi.org/10.1007/s100670050113

[59] D. W. Carlson and D. R. Finger, "Beaver Fever Arthritis," *Journal of Clinical Rheumatology*, Vol. 10, No. 2, 2004, pp. 86-88.

http://dx.doi.org/10.1097/01.rhu.0000120979.11380.16

[60] A. Sing, S. Bechtold, J. Heesemann, B. H. Belohradsky and H. Schmidt, "Reactive Arthritis Associated with Prolonged *Cryptosporidial* Infection," *Journal of Infection*, Vol. 47, No. 2, 2003, pp. 181-184.
http://dx.doi.org/10.1016/S0163-4453(03)00035-5

[61] B. Tejera, D. Grados, M. Martinez-Morillo and S. Roure, "Reactive Arthritis Caused by *Blastocystis hominis*," *Reumatología Clínica*, Vol. 8, No. 1, 2012, pp. 50-51.

[62] K. Granfors, R. Merilahti-Palo, R. Luukkainen, T. Mottonen, R. Lahesmaa, P. Probst, E. Marker-Hermann and P. Toivanen, "Persistence of *Yersinia* Antigens in Peripheral Blood Cells from Patients with *Yersinia enterocolitica* O:3 Infection with or without Reactive Arthritis," *Arthritis & Rheumatism*, Vol. 41, No. 5, 1998, pp. 855-862.
http://dx.doi.org/10.1002/1529-0131(199805)41:5<855:: AID-ART12>3.0.CO;2-J

[63] J. A. Curfs, J. G. Meis, H. L. Van Der Lee, J. Mulder, W. G. Kraak and J. A. Hoogkamp-Korstanje, "Persistent *Yersinia enterocolitica* Infection in Three Rat Strains," *Microbial Pathogenesis*, Vol. 19, No. 1, 1995, pp. 57-63.
http://dx.doi.org/10.1006/mpat.1995.0045

[64] M. Saarinen, L. J. Pelliniemi and K. Granfors, "Survival and Degradation of *Salmonella enterica* Serotype Enteritidis in Intestinal Epithelial Cells *in Vitro*," *Journal of Medical Microbiology*, Vol. 45, No. 6, 1996, pp. 463-471.
http://dx.doi.org/10.1099/00222615-45-6-463

[65] J. Braun, Z. Yin, I. Spiller, S. Siegert, M. Rudwaleit, L. Liu, A. Radbruch and J. Sieper, "Low Secretion of Tumor Necrosis Factor Alpha, but No Other Th1 or Th2 Cytokines, by Peripheral Blood Mononuclear Cells Correlates with Chronicity in Reactive Arthritis," *Arthritis & Rheumatism*, Vol. 42, No. 10, 1999, pp. 2039-2044.
http://dx.doi.org/10.1002/1529-0131(199910)42:10<2039 ::AID-ANR3>3.0.CO;2-6

[66] I. Butrimiene, S. Jarmalaite, J. Ranceva, A. Venalis, L. Jasiuleviciute and A. Zvirbliene, "Different Cytokine Profiles in Patients with Chronic and Acute Reactive Arthritis," *Rheumatology*, Vol. 43, No. 10, 2004, pp. 1300-1304.
http://dx.doi.org/10.1093/rheumatology/keh323

[67] H. Shen, J. C. Goodall and J. S. Gaston, "Frequency and Phenotype of T Helper 17 Cells in Peripheral Blood and Synovial Fluid of Patients with Reactive Arthritis," *Journal of Rheumatology*, Vol. 37, No. 10, 2010, pp. 2096-2099. http://dx.doi.org/10.3899/jrheum.100146

[68] R. J. Eliçabe, E. Cargnelutti, M. I. Serer, P. W. Stege, S. R. Valdez, M. A. Toscano, G. A. Rabinovich and M. S. Di Genaro, "Lack of TNFR p55 Results in Heightened Expression of IFN-γ and Il-17 During the Development of Reactive Arthritis," *Journal of Immunology*, Vol. 185, No. 7, 2010, pp. 4485-4495.
http://dx.doi.org/10.4049/jimmunol.0902245

[69] E. Cargnelutti, J. L. Arias, S. R. Valdez, G. A. Rabinovich and M. S. Di Genaro, "TNFR p55 Controls Regulatory T Cell Responses in *Yersinia*-Induced Reactive Arthritis," *Immunology and Cell Biology*, Vol. 91, No. 2, 2013, pp. 159-166.
http://dx.doi.org/10.1038/icb.2012.65

[70] J. Sieper, J. Braun, P. Wu and G. Kingsley, "T Cells Are

Responsible for the Enhanced Synovial Cellular Immune Response to Triggering Antigen in Reactive Arthritis," *Clinical & Experimental Immunology*, Vol. 91, No. 1, 1993, pp. 96-102. http://dx.doi.org/10.1111/j.1365-2249.1993.tb03361.x

[71] C. Alvarez-Navarro, J. J. Cragnolini, H. G. Dos Santos, E. Barnea, A. Admon, A. Morreale and J. A. López De Castro, "Novel HLA-B27-Restricted Epitopes from *Chlamydia trachomatis* Generated Upon Endogenous Processing of Bacterial Proteins Suggest a Role of Molecular Mimicry in Reactive Arthritis," *Journal of Biological Chemistry*, Vol. 288, No. 36, 2013, pp. 25810-25825. http://dx.doi.org/10.1074/jbc.M113.493247

[72] R. Benjamin and P. Parham, "Guilt by Association: HLA-B27 and Ankylosing Spondylitis," *Immunology Today*, Vol. 11, No. 4, 1990, pp. 137-142. http://dx.doi.org/10.1016/0167-5699(90)90051-A

[73] W. Kuon, H. G. Holzhutter, H. Appel, M. Grolms, S. Kollnberger, A. Traeder, P. Henklein, E. Weiss, A. Thiel, R. Lauster, P. Bowness, A. Radbruch, P. M. Kloetzel and J. Sieper, "Identification of HLA-B27-Restricted Peptides from the *Chlamydia trachomatis* Proteome with Possible Relevance to HLA-B27-Associated Diseases," *Journal of Immunology*, Vol. 167, No. 8, 2001, pp. 4738-4746.

[74] E. May, M. L. Dorris, N. Satumtira, I. Iqbal, M. I. Rehman, E. Lightfoot and J. D. Taurog, "CD8 Alpha Beta T Cells Are Not Essential to the Pathogenesis of Arthritis or Colitis in HLA-B27 Transgenic Rats," *Journal of Immunology*, Vol. 170, No. 2, 2003, pp. 1099-1105.

[75] J. D. Taurog, M. L. Dorris, N. Satumtira, T. M. Tran, R. Sharma, R. Dressel, J. Van Den Brandt and H. M. Reichardt, "Spondylarthritis in HLA-B27/Human Beta2-Microglobulin-Transgenic Rats Is Not Prevented by Lack of CD8," *Arthritis & Rheumatism*, Vol. 60, No. 7, 2009, pp. 1977-1984. http://dx.doi.org/10.1002/art.24599

[76] M. A. Whelan and J. R. Archer, "Chemical Reactivity of an HLA-B27 Thiol Group," *European Journal of Immunology*, Vol. 23, No. 12, 1993, pp. 3278-3285. http://dx.doi.org/10.1002/eji.1830231233

[77] R. A. Colbert, T. M. Tran and G. Layh-Schmitt, "HLA-B27 Misfolding and Ankylosing Spondylitis," *Molecular Immunology*, Vol. 57, No. 1, 2014, pp. 44-51. http://dx.doi.org/10.1016/j.molimm.2013.07.013

[78] L. H. Boyle, J. C. Goodall, S. S. Opat and J. S. Gaston, "The Recognition of HLA-B27 by Human CD4(+) T Lymphocytes," *Journal of Immunology*, Vol. 167, No. 5, 2001, pp. 2619-2624.

[79] J. D. Reveille, "Genetics of Spondyloarthritis-Beyond the MHC," *Nature Reviews Rheumatology*, Vol. 8, No. 5, 2012, pp. 296-304. http://dx.doi.org/10.1038/nrrheum.2012.41

[80] J. D. Carter, H. C. Gerard, J. A. Whittum-Hudson and A. P. Hudson, "Combination Antibiotics for the Treatment of *Chlamydia*-Induced Reactive Arthritis: Is a Cure in Sight?" *International Journal of Clinical Rheumatology*, Vol. 6, No. 3, 2011, pp. 333-345. http://dx.doi.org/10.2217/ijr.11.20

[81] J. Sieper, "Developments in Therapies for Spondyloarthritis," *Nature Reviews Rheumatology*, Vol. 8, No. 5, 2012, pp. 280-287. http://dx.doi.org/10.1038/nrrheum.2012.40

[82] A. Toivanen, "Managing Reactive Arthritis," *Rheumatology*, Vol. 39, No. 2, 2000, pp. 117-119. http://dx.doi.org/10.1093/rheumatology/39.2.117

[83] M. Dougados, "Current Therapy for Seronegative Arthritides (Spondyloarthritis)," *Bulletin of the NYU Hospital for Joint Diseases*, Vol. 69, No. 3, 2011, pp. 250-252.

[84] D. Flores, J. Marquez, M. Garza and L. R. Espinoza, "Reactive Arthritis: Newer Developments," *Rheumatic Disease Clinics of North America*, Vol. 29, No. 1, 2003, pp. 37-59. http://dx.doi.org/10.1016/S0889-857X(02)00081-9

[85] D. O. Clegg, D. J. Reda, M. H. Weisman, J. J. Cush, F. B. Vasey, H. R. Schumacher Jr., E. Budiman-Mak, D. J. Balestra, W. D. Blackburn, G. W. Cannon, R. D. Inman, F. P. Alepa, E. Mejias, M. R. Cohen, R. Makkena, M. L. Mahowald, J. Higashida, S. L. Silverman, N. Parhami, J. Buxbaum, C. M. Haakenson, R. H. Ward, B. J. Manaster, R. J. Anderson, W. G. Henderson, *et al.*, "Comparison of Sulfasalazine and Placebo in the Treatment of Reactive Arthritis (Reiter's Syndrome). A Department of Veterans Affairs Cooperative Study," *Arthritis & Rheumatism*, Vol. 39, No. 12, 1996, pp. 2021-2027. http://dx.doi.org/10.1002/art.1780391211

[86] L. Goh and A. Samanta, "Update on Biologic Therapies in Ankylosing Spondylitis: A Literature Review," *International Journal of Rheumatic Diseases*, Vol. 15, No. 5, 2012, pp. 445-454. http://dx.doi.org/10.1111/j.1756-185X.2012.01765.x

[87] S. D. Flagg, R. Meador, E. Hsia, T. Kitumnuaypong and H. R. Schumacher, "Decreased Pain and Synovial Inflammation after Etanercept Therapy in Patients with Reactive and Undifferentiated Arthritis: An Open-Label Trial," *Arthritis Care & Research*, Vol. 53, No. 4, 2005, pp. 613-617. http://dx.doi.org/10.1002/art.21323

[88] R. Meador, E. Hsia, T. Kitumnuaypong and H. R. Schumacher, "TNF Involvement and Anti-TNF Therapy of Reactive and Unclassified Arthritis," *Clinical and Experimental Rheumatology*, Vol. 20, No. 6, 2002, pp. S130-S134.

[89] A. Meyer, E. Chatelus, D. Wendling, J. M. Berthelot, E. Dernis, E. Houvenagel, J. Morel, O. Richer, T. Schaeverbeke, J. E. Gottenberg and J. Sibilia, "Safety and Efficacy of Anti-Tumor Necrosis Factor Alpha Therapy in Ten Patients with Recent-Onset Refractory Reactive Arthritis," *Arthritis & Rheumatism*, Vol. 63, No. 5, 2011, pp. 1274-1280. http://dx.doi.org/10.1002/art.30272

[90] K. S. Oili, H. Niinisalo, T. Korpilahde and J. Virolainen, "Treatment of Reactive Arthritis with Infliximab," *Scandinavian Journal of Rheumatology*, Vol. 32, No. 2, 2003, pp. 122-124. http://dx.doi.org/10.1080/03009740310000157

[91] M. Rihl, A. Klos, L. Kohler and J. G. Kuipers, "Infection and Musculoskeletal Conditions: Reactive Arthritis," *Best Practice & Research Clinical Rheumatology*, Vol. 20, No. 6, 2006, pp. 1119-1137. http://dx.doi.org/10.1016/j.berh.2006.08.008

[92] M. D. Schafranski, "Infliximab for Reactive Arthritis Secondary to *Chlamydia trachomatis* Infection," *Rheuma-

tology International, Vol. 30, No. 5, 2010, pp. 679-680. http://dx.doi.org/10.1007/s00296-009-0965-9

[93] R. J. Eliçabe, J. L. Arias, G. A. Rabinovich and M. S. Di Genaro, "TNFRp55 Modulates IL-6 and Nitric Oxide Responses Following *Yersinia* Lipopolysaccharide Stimulation in Peritoneal Macrophages," *Immunobiology*, Vol. 216, No. 12, 2011, pp. 1322-1330. http://dx.doi.org/10.1016/j.imbio.2011.05.009

[94] A. Gottlieb, A. Menter, A. Mendelsohn, Y. K. Shen, S. Li, C. Guzzo, S. Fretzin, R. Kunynetz and A. Kavanaugh, "Ustekinumab, a Human Interleukin 12/23 Monoclonal Antibody, for Psoriatic Arthritis: Randomised, Double-Blind, Placebo-Controlled, Crossover Trial," *Lancet*, Vol. 373, No. 9664, 2009, pp. 633-640. http://dx.doi.org/10.1016/S0140-6736(09)60140-9

[95] I. B. Mcinnes, J. Sieper, J. Braun, P. Emery, D. Van Der Heijde, J. D. Isaacs, G. Dahmen, J. Wollenhaupt, H. Schulze-Koops, J. Kogan, S. Ma, M. M. Schumacher, A.

P. Bertolino, W. Hueber and P. P. Tak, "Efficacy and Safety of Secukinumab, a Fully Human Anti-Interleukin-17A Monoclonal Antibody, in Patients with Moderate-to-Severe Psoriatic Arthritis: A 24-Week, Randomised, Double-Blind, Placebo-Controlled, Phase II Proof-of-Concept Trial," *Annals of the Rheumatic Diseases*, 2013.

[96] M. Leirisalo-Repo, P. Helenius, T. Hannu, A. Lehtinen, J. Kreula, M. Taavitsainen and S. Koskimies, "Long-Term Prognosis of Reactive *Salmonella* Arthritis," *Annals of the Rheumatic Diseases*, Vol. 56, No. 9, 1997, pp. 516-520. http://dx.doi.org/10.1136/ard.56.9.516

[97] M. Leirisalo-Repo and H. Suoranta, "Ten-Year Follow-up Study of Patients with *Yersinia* Arthritis," *Arthritis & Rheumatism*, Vol. 31, No. 4, 1988, pp. 533-537. http://dx.doi.org/10.1002/art.1780310410

[98] E. Sairanen, I. Paronen and H. Mähönen, "Reiter's Syndrome: A Follow-up Study," *Acta Medica Scandinavica*, Vol. 185, No. 1-6, 1969, pp. 57-63.

Bilateral nephromegaly and arthritis: A rare presentation of acute lymphoblastic leukemia[*]

Tapas Kumar Sabui[1#], Syamal Sardar[2], Sumanta Laha[3], Abhishek Roy[4]

[1]Department of Pediatrics & Neonatology, Institute of Post Graduate Medical Education & Research, Kolkata, India
[2]Department of Neonatology, Institute of Post Graduate Medical Education & Research, Kolkata, India
[3]Department of Pediatrics, Burdwan Medical College & Hospital, Burdwan, India
[4]Department of Pediatrics, North Bengal Medical College & Hospital, Darjeeling, India
Email: [#]tsabui@gmail.com

ABSTRACT

A 2.5-year-old boy presented with fever, intermittent small joint arthritis of hands and feet, bilateral nephromegaly with normal hemogram and uric acid level. Bone marrow aspiration revealed pre-B acute lymphoblastic leukemia without leukemic infiltration of kidneys. Leukemia should be suspected in any patient with arthritis and nephromegaly.

Keywords: Acute Lymphoblastic Leukemia; Nephromegaly; Arthritis

1. INTRODUCTION

Acute lymphoblastic leukemia (ALL) is a common disease and occasionally presents with rare features. However, bilateral kidney enlargement and intermittent small joint arthritis is extremely rare and this combination has never been described in literature till date. Hereby we report such a case with small joint arthritis and nephromegaly as an initial manifestation of ALL.

2. CASE REPORT

A 2.5-year-old male child born out of non consanguineous marriage was referred to our Pediatric Rheumatology clinic for opinion with history of fever for a short duration and intermittent arthritis of small joints of both hands and feet. He had two similar episodes of arthritis of hands, feet and ankle joint in last 3 months. It was treated by local pediatrician and he responded well to analgesics. He was clinically asymptomatic in between these acute illnesses.

His anthropometric measurements were within normal

limits. He was febrile and his interphalangeal, meta-carpo-phalangeal joints of hands (**Figure 1**) and small joints of feet were tender and inflamed. Abdominal examination revealed bilateral palpable renal masses (left more than right). There was no pallor, hepatosplenomegaly or muco-cutaneous haemorrhagic spots. The child was normotensive and examination of others systems were within normal limit.

Complete hemogram showed hemoglobin of 14.6 gm/dl, total leucocyte count of 8400/mm^3, neutrophil 48%, lymphocyte 50%, eosinophil 2%, platelet count 2.4 lacs/mm^3 and normocytic normochromic RBC. His ESR and ASO titer were 28 mm in 1st hour and 400 IU/ml respectively. Biochemical parameters including uric acid level, renal function and hepatic function tests were within normal limits. An increased uric acid value of 13.5 mg/dl was documented later during hospital stay. X-ray of both hands and feet were normal. Bilaterally enlarged kidneys were documented with ultrasonography of abdomen. The size of right and left kidney was 11.2 cm × 5.5 cm and 12 cm × 6 cm respectively. There was loss of cortico-medullary differentiation. CT abdomen revealed diffusely enlarged and bulky kidneys with delayed contrast excretion and no focal mass lesion (**Figure 2**). Kidney biopsy showed hyperplasia and hypertrophy of parenchymal cells with infiltration of the interstitium by round cells with normochromatic nuclei. There was no definite evidence of leukemic infiltration. Bone marrow examination revealed markedly hypercellular marrow packed with blast cells which were cytomorphologically lymphoblasts. The blast cells were Periodic Acid Schiff (PAS) positive but negative for Sudan Black and Myeloperoxidase (MPO). On flow cytometric analysis, the blast cells expressed cCD79a, CD19 and CD10. CD19/CD10 co-expression was present in 95% of these cells. CD20, CD34, HLADR, Kappa and Lambda

---
[*]Conflict of interest: Nil.
[#]Corresponding author.

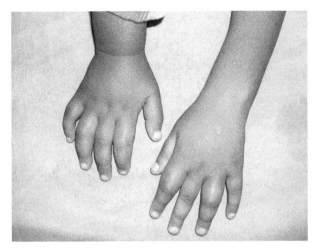

Figure 1. Hands of the child showing inflammed, swollen metacarpo-phalangeal and interphalangeal joints.

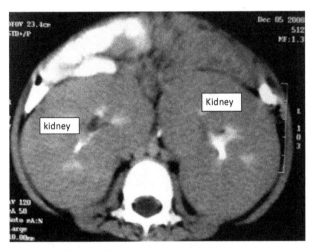

Figure 2. Contrast CT scan of abdomen showing grossly enlarged and diffuse bulky kidneys.

monoclonal light chains, T cell and myeloid markers were absent suggesting pre-B ALL. Cerebrospinal fluid examination did not reveal any evidence of meningeal infiltration. The final diagnosis was Pre-B acute lymphoblastic leukemia.

Hospital course: He was subjected to ALL BFM90 regime after confirmation of the diagnosis [1]. He received 12.5 mg intrathecal methotrexate on Day 1, oral prednisolone (60 mg/m^2/day) daily for 7 days and intravenous fluid during pre-induction phase. Thereafter phase 1 induction was started with intravenous vincristine (1.4 mg/m^2), doxorubicine (30 mg/m^2), deep intramascular l-asparaginase (10000 u/m^2), intrathecal methotrexate (12.5 mg) and oral prednisolone (60 mg/m^2) according to the BFM90 protocol. We noticed dramatic response during the induction phase and the kidneys became non palpable within 10 days after starting chemotherapy. Repeat USG abdomen revealed normal size kidneys 4 wk later. Elevated uric acid level (13.5 mg/dl) was de-

tected during his hospital stay. It was treated with adequate intravenous fluid, alkalization of urine and oral allopurinol. The joint symptoms subsided with normalization of uric acid level. The child had just completed the phase 1 induction chemotherapy at the time of reporting it and was doing well.

3. DISCUSSION

The unique combination of nephromegaly and transient intermittent arthritis of small joints in ALL has not been described in literature till date to the best of our knowledge. Children with ALL characteristically present with fever, pallor, bleeds, lymphadenopathy and organomegaly. Although renal infiltration is relatively frequent in acute lymphoblastic leukemia, clinically palpable renal enlargement occurs only in 2% - 5% of cases. Isolated renal enlargement as a primary presenting feature of ALL is extremely rare [2-5]. Renal enlargement in a case of leukemia may be due to leukemic infiltration or simple hypertrophy or hyperplasia of cells [6]. Enlarged kidneys do not always indicate leukemic involvement as shown in a study by Frei *et al.* [6], where, as many as 30% of the kidneys in leukemic patients were free of malignant cells on autopsy. Therefore, kidney mass oriented approach for confirmation of diagnosis leaving aside bone marrow examination may lead to high possibility of missing the correct diagnosis. Nephromegaly without any leukemic infiltration is generally associated with heaptosplenomagaly [6]. The index patient presented only with nephromegaly. Renal functions are usually well preserved in such a situation as in the present case and only a few cases of renal failure secondary to a diffuse bilateral parenchymal infiltration are reported in the literature [7]. Although the role of radiotherapy in the treatment of leukemic infiltrates has been studied in the past, currently systemic chemotherapy remains the basic treatment even with leukemic infiltrates. Enlarged kidneys in ALL are thought to be an unfavourable sign. The index patient, however, responded well to chemotherapy and follow up ultrasound revealed normal size kidneys.

Joint involvement as an initial presentation of acute leukemia in children has been described in literature [8-11]. About 15% to 30% of ALL patients manifest with osteoarthritic symptoms, some of which may mimic juvenile idiopathic arthritis (JIA) [11]. However, the interesting fact was that the arthritis here was transient and intermittent. The exact mechanism of this transient arthritis was not clear. Although high uric acid, end product of leukocyte nucleic acid breakdown, causes arthritis it seems that it is not a causative agent here as it is normal to begin with the disease. A ten years survey in paediatric rheumatology clinic conducted by Trapani *et al.* [8] found 6 cases of ALL with arthritis out of 1254 patients. JIA was the most frequent provisional diagnosis and monoarticular arthritis of large joint was the commonest mode of presentation. Investigators from Europe, North and South America have reported a similar pattern of joint involvement in ALL patients with osteoarthritic manifestation [9].

In another study by Jung et al. [10], out of 30 children initially diagnosed as JIA, 3 were later diagnosed as acute leukemia (2 ALL, 1 AML) by bone marrow examination. Among these 3 patients, one had monoarticular arthritis of large joint, another had arthritis in 3 large joints and third patient had only arthralgia. All had absence of blasts in peripheral smear which was similar to our case. Robazzi et al. [11] observed arthritis in 26% occasions in a pool of 313 cases of ALL and it was mainly large joint arthritis. Marwaha et al. has reported an incidence of 16% of small joints involvement in a recently published article. There was no mention of transient intermittent arthritis [9]. The index case presented here with transient arthritis of small joints of hands and feet in contrast. The literature on comparison of children with ALL whose initial diagnosis was JIA, with other ALL patients, for the pattern of initial presentation, management, outcome, and prognostic factors is scant.

4. CONCLUSION

Bilateral enlargement of kidneys and arthritis in another normal child should raise the suspicion of acute leukemia and the patient should be subjected to bone marrow examination before ordering for other invasive tests.

REFERENCES

[1] Schrappe, M., Reiter, A., Ludwig, W.D., et al. (2000) Improved outcome in childhood acute lymphoblastic leukemia despite reduced use of anthracyclines and cranial radiotherapy: Results of trial ALL-BFM 90. Blood, 95, 3310-3322.

[2] Boueva, A. and Bouvier, R. (2005) B-cell lympholblastic leukemia as a cause of bilateral nephromegaly. Pediatric Nephrology, 20, 679-682. doi:10.1007/s00467-004-1740-5

[3] Basker, M., Scott, J.X., Ross, B., et al. (2002) Renal enlargement as primary presentation of acute lymphoblastic leukemia. Indian Journal of Cancer, 39, 154-156.

[4] Rudramurthy, P., Madhumathi, S.D., et al. (2008) Bilateral nephromegaly simulating wilms tumour: A rare initial manifestation of acute lymphoblastic leukemia. Journal of Pediatric Hematology/Oncology, 30, 471-473. doi:10.1097/MPH.0b013e318168e7b3

[5] Ali, S.H., Yacoub, F.M. and Al Matar, E. (2008) Acute lymphoblastic leukemia presenting as bilateral renal enlargement in a child. Medical Principles and Practice, 17, 504-506. doi:10.1159/000151576

[6] Frei III, E., Fritz, R.D., Price, E., et al. (1963) Renal and hepatic enlargement in acute leukemia. Cancer, 16, 1089-1092. doi:10.1002/1097-0142(196308)16:8<1089::AID-CNCR2820160817>3.0.CO;2-1

[7] Glicklich, D., Sung, M.V. and Frey, M. (1986) Renal failure due to lymphomatous infiltration of the kidneys. Cancer, 58, 748-753. doi:10.1002/1097-0142(19860801)58:3<748::AID-CNCR2820580323>3.0.CO;2-U

[8] Trapani, S., Grisolia, F., Simonini, G., et al. (2000) Incidence of occult cancer in children presenting with musculoskeletal symptoms: A 10 yr survey in pediatric rheumatology unit. Semin Arthritis Rheum, 29, 348-359. doi:10.1053/sarh.2000.5752

[9] Marwaha, R.K., Kulkarni, K.P., Bansal, D. and Trehan, A. (2010) Acute lymphoblastic leukemia masquerading as juvenile rheumatoid arthritis: Diagnostic pitfall and association with survival. Annals of Hematology, 89, 249-254. doi:10.1007/s00277-009-0826-3

[10] Jung, A. and Nielsen, S.M. (1998) Arthritis as first symptom of leukemia in children. Ugeskrift for Laeger, 160, 2889-2890.

[11] Robazzi, T.C., Barreto, J.H., Silva, L.R., et al. (2007) Osteoarticular manifestations as initial presentation of acute leukemias in children and adolescents in Bahia, Brazil. Journal of Pediatric Hematology/Oncology, 29, 622-626.

Experience of Patients Undergoing Mini-Arthroscopy Compared to MRI in the Earliest Phases of Arthritis[*]

Maria J. H. de Hair[1#], Marleen G. H. van de Sande[1], Mario Maas[2], Danielle M. Gerlag[1], Paul P. Tak[1]

[1]Department of Clinical Immunology and Rheumatology, Academic Medical Center, University of Amsterdam, Amsterdam, The Netherlands; [2]Department of Radiology, Academic Medical Center, University of Amsterdam, Amsterdam, The Netherlands.
Email: [#]m.j.dehair@amc.uva.nl

ABSTRACT

Objective: To evaluate the expectations and experience of patients undergoing mini-arthroscopy compared to contrast enhanced MRI for research purposes. **Methods:** Seventeen patients with early, active arthritis (Group A) and 21 autoantibody-positive individuals without any evidence of arthritis upon physical examination (Group B) were included. All subjects underwent both contrast enhanced MRI and synovial biopsy sampling by mini-arthroscopy of the same joint within one week. At inclusion and after both procedures, subjects filled in questionnaires with items about expectations and experience with regard to the procedures. **Results:** Before procedures, subjects in group B had a higher fear of and reluctance to undergo mini-arthroscopy compared to MRI ($p < 0.0001$ and $p = 0.001$, respectively). Before procedures, 42% of the subjects preferred MRI, 11% of the subjects preferred mini-arthroscopy and 47% had no preference for either procedure. After both procedures, subjects preferences changed to 39% for MRI, 32% for mini-arthroscopy and 29% for no preference for one or the other procedure. When comparing Group A with Group B, there were no significant differences in preference before and after the procedures. **Conclusion:** Synovial biopsy sampling by mini-arthroscopy for analysis of synovial inflammation is a well-experienced procedure when compared to contrast enhanced MRI. These results support the use of mini-arthroscopy in a research setting from a patient perspective.

Keywords: Arthritis; Rheumatoid; Synovium; Arthroscopy; MRI

1. Introduction

Rheumatoid arthritis (RA) is a chronic autoimmune disease characterised by inflammation of synovial tissue leading to joint destruction and deformity [1]. Since the synovium is the main target tissue affected in RA, analysis of the features of the synovial inflammation is of major importance for pathogenetic studies. For analysis of synovial inflammation imaging but also histologic studies can be used. Analysis of the synovial tissue can be used to give insight into disease pathogenesis and to evaluate the effects of new treatments and the mechanisms of action of therapeutic compounds. Mini-arthroscopy, performed under local anaesthetics at the outpatient clinic, is a feasible means of synovial biopsy sampling. It has been used for research purposes and is generally well tolerated with low complication rates [2-4]. Still, mini-arthroscopy is regarded as a rather invasive procedure and only performed in a few specialised centres.

Imaging of synovial inflammation can be done making use of MRI. MRI gives information about the degree of synovial inflammation, and additionally the compartment surrounding the synovium can be evaluated, including the bone (marrow) and cartilage. In the current project we performed dynamic contrast enhanced (DCE) MRI, by injecting a contrast agent intravenously during and after which time-dependent changes in MRI signal can be registered. DCE-MRI clearly visualizes the degree of synovial inflammation [5], enables to study physiologic characteristics of the inflamed synovium, such as vessel

[*]This study was financially supported by the Dutch Arthritis Association (grant 06-1-303) and the European Community's FP6 funding (Autocure).
[#]Corresponding author.

permeability, and has been shown to be a sensitive tool to detect changes after treatment [6-11].

At international scientific meetings, when results from studies using synovial biopsy sampling by mini-arthroscopy are presented by researchers of our Department of Clinical Immunology and Rheumatology of the Academic Medical Center (AMC) Amsterdam, questions are raised concerning patient's experience of synovial biopsy sampling by mini-arthroscopy, especially in individuals without arthritis. It seems that there is a general idea that mini-arthroscopy is an invasive procedure and a burden for patients, which seems to hamper the use of mini-arthroscopic synovial biopsy sampling in some research centres. Patient expectations and experience of mini-arthroscopy have never been studied. Therefore, we investigated patient's expectations before and experience after mini-arthroscopic synovial biopsy sampling and compared those with expectations before and experience after undergoing dynamic contrast-enhanced MRI, which is generally seen as a non-invasive procedure.

2. Methods

2.1. Study Subjects

Group A consisted of early arthritis patients (arthritis duration less than 1 year) with an inflamed knee, ankle or wrist, who were disease modifying antirheumatic drug naive (AMC's "Synoviomics" program) [12]. Group B consisted of individuals at risk for developing RA, defined by the presence of IgM-rheumatoid factor and/or anti-citrullinated protein antibodies, but no evidence of arthritis upon physical examination [13] (AMC's "Pre-Synoviomics" program) [14]. The study was performed according to the principles of the Declaration of Helsinki, approved by the medical ethical committee of the AMC, and all study subjects gave written informed consent.

2.2. MRI

All study subjects underwent DCE-MRI as previously described [6]. In Group A, a clinically inflamed (swollen and painful) wrist, knee or ankle joint was examined and in Group B an arbitrarily chosen knee joint was examined in all cases. Briefly, images were acquired on either a closed (1.5 Tesla GE Signa Horizon Echospeed, LX9.0, General Electric Medical Systems, Milwaukee, Wisconsin, USA) or open (Panorama 1 Tesla Open, Philips, Best, the Netherlands) MRI scanner, depending on the availability of the machine. Three scans were performed after which a contrast agent gadolinium (Magnevist, Schering, Berlin, Germany) was injected intravenously and 2 additional scans were performed. Total duration of the procedure was 60 minutes.

2.3. Synovial Biopsy Sampling by Mini-Arthroscopy

Within one week after the MRI, synovial biopsy sampling was performed at the outpatient clinic by means of mini-arthroscopy under local anaesthetics, as previously described [2,15]. The same joint was chosen for both procedures. For each study group 24 up to 32 synovial tissue biopsies were obtained during one procedure. The duration of the total procedure was 45 to 60 minutes.

2.4. Questionnaires

Before and after both procedures, subjects filled in questionnaires with items about expectations and the experience they had with regard to the procedures. Questions asked were 1) Do you have preference for MRI or mini-arthroscopy or do you have "no preference"? 2) Please mark how well you think you are prepared for (a) MRI and (b) mini-arthroscopy 3) Please mark the level of fear you experience of (a) MRI and (b) mini-arthroscopy? 4) Please mark if you are reluctant to undergo (a) MRI and (b) mini-arthroscopy. The first question was multiple choice; the latter three questions were depicted on a visual analogue scale (VAS) of 0 - 100 mm. In addition, study subjects could comment their choice of preference for one of the procedures. The first questionnaire was completed and handed in before and the second questionnaire was filled in after both procedures.

2.5. Statistical Analysis

We describe preference for either of the procedures before and after the procedures or compared preference in Group A with Group B using Chi-square test. In addition, differences in baseline emotional aspects with respect to both procedures and differences in preference after procedures compared to baseline were analysed using Wilcoxon signed rank test for related samples. P-value < 0.05 was considered statistically significant. Statistical analysis was performed using PASW Statistics 18 (SPSS Inc., Chicago, IL).

3. Results

Of 38 subjects baseline and follow-up questionnaires were available: 17 from Group A and 21 from Group B. **Table 1** shows the disposition of study subjects with regard to type of joint examined and MRI machine used.

3.1. Emotional Aspects

With respect to emotional aspects subjects generally felt well prepared for both procedures. In Group B scores for fear and reluctance were higher for mini-arthroscopy compared to MRI, see **Table 2**. This was not the case for

Table 1. Disposition of study subjects.

Group A*	Open MRI	Closed MRI
Wrist	0	1
Knee	2	10
Ankle	1	3
Group B*	Open MRI	Closed MRI
Knee	6	15

*Group A represents early arthritis patients; *Group B represents autoantibody-positive individuals without arthritis at risk for developing RA.

Table 2. Emotional aspects regarding DCE-MRI and mini-arthroscopy at baseline.

Group A*	Mini-arthroscopy	DCE-MRI	P-value
Preparation for procedure	85 (52 - 91)	82 (60 - 94)	0.504
Fear of procedure	25 (6 - 46)	5 (0 - 51)	0.084
Being reluctant to undergo procedure	18 (6 - 31)	4 (0 - 43)	0.248
Group B*	Mini-arthroscopy	DCE-MRI	P-value
Preparation for procedure	90 (59 - 96)	89 (62 - 96)	0.316
Fear of procedure	21 (7 - 57)	3 (0 - 7)	**0.000**
Being reluctant to undergo procedure	16 (4 - 47)	1 (0 - 5)	**0.001**

DCE-MRI: dynamic contrast enhanced MRI; All items measured on a visual analogue scale of 0 - 100 mm; Results depicted as median (IQR); *Group A represents early arthritis patients; *Group B represents autoantibody-positive individuals without arthritis at risk for developing RA.

Group A. However, there were no statistically significant differences between Groups A and B at baseline for individual emotional aspects (**Table 3**).

3.2. Experience of Mini-Arthroscopy and DCE-MRI

In the total study population, before undergoing both procedures 42% of the subjects preferred MRI, 11% preferred mini-arthroscopy and 47% had no preference for either procedure. After both procedures subjects preference changed to 39% preferring MRI, 32% mini-arthroscopy and 29% having no preference for one of the procedures for studying synovitis. This shows that there was not a clear preference for one of the procedures. In addition, preference after both procedures was not significantly different from baseline preference (P = 0.602).

When focusing on the subgroups, within Group A preference was as follows: at baseline 47% of the subjects did not have preference for either procedure, 35% preferred MRI and 18% preferred mini-arthroscopy. After both procedures 29% did not have preference, 24% preferred MRI and 47% preferred mini-arthroscopy (no difference was observed between preference after both procedures and before, p = 0.755).

Table 3. A comparison of emotional aspects regarding DCE-MRI and mini-arthroscopy at baseline between group A and group B.

	Group A*	Group B*	P-value
Preparation for MRI	82 (60 - 94)	89 (62 - 96)	0.521
Preparation for mini-arthroscopy	85 (52 - 91)	90 (59 - 96)	0.293
Fear of MRI	5 (0 - 51)	3 (0 - 7)	0.318
Fear of mini-arthroscopy	25 (6 - 46)	21 (7 - 57)	0.751
Being reluctant to undergo MRI	4 (0 - 43)	1 (0 - 5)	0.237
Being reluctant to undergo mini-arthroscopy	18 (6 - 31)	16 (4 - 47)	0.894

DCE-MRI: dynamic contrast enhanced MRI; All items measured on a visual analogue scale of 0 - 100 mm; Results depicted as median (IQR); *Group A represents early arthritis patients; *Group B represents autoantibody-positive individuals without arthritis at risk for developing RA.

Within group B, at baseline, 38% did not have preference for either procedure, 57% preferred MRI and 5% preferred mini-arthroscopy. After both procedures, these percentages were, 29%, 52% and 19%, respectively (no difference was observed between preference after both procedures and before (P = 0.715). In addition, comparing study groups, there was no difference in preference between Groups A and B at baseline (P = 0.271) or after both procedures (P = 0.115).

Of importance, after both procedures, 6 individuals of Group A who did not have preference (n = 2) or preferred MRI (n = 4) at baseline changed to preference for mini-arthroscopy. Four of the individuals of Group B changed towards preference for mini-arthroscopy, of which 3 individuals preferred MRI at baseline. In both groups, none of the subjects who preferred mini-arthroscopy at baseline changed to MRI and, of those, only 1 individual changed to "no preference". See **Figure 1** for preference at baseline, after both procedures and change in preference.

Of subjects who underwent MRI in the open scanner, nobody changed to preference for MRI afterwards. Main remarks with regard to DCE-MRI were complaints about the noise coming from the MRI machine and being immobile for a long period of time, the latter in particular in patients with arthritis. Some patients indicated that mini-arthroscopy was better tolerated than expected, but two subjects complained about having more joint complaints until a few days after mini-arthroscopy. All study subjects were contacted by telephone one week after the procedures or consulted their rheumatologist within 3 weeks time and otherwise the procedures were well tolerated; no complications were reported.

4. Discussion

In this small study, we show that synovial biopsy sam-

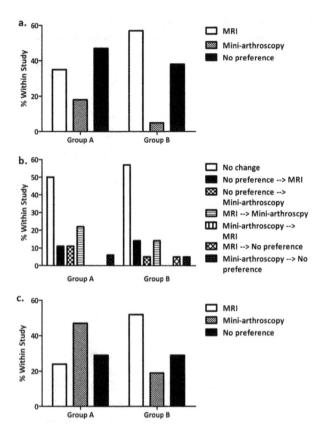

Figure 1. Preference of mini-arthroscopy or dynamic contrast enhanced MRI. Preference at baseline a, change in preference b and preference after both procedures c. Results are depicted as percentage within study Group A or B. Group A represents early arthritis patients; Group B represents autoantibody-positive individuals without arthritis at risk for developing RA.

pling by means of mini-arthroscopy is well experienced when compared to DCE-MRI for studying synovial inflammation, both in early arthritis patients and in individuals without arthritis at risk for developing RA. Interestingly, we observed an increase, although not statistically significant, in the percentage of early arthritis patients preferring mini-arthroscopy after both procedures. Although at baseline the group of autoantibody-positive individuals without arthritis had higher levels of fear of and reluctance to undergo mini-arthroscopy than MRI, in this group the percentage of individuals preferring mini-arthroscopy increased after procedures as well. Overall, these results refute assumptions that mini-arthroscopy would be a procedure not well-experienced by study subjects.

A factor that could be in favour of mini-arthroscopy may be that during mini-arthroscopy patients have direct contact with physicians and nurses, whereas during MRI they are completely on their own in a distinct room. After having undergone both procedures, most arthritis patients preferred mini-arthroscopy, which may be explained in

part by the more stringent need for immobilisation during MRI. In contrast to the arthritis group, most individuals without arthritis still favoured MRI, which might be due to a short period of relative rest necessary after mini-arthroscopy whereas after MRI no restrictions are imposed. Still, 19% of the subjects without arthritis favoured mini-arthroscopy after both procedures and none of these individuals preferring mini-arthroscopy at baseline changed to a preference for DCE-MRI. Of importance, the results of our study cannot be extrapolated to studies using conventional MRI, because scanning duration is generally longer for DCE-MRI and requires venipuncture in all cases, but do support the notion that mini-arthroscopy is generally well experienced, even in individuals without arthritis.

In summary, our results show the important observation that mini-arthroscopy, compared to DCE-MRI, is well experienced in patients with early arthritis as well as in autoantibody-positive individuals without arthritis who are at risk of developing RA. These results support the use of mini-arthroscopy in a research setting from a patient perspective, which, together with the low complication rates [2-4] should help to start using mini-arthroscopy in additional research centres.

5. Acknowledgements

We thank our study subjects for participation in the study and the AMC mini-arthroscopy team for synovial biopsy sampling. We thank the Dutch Arthritis Association (grant 06-1-303) and the European Community's FP6 funding (Autocure) for financial support.

REFERENCES

[1] P. P. Tak and B. Bresnihan, "The Pathogenesis and Prevention of Joint Damage in Rheumatoid Arthritis: Advances from Synovial Biopsy and Tissue Analysis," *Arthritis & Rheumatism*, Vol. 43, No. 12, 2000, pp. 2619-2633.
http://dx.doi.org/10.1002/1529-0131(200012)43:12<2619::AID-ANR1>3.0.CO;2-V

[2] D. M. Gerlag and P. P. Tak, "How to Perform and Analyse Synovial Biopsies," *Best Practice & Research Clinical Rheumatology*, Vol. 23, No. 2, 2009, pp. 221-232. http://dx.doi.org/10.1016/j.berh.2009.01.006

[3] D. Kane, D. J. Veale, O. Fitzgerald, *et al.*, "Survey of Arthroscopy Performed by Rheumatologists," *Rheumatology (Oxford)*, Vol. 41, No. 2, 2002, pp. 210-215. http://dx.doi.org/10.1093/rheumatology/41.2.210

[4] S. Vordenbaumen, L. A. Joosten, J. Friemann, *et al.*, "Utility of Synovial Biopsy," *Arthritis Research & Therapy*, Vol. 11, 2009, p. 256. http://dx.doi.org/10.1186/ar2847

[5] M. B. Axelsen, M. Stoltenberg, R. P. Poggenborg, *et al.*, "Dynamic Gadolinium-Enhanced Magnetic Resonance

Imaging Allows Accurate Assessment of the Synovial Inflammatory Activity in Rheumatoid Arthritis Knee Joints: A Comparison with Synovial Histology," *Scandinavian Journal of Rheumatology*, Vol. 41, No. 2, 2012, pp. 89-94. http://dx.doi.org/10.3109/03009742.2011.608375

[6] C. van der Leij, M. G. van de Sande and C. Lavini, *et al.*, "Rheumatoid Synovial Inflammation: Pixel-by-Pixel Dynamic Contrast-Enhanced MR Imaging Time-Intensity Curve Shape Analysis—A Feasibility Study," *Radiology*, Vol. 253, No. 1, 2009, pp. 234-240. http://dx.doi.org/10.1148/radiol.2531081722

[7] M. Navalho, C. Resende, A. M. Rodrigues, *et al.*, "Dynamic Contrast-Enhanced 3-T Magnetic Resonance Imaging: A Method for Quantifying Disease Activity in Early Polyarthritis," *Skeletal Radiology*, Vol. 41, No. 1, 2012, pp. 51-59. http://dx.doi.org/10.1007/s00256-011-1112-8

[8] B. Ejbjerg, E. Narvestad, E. Rostrup, *et al.*, "Magnetic Resonance Imaging of Wrist and Finger Joints in Healthy Subjects Occasionally Shows Changes Resembling Erosions and Synovitis as Seen in Rheumatoid Arthritis," *Arthritis & Rheumatism*, Vol. 50, 2004, pp. 1097-1106. http://dx.doi.org/10.1002/art.20135

[9] M. Ostergaard, I. Lorenzen and O. Henriksen, "Dynamic Gadolinium-Enhanced MR Imaging in Active and Inactive Immunoinflammatory Gonarthritis," *Acta Radiologica*, Vol. 35, No. 3, 1994, pp. 275-281.

[10] M. Ostergaard, M. Stoltenberg, P. Lovgreen-Nielsen, *et al.*, "Quantification of Synovistis by MRI: Correlation between Dynamic and Static Gadolinium-Enhanced Magnetic Resonance Imaging and Microscopic and Macroscopic Signs of Synovial Inflammation," *Magnetic Resonance Imaging*, Vol. 16, No. 7, 1998, pp. 743-754. http://dx.doi.org/10.1016/S0730-725X(98)00008-3

[11] A. L. Tan, S. F. Tanner, P. G. Conaghan, *et al.*, "Role of Metacarpophalangeal Joint Anatomic Factors in the Distribution of Synovitis and Bone Erosion in Early Rheumatoid Arthritis," *Arthritis & Rheumatism*, Vol. 48, No. 5, 2003, pp. 1214-1222. http://dx.doi.org/10.1002/art.10963

[12] M. J. de Hair, L. C. Harty, D. M. Gerlag, *et al.*, "Synovial Tissue Analysis for the Discovery of Diagnostic and Prognostic Biomarkers in Patients with Early Arthritis," *The Journal of Rheumatology*, Vol. 38, No. 9, 2011, pp. 2068-2072. http://dx.doi.org/10.3899/jrheum.110426

[13] D. M. Gerlag, K. Raza, L. G. van Baarsen, *et al.*, "EULAR Recommendations for Terminology and Research in Individuals at Risk of Rheumatoid Arthritis: Report from the Study Group for Risk Factors for Rheumatoid Arthritis," *Annals of the Rheumatic Diseases*, Vol. 71, No. 5, 2012, pp. 638-641. http://dx.doi.org/10.1136/annrheumdis-2011-200990

[14] M. G. van de Sande, M. J. de Hair, C. van der Leij, *et al.*, "Different Stages of Rheumatoid Arthritis: Features of the Synovium in the Preclinical Phase," *Annals of the Rheumatic Diseases*, Vol. 70, No. 5, 2011, pp. 772-777. http://dx.doi.org/10.1136/ard.2010.139527

[15] M. G. van de Sande, "Evaluating Antirheumatic Treatments Using Synovial Biopsy: A Recommendation for Standardisation to Be Used in Clinical Trials," *Annals of the Rheumatic Diseases*, Vol. 70, No. 3, 2011, pp. 423-427. http://dx.doi.org/10.1136/ard.2010.139550

5

Evaluation of Tuberculin Skin Test Response and Interfering Factors in Patients with Juvenile Idiopathic Arthritis

Işıl Eser Şimşek, Müferet Ergüven, Olcay Bilgiç Dağcı

Göztepe Teaching and Research Hospital, Istanbul, Turkey.
Email: olcaybilgic@yahoo.com

ABSTRACT

Juvenile idiopathic arthritis (JIA) is the most common rheumatologic disease in pediatric age group. Mycobacterium tuberculosis infection (TB) is an important cause of mortality and morbidity in patients with inflammatory rheumatologic disease. The objective of this study is to determine to what extent active disease and use of drugs in JIA affects response to PPD skin test and thus to investigate the significance of PPD skin test in the diagnosis of latent TB. 77 children diagnosed with JIA according to ILAR diagnostic criteria and routinely followed by our rheumatology clinic were included in the patient group. Patients were grouped according to subtypes of disease, activity status and drugs they used. Control group was formed from 58 healthy children. PPD skin test was applied to each subject and the number of BCG scars of all cases was recorded. We found no significant difference in PPD induration diameters between JIA and control group (p > 0.05). The number of BCG scar is similar in both groups. In the control group, age and number of BCG scars and PPD skin test diameter are positively correlated. But there is no such significant relationship in patients with JIA (p > 0.05). PPD induration diameter of patients with active disease is significantly shorter than patients in remission (p > 0.05). PPD induration diameter of patients treated with steroid and disease modifying anti-rheumatic drug (DMARD) and underwent remission were not significantly different from the control group. When compared with patients using other drugs, patients on remission using steroid and DMARD have shorter PPD induration diameter. Activity of disease and drugs used (steroid, DMARD) affects PPD response. In the diagnosis of latent TB, normal range of PPD diameter in healthy child changes in JIA patient with active disease. That the PPD diameter is shorter than normal range could indicate underlying TB infection. This fact should be considered in the follow-up of the patients with JIA.

Keywords: PPD; Juvenile Idiopathic Arthritis

1. Introduction

Juvenile idiopathic arthritis (JIA) is the most common rheumatologic disease of childhood. In the treatment of acute period control of inflammation, prevention of deformities and protection of joint functions is targeted, while limitation of complications of disease and treatment, to provide normal growth and development, rehabilitation of patient and education of family is purposed in a long period. Extra-articular involvement is common in JIA [1,2]. Th1 cells are predominant in its pathogenesis. Mycobacterium tuberculosis infection commonly seen in patients with inflammatory rheumatoid disease is an important cause of mortality and morbidity. Though the diagnostic techniques of tuberculosis proceed everyday

because of the fact that both these techniques are expensive and there is no consensus about the sensitivity, PPD is still important in the diagnosis of tuberculosis. PPD reaction is a typical delayed hypersensitivity reaction and its formation requires normal T cell functions. Since Th1 cells play an important role in JIA pathogenesis, JIA patients are expected to show higher PPD response with respect to healthy children. However, there are investigations on the suppression of delayed hypersensivity response in adults with rheumatoid arthritis (RA) [3], but there are no reports in the literature of similar studies in children with JIA. Immunosuppression due to disease or drugs used in the treatment of disease (steroid etc.) could interfere with the PPD reaction and cause difficulty in the detection of the infection.

In our study, we aimed to evaluate to what extent active disease and immunosuppressive drug use affect PPD response so to detect the role of PPD test in the diagnosis of latent tuberculosis.

2. Material and Method

2.1. Study Group

77 children (average age 11.9 ± 4.33) who are regularly followed in our rheumatology outpatient clinics because of JIA diagnosed according to ILAR criteria and 58 healthy children (average age 11.9 ± 4.33) followed by our healthy child outpatient clinic as a control group are taken into our study group. The children with JIA are categorized into three groups as remission without medication, remission with medication and active. There were 31 patients (40.3%) in the remission without medication group, 39 patients (50.6%) in the remission with medicateon and seven patients (9.1%) with active disease. The patients in the remission group are the one who do not have any JIA related complaints in the last six months and whose CHAQ scores were less than 0.5. The active patients had JIA related complaints in the last six months and their CHAQ scores were more than 0.5. The patients with JIA are grouped into subtypes of this disease: Seven of them had systemic JIA, 34 had oligoarticular JIA, 26 had polyarticular JIA and 10 had enthesitis related arthritis.

Besides that, the patients were categorized according to the medication they were taking. 26 of JIA patients were taking DMARD (disease modifying anti-rheumatic drugs), 17 both DMARD and steroid and 2 anti-TNF. Tuberculin skin test with the Mantoux method were applied intradermally to all cases and their number of BCG scars were recorded.

For this study ethical approval is taken from Ethic Committee of Goztepe Teaching and Research Hospital.

2.2. Tuberculin Skin Test

Tuberculin Skin Test was made by applying 5TU PPD intradermal solution to the volar surface of the left front arm with a tuberculin injector. For the sake of standardization, these tests were applied and evaluated by the same doctor. The emergence of 6 - 10 mm papule around the injection area was accepted as the sign of correct application of the test. The longest diameter of the endurance around the injection area was measured and recorded after 72 hours with the pencil method.

2.3. Statistical Analysis

The results of this study were evaluated using NCSS 2007 & PASS 2008 Statistical Software (Utah, USA). Since PPD measurements did not show normal distribution, Kruskall Wallis test was applied in the group comparisons besides descriptive statistical methods (average, standard deviation). In the detection of the differentiating group and evaluations according to two groups, Mann Whitney U test was used. In the PPD correlations, Spearman correlation analysis was utilized. In the quailtative data comparison, chi-square test was applied. The results were evaluated in the confidence range of 95% and significance $p < 0.05$ level.

3. Results

There was no significant difference in the age, gender and BMI of both groups. When PPD induration values of JIA and control groups were compared, no statistical significant difference was found ($p > 0.05$). The number of BCG scars showed similar distribution in both groups. In the healthy group, positive correlation and significant relation ($p < 0.05$) were seen between PPD induration, age and BCG scars. In the JIA group, the effect of age and number of BCG scars on PPD was not found. Moreover, there was not found a significant relation between PPD values, JIA subtypes and follow-up period ($p > 0.05$). According to disease activity state, PPD induration values showed significant difference. The significance was due to the active group. PPD values of the active group were significantly lower than the ones of the remission patients. The PPD values of the patients in remission who had been treated with the combination of DMARD and methylprednisolone were lower than the ones treated with other medication. Furthermore, the PPD values of the patients in remission and active patients who take both DMARD and methylprednisolone didn't show a significant difference ($p > 0.05$). The patients who take both DMARD and methylprednisolone even though they were in remission have lower PPD values similar to results of active patients.

4. Discussion

Tuberculosis with the incidence rate of 34/100,000 in Turkey is a common disease [4]. It is recommended that BCG vaccines be made at the early age and screening be conducted with PPD tests on the healthy children in the societies with high tuberculosis incidence [5]. PPD reaction is a typical delayed hypersensitivity reaction and its formation depends on the normal T cell functions. The most important feature of JIA is inflammatory synovitis. In the diseases with the defected T cell functions such as JIA, PPD reaction can be affected and it can cause low sensitivity in the detection of latent TB infection. Moreover, immunosuppressive treatment used in these patients creates an extra ambiguity in the PPD evaluation.

When the induration values of both JIA and healthy cases are compared in our study, a statistically significant difference was not detected. In the literature, a similar study was conducted to the rheumatoid arthritis cases by Wolfe *et al.* and the percent of PPD positivity was found as 9.2% [6]. When this rate is compared to the rates in the US population, it is found that PPD response didn't decrease in the rheumatoid arthritis patients. Many studies in the literature have shown that the infection rate increased in healthy children with the age [7,8]. Furthermore, the conducted studies found out that the vaccines in older ages caused larger indurations [9,10]. Many studies reported out that there is a positive correlation between PPD reaction and number of BCG scars [11-13]. In our study, similar to literature results PPD induration values went up in the control group as their age and number of BCG scars increased. On the contrary, the fact that PPD responses are not affected by these factors in patients with JIA can be caused by a possible defect in the late hypersensitivity reactions.

According to disease activity state (remission without medication, remission with medication and active), PPD induration diameter ratios show significant difference (p < 0.05). The significance was caused by the active group. PPD values of the active group were significantly lower than the ones of the remission patients (p < 0.05). There was no significant difference between PPD responses of patients in remission with medication and without medication. In the study of Waxman *et al.*, rheumatoid arthritis patients were grouped into anergic and reactive categories according to their responses to the skin test with specific allergens. During these tests, it was found that there was no difference in disease activity between these two groups but anergic patients had longer active disease period [14].

The purpose in the comparison of medication used by patients in remission is to determine the effects of medication and activation on the immune system while keeping the effect of the disease. The average PPD induration diameters of the remission cases treated with the combination of DMARD and methylprednisolone have statistically lower significance than the cases treated only with DMARD. The purpose of the comparison of the patients in remission using medication to the active patients is to explore the effect of activation of the disease on the immune system. The PPD induration values of the patients in remission with medication who take DMARD and methylprednisolone and active patients who take the same medication didn't show significant difference. We can deduce from our study that disease activation affects PPD response and the cases in which methylprednisolone and DMARD were taken even though they are in remission delayed hypersensitivity is affected as much as the effect of the disease activation.

In the literature, there are many publications with many different results which investigated the effects of immune suppressive medications especially methylprednisolone on the PPD response. In the Hoeyeraal's study where the patients who took 7.4 mg/day of methylprednisolone were investigated, the PPD responses of the patients who took methylprednisolone were compared to the ones who did not take it. That study did not find any significant difference [15]. In the Hayes *et al.* study, similarly the same results were found out for the RA patients taking prednisone [16]. On the contrary to these results, Helliwell *et al.* compared the PPD responses of 50 RA and 50 healthy cases and found out that immune suppressive treatment was used more often for the RA patients with anergic [17]. In E. Kiray's study, it was determined that neither the activity of the disease nor the use of corticosteroid and methotrexate affected the PPD response [18]. In I. Sezer's study, the PPD responses of RA patients who were followed up without treatment were significantly higher than healthy cases and RA patients who were taking DMARD and methylprednisolone. In addition to this exploration of that study, it detected that the factors which are responsible of pathogenesis of the disease suppressed the late hypersensitivity reaction independent from the treatment [19].

5. Conclusion

JIA is a chronic disease of childhood period. The activation of the disease and the medications used (steroid and DMARD combination) affect the PPD responses and cause difficulties in the evaluation of latent TB. PPD responses that are lower than cut-off values which are acceptable for the healthy children with and without vaccine can point out the underlying tuberculosis infection for the active JIA patients who are treated with methylprednisolone.

REFERENCES

[1]   T. J. Cassidy and R. E. Patty, "Juvenile Rheumatoid Arthritis. Textbook of Pediatric Rheumatology," 3rd Edition, W. B. Saunders, 1995, pp. 133-223.

[2]   R. N. Lipnick, G. C. Tsokov and D. B. Maglavy, "Immune Abnormalities in the Pathogenesis of Juvenile Rheumatoid Arthritis," *Rheumatic Disease Clinics of North America*, Vol. 17, 1991, pp. 703-859.

[3]   D. Ponce de Leon, E. Acevedo-Vasquez, A. Sanchez-Torres, *et al.*, "Attenuated Response to Purified Protein Derivative in Patients with Rheumatoid Arthritis: Study in a Population with a High Prevalence of Tuberculosis," *Annals of the Rheumatic Diseases*, Vol. 64, 2005, pp. 1360-1361.

http://dx.doi.org/10.1136/ard.2004.029041

[4]   Turkish Ministry of Health Division of Tuberculosis, "Incidence of Tuberculosis and Number of Cases over Years," 2000.

[5]   American Academy of Pediatrics, "Report of the Committee on Infectious Disease. Red Book," 24th Edition, 1997, p. 544.

[6]   F. Wolfe, K. Michaud, J. Anderson and K. Urbansky, "Tuberculosis Infection in Patients with Rheumatoid Arthritis and the Effect of Infliximab Therapy," *Arthritis & Rheumatism*, Vol. 2, 2004, pp. 372-379. http://dx.doi.org/10.1002/art.20009

[7]   H. Güvenç, A. Koç and O. Özkarakas, "PPD Skin Testing in Schoolchildren with and without BCG Vaccination," *Turkish Journal of Medical Research*, Vol. 11, No. 3, 1993, pp. 116-119.

[8]   A. Koç and T. Karagöz, "Tüberkülozda Epidemiyolojik Ölçütler ve Hasta Grubu Analizi," *Solunum Hastalıkları Dergisi*, Vol. 8, No. 4, 1997, pp. 621-634.

[9]   R. L. Sepulveda, X. Ferrer and R. U. Sorensen, "The Influence of Calmette Guerin Bacillus Immunization on the Booster Effect to Tuberculin Testing in Healthy Young Adults," *The American Review of Respiratory Disease*, Vol. 142, 1990, pp. 24-28. http://dx.doi.org/10.1164/ajrccm/142.1.24

[10]   G. W. Comstock, L. B. Edwards and X. T. Nabang, "Tuberculin Sensitivity Eight to Fifteen Years after BCG Vaccination," *The American Review of Respiratory Disease*, Vol. 103, 1971, pp. 572-575.

[11]   E. S. Uçan, C. Sevinç and Ö. Abadoglu, "Tüberkülin Testi Sonuçlarının Yorumlanması Ülkemiz Standartları ve yeni Gereksinimler," *Toraks Dergisi*, Vol. 1, 2000, pp. 25-29.

[12]   E. Bozkanat, F. Çiftci, M. Apaydın, Z. Kartaloglu, E. Tozkoparan, O. Deniz and O. Sezer, "Tuberculin Skin Test Screening in a Military School in Istanbul City Center."

[13]   A. Sakar, T. Göktalay, L. Dagyıldızı and A. C. Yıldırım, "Manisa Ilinde Tüberküloz Taraması," Toraks Dergisi, 2001.

[14]   J. Waxman, M. D. Lockshin, J. J. Schnapp and I. N. Doneson, "Cellular Immunity in Rheumatic Diseases I. Rheumatoid Arthritis," *Arthritis & Rheumatism*, Vol. 4, 1974, pp. 499-506.

[15]   H. M. Hoyeraal, "Impaired Delayed Hypersensitivity in Juvenile Rheumatoid Arthritis," *Annals of the Rheumatic Diseases*, Vol. 32, 1973, p. 331. http://dx.doi.org/10.1136/ard.32.4.331

[16]   J. R. Hayes, D. J. Ward and J. F. Jennings, "Studies on Cell-Mediated Hypersensitivity Responses in Rheumatoid Arthritis," *Proceedings of the Third Symposium*, 1970.

[17]   M. G. Helliwell, G. S. Panayi and A. Unger, "Delayed Cutaneous Hypersensitivity in Rheumatoid Arthritis: The Influence of Nutrition and Drug Therapy," *Clinical Rheumatology*, Vol. 1, 1984, pp. 39-45. http://dx.doi.org/10.1007/BF02715694

[18]   E. Kiray, O. Kasapcopur, V. Bas, *et al.*, "Purified Protein Derivative Response in Juvenile Idiopathic Arthritis," *Journal of Rheumatology*, Vol. 36, 2009, pp. 2029-2032. http://dx.doi.org/10.3899/jrheum.090173

[19]   I. Sezer, H. Kocabas, M. A. Melikoglu and M. Arman, "Positiveness of Purified Protein Derivatives in Rheumatoid Arthritis Patients Who Are Not Receiving Immunosuppressive Therapy," *Clinical Rheumatology*, Vol. 28, 2009, pp. 53-55. http://dx.doi.org/10.1007/s10067-008-0982-1

Abbreviations

JIA: Juvenile idiopathic arthritis
PPD: Purified Protein Derivative
RA: Rheumatoid Arthritis
ILAR: International League of Associations for Rheumatology
CHAQ: Childhood Health Assesment Questionnaire
DMARD: Disease Modifying Anti-rheumatic Drugs
TU: Turbidity Unit
BMI: Body Mass Index
BCG: Bacille Calmette-Guérin
TB: Tuberculosis

6

A Composite Endpoint Measure to Consolidate Multidimensional Impact of Treatment on Gouty Arthritis

Andrew J. Sarkin[1], Ari Gnanasakthy[2], Rachel S. Lale[1], Kyle J. Choi[1], Jan D. Hirsch[3]

[1]Health Services Research Center, University of California, San Diego, USA; [2]Novartis Pharmaceuticals Corporation, East Hanover, USA; [3]Skaggs School of Pharmacy and Pharmaceutical Sciences, University of California, San Diego, USA.
Email: asarkin@ucsd.edu

ABSTRACT

Objective: To create a multidimensional composite outcomes endpoint for gouty arthritis treatment in order to consolidate disparate measures of comparative effectiveness. **Methods:** One solution is to create a multidimensional composite endpoint that consolidates the complexity of outcomes into a single scale, as was done in this study. The psychometrics of the multidimensional scale and subgroup differences were investigated. **Results:** Cronbach's alpha for the multidimensional composite endpoint created in this study was 0.76, indicating good internal reliability. Similar results were found across age, race, and gender. Removing any single item did not increase Cronbach's alpha beyond 0.77, indicating that none of the items were interfering with the reliability of the scale. However, a reduction in serum urate levels was not significantly correlated with the overall multidimensional endpoint scale with that variable removed, $r = 0.03$, $p > 0.05$. **Conclusion:** This study demonstrated the feasibility and usefulness of creating a composite multidimensional endpoint for assessing treatment outcomes among individuals with gouty arthritis.

Keywords: Gout; Response Criteria; Composite Endpoint

1. Introduction

Obtaining a comprehensive assessment of treatment impact usually requires the use of multiple outcome measures such as self-reported pain, physical limitations, flare frequency, and biochemical markers, but the results of multiple measures can be challenging to consolidate. Gouty arthritis (GA) is one such disorder where different indicators of improvement can be challenging to interpret when there are different impacts on the multiple outcomes, and GA domains are not all impacted equally across all treatments and patients who experience improvement in gout symptoms. Management of GA involves medications and lifestyle modification to prevent flares (attacks) from occurring and medications to treat acute symptoms such as pain, inflammation, and swelling when a flare does occur [1-3]. Effectiveness of treatments varies among patients who may have marked response, poor response, no response, and/or adverse reactions to the medications themselves. Different levels of response or disagreement among multiple outcome measures complicates treatment decisions, therefore causing action decisions to be based on clinical experience or

pathophysiologic principles [4].

Because GA is a complex disorder that has multiple impacts on patients' quality of life [5,6] that differ by treatment type and individual patient characteristics, it would be useful to reflect this complexity by using multidimensional response criteria. Physicians and patients may not always agree on the relative importance of different outcomes [7]. In addition to the difficulties with interpretation that arise from disparate results from separate statistical tests of different response criteria, there is also an increase in the probability of making a Type I error, or a loss of statistical power if Type I error probability is kept constant by adjusting the significance criteria for the individual tests. Further, missing data can make these challenges even more complex if different patients are included in different analyses because of systematic biases in the patterns of missing data.

A possible solution is to create a composite scale measuring the multidimensional impact of treatment by combining the different outcome measures. Several studies have demonstrated the benefits of utilizing composite scale measures. To quantify and assess the multidimensional impact of asthma severity, this approach was employed to develop a Composite Asthma Severity Index (CASI), which accounts for disease symptoms and impairment, lung function, controller medication usage and frequency of hospitalizations with oral corticosteroid bursts. When validated using an independent sample, the CASI demonstrated a 32% greater magnitude of improvement within the treatment group compared with measuring symptom days alone [8]. Likewise, this approach was taken with hand osteoarthritis, where researchers combined the responsiveness of patient-reported measures (e.g. the Australian/Canadian osteoarthritis hand index [AUSCAN] and visual analogue pain subscale [VAS]), and counts of distal interphalangeal, proximal interphalangeal, metacarpophalangeal, and carpometacarpal joints to calculate patient activity and clinical disease activity composite scores. Researchers found the composite scores to be superior to the AUSCAN score in detecting the difference between the mean change in baseline values of pain, disability, and joint stiffness between the two treatment groups. The composite scores showed similar responsiveness to treatment effects as VAS pain single item measure; however, the use of composite indices appears to improve the ability to capture and quantitate multiple important aspects of disease impact and activity, and may be more sensitive to detect change over time [9]. Similarly, in a study of chronic obstructive pulmonary disease (COPD), researchers hypothesized that a multidimensional grading system that assessed the respiratory, perceptive, and systemic aspects of COPD would better predict risk of death due to COPD than the use of a single physiological variable, forced expiratory volume in one second (FEV1). This was done by assigning point values from 0 - 3 to four factors that predicted risk of death (body mass index, degree of airflow obstruction, dyspnea, and exercise capacity), and then adding up the points for each factor to create the composite index score. This study showed that the sensitivity and specificity of the composite index in classifying patients with COPD as either dying or surviving was greater than FEV1 alone [C statistic of 0.74, compared to 0.65 for FEV1 alone] [10].

Because different measures may use different metrics (e.g. serum urate levels versus categorical responses to self-reported pain measures), a common metric needs to be created. One way to do this is by categorizing outcomes into response criteria. For the current study, we used the dichotomous measure of whether there was a markedly important difference on each variable, using criteria previously defined in the literature. For example, a reduction of more than two points on a 10-point pain scale or a 25% reduction in urate levels could each be response criteria. A recent Outcome Measures in Rheumatology (OMERACT) meeting asked members to give input on multidimensional response criteria for gout [11].

Core-set domains such as serum uric acid, number of tophi, flare frequency, and health assessment questionnaire disability index (HAQ-DI) that were derived from prior work with patient profiles were examined using 1000Minds™ by two groups; the gout experts and the OMERACT registrants. In the present study, we created a multidimensional composite endpoint that is disease-specific for gout based on recommendations discussed in the OMERACT results [11].

2. Materials and Methods

2.1. Participants

This analysis used pooled data from the β-RELIEVED program, which included patients meeting the American College of Rheumatology (ACR) 1977 preliminary criteria for acute GA, and contraindicated, intolerant, or unresponsive to non-steroidal anti-inflammatory drugs (NSAIDs) and/or colchicine. Both core studies (β-RELIEVED [N = 228]; β-RELIEVED II [N = 226]) were 12-week, multiregional, active controlled, double-blind, parallel-group, double-dummy, phase 3 studies [12]. Patients were enrolled to receive a single dose canakinumab 150 mg s.c. or TA 40 mg i.m. to treat an acute GA attack and were re-dosed "on demand" on each new attack. Demographic characteristics of the participants are shown in **Table 1**.

Table 1. Demographic characteristics of the pooled sample.

Characteristic	Pooled Sample
Gender, n (%)	
Male	414 (91.2)
Female	40 (8.8)
Age, years	
Mean (SD)	53.0 (11.7)
Median (range)	53 (20 - 85)
Race, n (%)	
White	343 (75.6)
Black	50 (11.0)
Asian	25 (5.5)
Other	36 (7.9)
Ethnicity, n (%)	
Hispanic or Latino	30 (6.6)
Mixed Ethnicity	12 (2.6)
Weight (kg)	
Mean (SD)	98.0 (19.0)
Median (range)	95.5 (57.9 - 170.5)
Height (cm)	
Mean (SD)	175.5 (8.6)
Median (range)	176 (140.0 - 200.6)
BMI, kg/m^2	
Mean (SD)	31.7 (5.2)
Median (range)	30.9 (19.5 - 44.9)

2.2. Measures

In addition to clinical measures such as serum urate and recorded flares, patients also reported frequency of flares, number of flares during the past four weeks, and global treatment response. They also completed the Gout Impact Scales (GIS) and Short Form-36 v2 (SF-36; Acute Form). The SF-36 was completed only by patients who reported GA symptoms in their lower extremities. Due to the lack of available translations required for all the study centers, the GIS was completed by participants where their preferred language was available. In addition to the two questionnaires, patients also responded to the separate questions pertaining to their overall experience of gout shown in **Table 2**.

2.2.1. Gout Impact Scales (GIS)

The GIS contains five scales; three assessing the impact of GA overall (Gout Concern Overall, Gout Medication Side Effects, Unmet Gout Treatment Need) and two assessing the impact of GA during an attack [13]. Response options for GIS items are on a five-point Likert scale (*i.e.*, from strongly agree to strongly disagree or all of the time to none of the time). GIS scales are scored from 0 to 100, with higher scores on each scale indicating "worse condition" or "greater gout impact".

2.2.2. Short Form-36 (SF-36)

The SF-36 v2 (Acute Form) is a widely used measure in clinical trials assessing health-related quality of life by assessing recent function and symptoms, including pain. Normative based scoring is used with a scale range between 0 and 100, where higher scores indicate higher levels of well-being [14].

2.3. Procedures

The composite response endpoint representing overall change in GA related health outcomes from baseline to 12 weeks included clinical markers (serum urate and flare activity), patient-reported data from the Gout Impact Scale (GIS) of the Gout Assessment Questionnaire 2.0 (including 6 items related to pain and quality of life), and the SF-36 bodily pain scale. Variables were chosen based on expert opinion, including the published literature and the results of the OMERACT meeting [11]. The 12 items representing five domains are shown in **Table 3** along with the criteria used as the responder definition. For each variable, the markedly important difference was determined based on published research and/or expert opinion [15-17].

A total score was calculated in two ways for each patient. One composite score was calculated as the percentage of all response criteria met out of the total number of response criteria. However, patients who could not be evaluated on each response criteria because of missing values would have scores that might underestimate their true improvement using this first method. Thus, a second composite was calculated as the percentage of response criteria for which data were available for each patient. This second method of calculating the score is less likely to be influenced by missing data, assuming that the amount and nature of missing data is the same between treatment groups. Reliability of the whole scale including all response criteria was measured by Cronbach's alpha, which was also calculated with each criterion removed. Corrected item-total correlations were also calculated as the relationship between each variable and the total number of other criteria met, in order to evaluate how the variables related to the overall construct of GA improvement.

3. Results

The correlation between the two ways of handling missing data when calculating the composite scale was 0.63

Table 2. Self-report questions related to patient's overall experience and impact of gout symptoms.

Item/Question	Response Options					
Because of your gout, how would you rate your <u>physical health</u> in the past 4 weeks?	Very Poor O	Poor O	Fair O	Good O	Very Good O	Excellent O
Because of your gout, how would you rate your <u>quality of life</u> in the past 4 weeks?	Very Poor O	Poor O	Fair O	Good O	Very Good O	Excellent O
Because of your gout, how would you rate your <u>mental health</u> in the past 4 weeks?	Very Poor O	Poor O	Fair O	Good O	Very Good O	Excellent O
Considering all the ways gout affects you, circle a number on the scale for how well you have been doing for the past 4 weeks.	No Disease Activity 1	2 3 4	5 6	7 8 9	10	Severe Disease Activity
Circle a number on the scale indicating the severity of pain you have experienced within the past 4 weeks.	No Pain 1	2 3 4	5 6	7 8 9	10	Severe Pain

(n = 454). Cronbach's alpha for the multidimensional composite endpoint was 0.76 for the 93 participants who had no missing data on any of the response criteria, indicating good internal reliability despite the breadth of the measure.

As shown in **Table 3**, removing any single item did not increase Cronbach's alpha beyond 0.77, indicating that none of the items were interfering with the reliability of the scale by not belonging with the others. However, **Table 3** shows that a reduction in serum urate levels was not significantly correlated with the overall multidimensional endpoint scale with that variable removed (r = 0.03, p > 0.05), indicating that reduction in urate levels was not associated with changes in other outcome measures used in this study.

Cronbach's alpha was similar for subgroups, showing that reliability was consistent across age, race, and gender. People older than 53 (the mean and median for age) demonstrated a reliability of 0.77 while people up to 53 had a reliability of 0.76. The reliabilities of Caucasian, Black, and Asian people were 0.76, 0.80, and 0.79, respectively. Cronbach's alpha indicated that the reliability was 0.76 for males and 0.66 for females.

4. Discussion

This analysis supports the creation of a multidimensional composite outcomes endpoint for GA treatment in order to consolidate disparate measures of comparative effectiveness. The multidimensional scale was reliable across age, race, and gender groups. By defining dichotomous endpoints based on markedly important differences and combining them into a scale, a single metric is created for judging the difference between treatments, thus addressing the confusion that may arise when outcome measures show varying levels of evidence of treatment impact. Consolidation enhances the ability to summarize, interpret, and communicate the overall treatment impact.

Items making up the composite measure were chosen based on expert opinion, mostly drawing from recommendations of the OMERACT consensus project [11], providing face validity for the multidimensional scale. The scale also showed good internal reliability. Although less related to the overall scale in this study, serum urate level change is probably still an important part of any multidimensional assessment of GA, despite its lack of relationship to the overall multidimensional composite endpoint scale in this study. The treatment in this study was not designed to have its main mechanism through serum urate levels, but many important GA treatments do have their impact through serum urate levels and this was one of the key indicators that came from the OMERACT participants. It is debatable whether the scale should include serum urate, which is more of a medication "process outcome" that mediates the effect of treatment rather than a "health outcome" that is experienced by the patient. In this case, very few patients (7.7%) had a change in serum urate. Indeed, the best future treatment for GA may not involve lowering serum urate, but rather making sure excess urate does not impact health by causing GA.

Table 3. Response criteria, item-total correlations, and Cronbach's alpha with criteria removed for the multidimensional composite endpoint.

Domain	Variable	Response Criterion	Overall % responder	Cronbach's alpha if item removed*	Corrected item-total correlation
Urate	Serum urate	>25% reduction	7.7 (n = 403)	0.77	0.03
	Flare past 4 weeks	No	79.1 (n = 225)	0.74	0.49
Flare frequency	New flare during trial	No	61.2 (n = 454)	0.77	0.24
	Use of rescue medications	No	48.5 (n = 454)	0.77	0.20
Pain	Gout pain severity past 4 weeks (GIS, 1 - 10 scale)	>2 point reduction	79.6 (n = 226)	0.73	0.50
	Bodily pain (SF-36, 0 - 100 scale)	>10 point reduction	62.5 (n = 373)	0.72	0.57
	How well doing past 4 weeks (GIS, 1 - 10 scale)	>2 point reduction	63.7 (n = 226)	0.74	0.47
Patient global response	Global treatment response	Acceptable, good, or excellent	89.9 (n = 424)	0.74	0.42
	GIS Global Control Scale (GIS, 0 - 100)	>8 points	75.8 (n = 227)	0.76	0.28
HRQoL (Disease specific)	Gout related quality of life	>1 point improvement	28.7 (n = 150)	0.73	0.56
	Gout related physical health	>1 point improvement	24.5 (n = 143)	0.74	0.45
(GIS, very poor - excellent)	Gout related mental health	>1 point improvement	19.4 (n = 139)	0.73	0.53

*Cronbach's alpha for the whole scale is 0.76

When studies do not have sufficient power to show significance for all endpoints, different conclusions may be drawn for different endpoints, and this can be exacerbated by the presence of missing data. Creating a multidimensional composite endpoint in this way improves handling of missing data as well as facilitates interpretation and communication of findings. For example, the presence of missing data could have been problematic in this study where different measures were given to different participants, but the composite endpoint allowed inclusion of all participants despite missing data points, and enabled the interpretation and communication of the treatment much more efficiently and effectively. When using this method to compare treatments, it is important to verify that the amount and nature of missing data do not vary by treatment group assignment. Even with random assignment, the treatment differences could be related to differential attrition [18]. If some response criteria are more difficult to meet because of missing data, then missing data can still bias scores.

The primary strength of this method is the ability to consolidate disparate results across multiple outcome measures. A limitation of this study was reliance on a single sample of patients receiving a specific type of treatment; results may differ in other patient groups. Like many instruments, this multidimensional index has multiple measures of some domains. In order to confirm that the results are not driven by any single domain, results can be checked by eliminating any item or domain. Decisions to give all items in the composite endpoint the same weight and to include only disease-specific quality of life measures are areas open to further investigation.

5. Conclusion

In summary, creation of composite multidimensional endpoints should be useful for existing data, ongoing studies, and future study designs. GA researchers usually obtain responses to these items and there is minimal burden for calculating the response criteria. The score could be calculated retrospectively in existing databases allowing for new analyses, especially when results were difficult to interpret. Future studies should explore better determination and weighting of the criteria and possible inclusion of other measures. Although there may be aspects of GA that were not represented, this study demonstrated the usefulness of calculating a composite endpoint as a way to examine the multidimensional impact of treatments in clinical trials, and as an individual clinical indicator of treatment success in healthcare settings.

6. Acknowledgements

The authors acknowledge Erik Groessl, Theodore Ganiats, Poorva Nemlekar, Kimberly Center, and Jennalee Woolbridge for contributions to editing the manuscript and Novartis Pharmaceuticals for funding the study.

REFERENCES

[1] K. M. Jordan, J. S. Cameron, M. Snaith, W. Zhang, M. Doherty, J. Seckl, A. Hingorani, R. Jaques and G. Nuki, "British Society for Rheumatology and British Health Professionals in Rheumatology Guideline for the Management of Gout," *Rheumatology*, Vol. 46, No. 8, 2007, pp. 1372-1374. doi:10.1093/rheumatology/kem056a

[2] W. Zhang, M. Doherty, T. Bardin, E. Pascual, V. Basrkova, P. Conghan, P. J. Gerster, J. Jacobs, B. Leeb, F. Lioté, G. McCarthy, P. Netter, G. Nuki, F. Perez-Ruiz, A. Pignone, J. Pimentão, L. Punzi, E. Roddy, T. Uhliq and I. Zimmermann-Gòrska, "EULAR Evidence Based Recommendations for Gout. Part II: Management. Report of a Task Force of the EULAR Standing Committee for International Clinical Studies Including Therapeutics (ESCISIT)," *Annals of Rheumatic Diseases*, Vol. 65, No. 10, 2006, pp. 1312-1324. doi:10.1136/ard.2006.055269

[3] T. Neogi, "Clinical Practice. Gout," *New England Journal of Medicine*, Vol. 364, No. 5, 2011, pp. 443-452. doi:10.1056/NEJMcp1001124

[4] H. El-zawawy and B. F. Mandell, "Managing Gout: How Is It Different in Patients with Chronic Kidney Disease?" *Cleveland Clinic Journal of Medicine*, Vol. 77, No. 12, 2010, pp. 919-928. doi:10.3949/ccjm.77a.09080

[5] S. J. Lee, R. Terkeltaub, D. Khannam, J. A. Singhm A. J. Sarkin and A. Kavanaugh, "Perceptions of Disease and Health-Related Quality of Life among Patients with Gout," *Rheumatology*, Vol. 48, No. 5, 2009, pp. 582-586. doi:10.1093/rheumatology/kep047

[6] J. D. Hirsch, R. Terkeltaub, D. Khanna, J. Singh, A. Sarkin, M. Shieh, A. Kavanaugh and S. J. Lee, "Impact of Gout on Health Related Quality of Life and the Relationship to Gout Characteristics," *Patient Related Outcome Measures*, Vol. 1, 2010, pp. 1-8. doi:10.2147/PROM.S8310

[7] J. Sarkin, A. E. Levack, M. M. Shieh, A. F. Kavanaugh, D. Khanna, J. A. Singh, R. A. Terkeltaub, S. J. Lee and J. D. Hirsch, "Predictors of Doctor-Rated and Patient-Rated Gout Severity: Gout Impact Scales Improve Assessment," *Journal of Evaluation in Clinical Practice*, Vol. 16, No. 6, 2010, pp. 1244-1247. doi:10.1111/j.1365-2753.2009.01303.x

[8] J. J. Wildfire, P. J. Gergen, C. A. Sorkness, H. E. Mitchell, A. Calatroni, M. Kattan, S. J. Szefler, S. J. Teach, G. R. Bloomberg, R. A. Wood, A. H. Liu, J. A. Liu, J. A. Pongracic, J. F. Chmiel, K. Conroy, Y. Rivera-Sanchez, W. W. Busse and W. J. Morgan, "Development and Validation of the Composite Asthma Severity Index—An Outcome Measure for Use in Children and Adolescents," *Journal of Allergy and Clinical Immunology*, Vol. 129, No. 3, 2012, pp. 694-701. doi:10.1016/j.jaci.2011.12.962

[9] I. K. Haugen, B. Slatkowsky-Christensen, J. Lessem and T. K. Kvien, "The Responsiveness of Joint Counts, Patient-Reported Measures and Proposed Composite Scores in Hand Osteoarthritis: Analyses from a Placebo-Con-

trolled Trial," *Annals of Rheumatic Diseases*, Vol. 69, No. 8, 2010, pp. 1436-1440. doi:10.1136/ard.2008.100156

[10] B. R. Celli, C. G. Cote, J. M. Marin, C. Casanova, M. Montes de Oca, R. A. Mendez, V. P. Plata and H. J. Cabral, "The Body-Mass Index, Airflow Obstruction, Dyspnea, and Exercise Capacity Index in Chronic Obstructive Pulmonary Disease," *New England Journal of Medicine*, Vol. 350, No. 10, 2004, pp. 1005-1012. doi:10.1056/NEJMoa021322

[11] W. J. Taylor, J. A. Singh, K. G. Saag, N. Dalbeth, P. A. MacDonald, N. L. Edwards, L. S. Simon, L. K. Stamp, T. Neogi, A. L. Gaffo, P. P. Khanna, M. A. Becker and H. R. Schumacher, "Bringing It All Together: A Novel Approach to the Development of Response Criteria for Chronic Gout Clinical Trials," *Journal of Rheumatology*, Vol. 38, No. 7, 2011, pp. 1467-1470. doi:10.3899/jrheum.110274

[12] N. Schlesinger, R. E. Alten, T. Bardin, H. R. Schumacher, M. Bloch, A. Gimona, G. Krammer, V. Murphy, D. Richard and A. K. So, "Canakinumab for Acute Gouty Arthritis in Patients with Limited Treatment Options: Results from Two Randomised, Multicentre, Active-Controlled, Double-Blind Trials and Their Initial Extensions," *Annals of Rheumatic Diseases*, Vol. 71, No. 11, 2012, pp. 1839-1848. doi:10.1136/annrheumdis-2011-200908

[13] J. D. Hirsch, S. J. Lee, R. Terkeltaub, D. Khanna, J. Singh, A. Sarkin, J. Harvey and A. Kavanaugh, "Evaluation of an Instrument Assessing Influence of Gout on Health-Related Quality of Life," *Journal of Rheumatology*, Vol. 35,

No. 12, 2008, pp. 2406-2414. doi:10.3899/jrheum.080506

[14] J. E. Ware, "SF-36 Health Survey Update," *Spine*, Vol. 25, No. 24, 2000, pp. 3130-3139. doi:10.1097/00007632-200012150-00008

[15] M. Kosinski, S. Z. Zhao, S. Dedhiya, J. T. Osterhaus and J. E. Ware, "Determining Minimally Important Changes in Generic and Disease-Specific Health-Related Quality of Life Questionnaires in Clinical Trials of Rheumatoid Arthritis," *Arthritis & Rheumatism*, Vol. 43, No. 7, 2000, pp. 1478-1487. doi:10.1002/1529-0131(200007)43:7<1478::AID-ANR10>3.0.CO;2-M

[16] D. Khanna, A. J. Sarkin, P. P. Khanna, M. M. Shieh, A. F. Kavanaugh, R. A. Terkeltaub, *et al.*, "Minimally Important Differences of the Gout Impact Scale in a Randomized Controlled Trial," *Rheumatology (Oxford)*, Vol. 50, No. 7, 2011, pp. 1331-1336. doi:10.1093/rheumatology/ker023

[17] B. Bruce and J. F. Fries, "The Stanford Health Assessment Questionnaire: A Review of Its History, Issues, Progress, and Documentation," *Journal of Rheumatology*, Vol. 30, No. 1, 2003, pp. 167-178.

[18] A. J. Sarkin, S. R. Tally, T. A. Cronan, G. E. Matt and H. W. Lyons, "Analyzing Attrition in a Community-Based Literacy Program," *Evaluation and Program Planning*, Vol. 20, No. 4, 1997, pp. 421-431. doi:10.1016/S0149-7189(97)00023-2

7

Dystrophic Calcinosis in the Hands of a Patient with Rheumatoid Arthritis and Secundary Sjögren's Syndrome

Daniel Jaramillo-Arroyave*, **Gerardo Quintana, Federico Rondon-Herrera, Antonio Iglesias-Gamarra**

Internal Medicine, Rheumatology, Department of Internal Medicine, Rheumatology Unit, Universidad Nacional de Colombia, Bogotá, Colombia.
Email: *dajaramilloar@unal.edu.co, *kenkorva@yahoo.com.ar, ge_quintana@yahoo.com, federicorondonh@hotmail.com, iglesias.antonio1@gmail.com

ABSTRACT

Salts of calcium phosphate and inorganic phosphate are normally found in serum and extracellular fluids, balancing through poorly understood factors that prevent abnormal tissue deposition of these minerals. However, in those tissues that are injured, especially due to chronic inflammatory processes, a predisposition to the deposition of these minerals is developed, triggering what has been called Dystrophic Calcinosis (DC), common in different Connective Tissue Diseases (CTD), especially dermatomyositis and scleroderma, but there is no a frecuent association with diseases like Rheumatoid Arthritis (RA) and Sjögren Syndrome (SS). We report a case of a female patient of 63 years old with RA and Secundary SS who presents with DC in the hands and no evidence of other connective tissue.

Keywords: Dystrophic Calcinosis; Rheumatoid Arthritis; Sjögren Syndrome

1. Case Presentation

The patient, who lives in Bogotá—Colombia, diagnosed with early RA at 56's with 6 months history polyarthritis at the time of consultation and without other significant medical history. During her first visit in June of 2005 she was included in the protocol of early arthritis at the *Universidad Nacional de Colombia*, where tests was performed: ESR 32 mm/h, CRP 1.0 mg/dL, RF 60.1 U/mL (0 - 30 U/mL, by Nephelometry), ACPA 6.4 (negative), ANA by IIF 1/160 Speckled Pattern, genotype HLADR1 *0301 - *0407, TNF Alpha Polymorphism: −308 G/A.

Initial Sharp Van de Heidje 41/448. RA diagnosis was made and immediately she started to take methotrexate 15 mg/week, folic acid 12 mg/week, prednisolone 7.5 mg/day, with excellent response from clinical and laboratory standpoint. In May of 2009, in a control MCP synovitis was found in 2 - 3 in both hands, x-ray was made, finding periarticular calcification at the PIP, MCP (bilateral) and feet without clinical evidence of Raynaud's phenomenon, acroosteolisis, muscle weakness, skin compromise (mRSS = 0, no rash), dysphagia or another CTD sign or symptom. She begins at the same time with sicca, with out fever, parotid enlargement, lymphadenopathy or vasculitis. New anti-antibody requested (June 2009) found ANA 1/1280 Nucleolar pattern, SSA/RO 188.9, SM 5.1, RNP 8.7, RA test IgG 85.2, RA test

IgA 120, RA test IgM 625 , ACPA 6.8, Alkaline phosphatasa, PTH, 25 (OH) vit D, Serum Calcium, phosphorrus inorganic, 24 h urine calcium, 24 h urine phosphorrus were all normal; Minor salivar gland biopsy with Chisholm-Mason Class IV, serum protein electrophoresis with polyclonal gamma pathy and video capillaroscopy with a nonspecific pattern of scleroderma, DM o MCTD. Diagnosis of DC associated with RA and secondary SS was made and further clinical and laboratory monitoring was performed. The patient its in clinical remission of RA and without sicca simptoms, the pain secondary to her DC has improved with RA treatment and addition of colchicine (MTX 15 mg/week; prednisone 5 mg QD, folic acid 12 mg/week, colchicine 0.5 mg QD), **Figure 1**.

2. Discussion

Calcinosis cutis is characterized by the deposition of insoluble calcium salts in the skin and subcutaneous tissue and is the result of local tissue damage, with levels of calcium, phosphorus, vitamin D and normal parathormone. It is classified into 5 groups: dystrophic, tumor, metastatic, idiopathic and iatrogenic [1,2,3].

In Dystrophic Calcinosis, tissue damage predisposes to precipitation of calcium salts at the extra skeletal. Is clearly unknown what factors predispose this local precipitation but could be considered that the calcium/phosphorus ratio is increasing extracellular fluid associated

---

*Corresponding author.

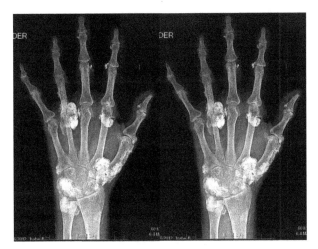

Figure 1. Dystrophic Calcinosis (DC) of the hands associated with RA and SS.

with local inflammatory factors that facilitate the development this illness.

From the pathophysiological point of view the DC occurs in tissues which have somehow had a change that promotes calcification although there is, in theory, a normal level of calcium and phosphorus. Factors that promote calcification have been described and are often found in patients with rheumatic diseases such as hypervascularity with secondary hypoxia, tissue structural damage, and tissue changes associated with age. However, it is important to consider the role of local inflamematory activity specifically mediated by macrophages and cytokines related to this (IL1-β, IL6, TNF-α), which found elevated locally at the site of calcinosis and less frequently in systemic levels (IL1-β) [4]. It has also been shown that at mitochondria level, an unusual increase of calcium salts and phosphate is observed, forming crystal deposits, tissue necrosis, foreign body reactions and fibrosis, generating an acidic microenvironment that interferes with endogenous inhibitors of calcification [3-5].

Other factors that become important for being therapeutic targets are the high levels of Calcium-Binding Amino Acid (CBAA) and the Gamma Carboxy Glutamic Acid (GCGA), modified from the pharmacological point of view by warfarin, with clinical improvement after decreasing its concentration at the site of calcinosis [6].

Dystrophic Calcinosis (DC) is the most common form of calcinosis cutis. This almost always in association with inflammatory diseases such as connective tissue diseases like dermatomyositis, juvenile dermatomyositis, Systemic Sclerosis, Systemic Lupus Erythematosus, mixed connective tissue disease and a lesser extent, with unknown explanation, in polymyositis [4,5]. As for the relationship between DC and RA, their concomitance is extremely rare, to date, there are only two reported cases of DC, both in buttocks [6,7], but no information on these cases involving hands and feet. Also, the associa-

tion with SS is exotic, with one case reported in the literature [8].

With regard to treatment, there is no drug that has shown strong effectiveness in the management of patients with DC, but some drugs have shown mild pharmacological effects that may help somewhat to control the disease like warfarin, colchicine, probenecid, bisphosphonates, diltiazem, aluminum hydroxide, minocycline, intralesional corticosteroids, surgery and CO_2 laser [2,4].

3. Conclusion

In conclusion, we present the first case of DC of the hands and feets in a patient with RA (the third case associated with this disease) simulating articular activity and the second case associated with SS. There are no evidence of another CTD that explains this manifestation. The objective of presenting this case is to inform the association described as an unusually rare even more mimicking RA activity and that despite the medical knowledge, we have not been able to figure out the pathogenesis or the treatment of DC.

REFERENCES

[1] N. Reiter, L. El-Shabrawi, et al., "Calcinosis Cutis: Part I. Diagnostic Pathway," Journal of the American Academy of Dermatology, Vol. 65, No. 1, 2011, pp. 1-12. doi:10.1016/j.jaad.2010.08.038

[2] N. Reiter, L. El-Shabrawi, B. Leinweber, A. Berghold and E. Aberer, "Calcinosis Cutis, Part II: Treatment Options," Journal of the American Academy of Dermatology, Vol. 65, No. 1, 2011, pp. 15-24. doi:10.1016/j.jaad.2010.08.039

[3] J. S. Walsh and J. A. Fairley, "Calcifying Disorders of the Skin," Journal of the American Academy of Dermatology, Vol. 33, No. 5, 1995, pp. 693-710. doi:10.1016/0190-9622(95)91803-5

[4] N. Boulman, G. Slobodin, M. Rozenbaum and I. Rosner, "Calcinosis in Rheumatic Diseases," Seminars in Arthritis and Rheumatism, Vol. 34, No. 6, 2005, pp. 805-812. doi:10.1016/j.semarthrit.2005.01.016

[5] S. Y. Kim, H. Y. Choi, K. B. Myung and Y. W. Choi, "The Expression of Molecular Mediators in the Idiopathic Cutaneous Calcification and Ossification," Journal of Cutaneous Pathology, Vol. 35, No. 9, 2008, pp. 826-831. doi:10.1111/j.1600-0560.2007.00904.x

[6] K. Harigane, Y. Mochida, K. Ishii, S. Ono, N. Mitsugi and T. Saito, "Dystrophic Calcinosis in a Patient with Rheumatoid Arthritis," Modern Rheumatology, Vol. 21, No. 1, 2011, pp. 85-88. doi:10.1007/s10165-010-0344-0

[7] S. Balin, D. Wetter, L. Andersen and M. Davis, "Calcinosis Cutis Occurring in Association with Autoimmune Connective Tissue Disease the Mayo Clinic Experience with 78 Patients, 1996-2009," Archives of Dermatology, Vol. 148, No. 4, 2011, pp. 455-462.

[8]   M. Llamas-Velasco, C. Eguren, D. Santiago, C. Gasrcía-García, J. Fraga and A. García-Diez, "Calcinosis Cutis and Sjögren's Syndorme," *Lupus*, Vol. 19, No. 6, 2010, pp. 762-764.

8

The difficult management of systemic-onset juvenile rheumatoid arthritis. Level of serum ferritin as aspecific diagnostic finding[*]

Maria Giovanna Colella[1#], Giuseppe Buttaro[1], Lucia Masi[1], Elena Palma[1], Raffaele Amelio[1], Alexander Vallone[2]

[1]Pediatric Unit, "Dono Svizzero" Hospital, Formia, Italy
[2]Faculty of Medicine and Surgery, Università Cattolica, Rome, Italy
Email: [#]mgcolella@hotmail.it

ABSTRACT

Systemic-onset JRA is characterized by spiking fevers lasting more than two weeks, typically occurring once, twice each day, with temperature returning to the normal or below normal. There are no specific diagnostic tests for systemic JRA. High level of serum ferritin is the most important, no specific, diagnostic finding associated.

Keywords: Fever of Unknown Origin; Juvenile Rheumatoid Arthritis; Ferritin

1. INTRODUCTION

Juvenile idiopathic arthritis (JIA) is the term used to describe a group of inflammatory joint diseases of unknown etiology, with onset before the age of 16, with a duration longer than 6 weeks [1,2]. The definition of JIA has been chosen to indicate the absence of a known mechanism responsible for the disease and to stress the need to exclude other forms of arthritis that occur in association with other diseases (especially arthritis is associated with diseases hematology-oncology, inflammatory and infectious diseases). Systemic-onset juvenile rheumatoid arthritis representing about 10% of JIA is characterized by spiking fevers lasting more than two weeks, typically occurring once or twice each day, at about the same time of day, with temperature returning to the normal or below normal [3,4] The fever pattern is very useful because infections, Kawasaki desease, and malignancy do not have such a predictable pattern [5].

We present two cases of systemic juvenile rheumatoid arthritis at the onset that presented fever of unknown origin, characterized by arthralgias migrants, evanescent rash and splenomegaly. The diagnosis was suggested by these findings in association with a double quotidian fever and a highly elevated serum ferritin level.

2. CASE 1

Child of 12 years old came to our observation for five days of persistent high fever, muscle pain, leg weakness and difficulty in walking which worsens with increasing temperature.

Family and past personal history were not contributory. In the month before the hospitalization, the parents referred complaining pain in the right temporo mandibular joint and than, after two weeks, deficit in walking on the morning after the use of rotating carpet. This problem was resolved with a single dose of paracetamol. In the following week he presented diarrhea for two days, slight increase in temperature and wearying. The parents also reported use of home-made eggs to eat and contact with family pets in occasion of visits to his grandmother who lived in the countryside.

At admission, physical examination was not contributory. But because he showed signs of leg pain and back pain, a lumbar puncture ruled out problems with meningeal involvement.

During hospitalization, his medical history showed intermittent fever, with at least two episodes a day for eighteen days, spine arthralgia (especially cervical and lumbosacral) and hip joint articulation, associated with functional impotence of the lower limbs, especially in the morning and during the peak of the fever; the tendon reflexes were symmetric and vivid, always. On three occasions, a pink salmon rash appeared on the neck, trunk and upper limbs, in association with fever (**Figure 1**). No improvement in clinical and laboratory response to broad-spectrum antibiotic therapy given for ten days he showed leukocytosis, persistently inflammatory markers (CRP, ESR) elevated, mild anemia, modest ele-

[*]Conflict of interest declarations.
The authors have no conflicts of interest relevant to this article to disclose.
[#]Corresponding author.

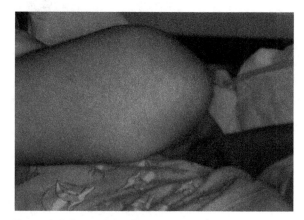

Figure 1. Salmon-pink rash on the limb.

Table 1. Values of white blood cells, inflammatory markers and serum ferritin in relation to days of hospitalization—Case 1.

	14/10/10	19/10/10	25/10/10	29/10/10	02/11/10
WBC $10^3/\mu l$	13870	30490	31330	25880	17250
ESR mm/hr	70	108	104	105	80
CRP mg/dl	13.58	15.45	8.71	13.76	6.32
Ferritin ng/ml	\	3066	4360	12461	8263
D-Dimers mg/l (v.n. 0.60mg/l)			7.55	5.14	

vation of transaminases and lactate dehydrogenase, normocomplementemia; serum ferritin level increased gradually from value of 1389 ng/ml to 12.000 (**Table 1**). An infectious workup was negative, including stool ova and parasites.

Antibodies for common autoimmune diseases were in the norm repeated twice. General coltural tests and blood coltures were negative, repeated several times.

A peripheral blood smear and then a bone marrow excluded malignancies; lymphocyte subpopulations were normal. Fundus examination was normal. An echo handwriting abdomen, followed by a CAT scan chest, abdomen and skull showed splenomegaly (splenic diameter: 14.5 cm). Magnetic resonance imaging of the brain excluded an issue of acute inflammatory neurologic disease. No coronaropathy and valvulopathy reperted.

The persistence of high values of inflammatory markers, in association with further raising of serum ferritin levels and the fever profile diagnosed of systemic onset JRA. Arthritis was not present yet, but there were diffuse arthralgias and with time the child was not able to use his thumb to play games. A complicating MAS has considered and then excluded [5,6].

Beacause child was not responsive to ibuprofen therapy, after a second negative bone marrow examination, he started prednisone treatment with significant improvement of clinical conditions.

3. CASE 2

Girl of 9 years was under our observation for persistent fever for five days and asthenia unresponsive to antibiotic and occasionally treatment with bethametasone. At admission, general conditions were expired; she presented a widespread multiforme erythema, right ankle swelling and edema of small phalanges of the hands (**Figure 2**). A diffuse arthralgia above the upper limbs and column was reported.

Personal history was not contributive. The father was affected from vitiligo; the mother had an autoimmune

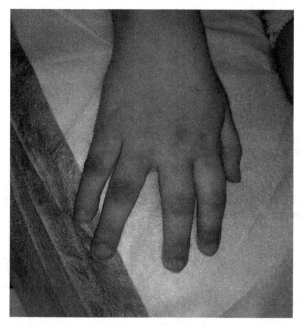

Figure 2. Multiforme erythema and edema of small phalanges of the hands.

tyroiditis. Her brother was suffering from allergic asthma.

Laboratory tests were characterized by elevated erythrocyte sedimentation rate, high level of serum ferritin and positive C-reactive protein (**Table 2**).

An infectious workup was negative. Antibodies for common autoimmune were in the norm. The echocardiogram, chest radiograph were normal. Abdominal ultrasound showed mild splenomegaly. An examination of the fundus was normal. General coltural tests and blood coltures, peripheral blood smear were negative. Serum ferritin level increased gradually to value of 5881 ng/ml.

The fever was intermittent at least two daily peaks; the rash seemed to coincide with the rise in body temperature. The course of the fever, the association with arthralgia, ankle edema and erythema and phalanges with high value of ferritin.suggested systemic-onset JRA. After a sample of bone marrow to rule out malignancy, it has been initiated treatment with prednisone with remission of symptoms and levels of ferritin .The therapy with ibuprofen was inefficay.

Table 2. Values of white blood cells, inflammatory markers and serum ferritin in relation to days of hospitalization before and after beginning of cortisonic terapy—Case 2.

	26/04/11	28/04/11	Beginning of therapy 02/05/11	After therapy 07/05/11	After therapy 13/05/11
WBC $10^3/\mu l$	10.060	15.840		7.520	9678
ESR mm/hr	65	45		49	18
CRP mg/dl	6.4	5.75		2.23	0.18
Ferritin ng/ml	4723	5881		934	267
D-Dimers mg/l v.n. 0.60 mg/l	2.03	4.15		0.58	0.44

4. DISCUSSION

There are no specific diagnostic tests for sistemic JRA, which commonly presents as prolonged fever that is not easily diagnosed (*i.e.*, FUO) [6]. Typically, patients with JRA present with liver/spleen involvement, pauci-articular arthritis, arthralgias and myalgias,ocular involvement, and evanescent salmon-colored truncal rash. Arthralgia occurs in other disorders [6,7]. Serum ferritin levels may be elevated in infections, malignancies (leukaemia, lymphomas), liver diseases and haemochromatosis. However, in these conditions serum ferritin concentrations rarely exceed values of >3000 ng/ml. High level of serum ferritin is the most important, non specific, diagnostic finding associated with JRA [8-10]. Clinicians should appreciate the diagnostic significance of fever patterns and the diagnostic significance of elevated serum ferritin levels in patients with FUO.

REFERENCES

[1] Petty, R.E., Southwood, T.R., Manners, P., *et al.* (2004) International league of associations for rheumatology classification of juvenile idiopathic arthritis: Second revision, Edmonton, 2001. *Journal of Rheumatology*, **31**, 390-392.

[2] Berntson, L., Andersson Gäre, B., Fasth, A., *et al.* (2003) Incidence of juvenile idiopathic arthritis in the Nordic countries. A population based study with special reference to the validity of the ILAR and EULAR criteria. Nordic Study Group. *Journal of Rheumatology*, **30**, 2275-2282.

[3] Riise, Ø.R., Handeland, K.S., Cvancarova, M., *et al.* (2008) Incidence and characteristics of arthritis in Norwegian children: A population-based study. *Pediatrics*, **121**, e299-e306. doi:10.1542/peds.2007-0291

[4] Woo, P. (2006) Systemic juvenile idiopathic arthritis: Diagnosis, management and outcome. *Nature Reviews Rheumatology*, **2**, 28-34. doi:10.1038/ncprheum0084

[5] Ravelli, A., Magni-Manzoni, S., Pistorio, A., *et al.* (2005) Preliminary diagnostic guidelines for macrophage activation syndrome complicating systemic juvenile idiopathic arthritis. *Journal of Pediatrics*, **146**, 598-604. doi:10.1016/j.jpeds.2004.12.016

[6] Insalaco, A. (2006) Macrophage activation syndrome in juvenile idiopathic arthritis. *Acta Paediatrica*, **95**, 38-41.

[7] Lomater, C., Gerloni, V., Gattinara, M., *et al.* (2000) Systemic onset juvenile idiopathic arthritis: A retrospective study of 80 consecutive patients followed for 10 years. *Journal of Rheumatology*, **27**, 491-496.

[8] Yao, T.C., Kuo, M.L., See, L.C., Ou, L.S., Lee, W.I., Chan, C.K. and Huang, J.L. (2006) RANTES and monocyte chemoattractant protein 1 as sensitive markers of disease activity in patients with juvenile arthritis: A six-year longitudinal study. *Arthritis & Rheumatism*, **54**, 2585-2593.

[9] Meijvis, H., Endeman, A.B.M., Geers, E.J. and Borg, E.J. (2007) Extremely high serum ferritin levels as diagnostic tool in adult-onset still's disease. *The Netherland Journal of Medicine*, **65**, 212-214.

[10] Jandus, P., Wang, W., Seitz, M., *et al.* (2010) High serum ferritin in adult-onset still's disease. *International Journal of Clinical Medicine*, **1**, 81-83.

ABBREVIATIONS USED

JRA: Juvenile Rheumatoid Arthritis
CRP: C-Reactive Protein
ESR: Erythro-Sedimentation-Rate
CAT: Computed Axial Tomography
MAS: Macrophage Activation Syndrome
FUO: Fever of Unknown Origin

9

Diagnostic Value of Antibodies against a Modified Citrullinated Vimentin in Rheumatoid Arthritis

Sahar Abou El-Fetou[1], Hanan S. Abozaid[2]

[1]Department of Clinical Pathology, Faculty of Medicine, Sohag University, Sohag, Egypt; [2]Department of Rheumatology and Rehabilitation, Faculty of Medicine, Sohag University, Sohag, Egypt.
Email: rmhamdy@yahoo.com

ABSTRACT

Aim of Work: To investigate the value of the detection of antibodies against modified citrullinated vimentin antibodies (anti-MCV) in comparison with anti-CCP2- for the diagnosis of rheumatoid arthritis (RA). *Patients and Methods*: The study Included Forty patients with Rheumatoid arthritis (RA). They under went assessment by the disease activity score (DAS-28), visual analogue scale (VAS) and health assessment questionnaire (HAQ). Thirty healthy subjects matched for age and sex served as a control group. Blood samples were obtained from patients and controls for erythrocyte sedimentation rate (ESR), C reactive protein (CRP), rheumatoid factor (RF). Anti-CCP2 and anti-MCV were determined using ELISA technique. *Results*: Estimated serum levels of anti-CCP2 and anti-MCV were significantly higher in patients compared to controls ($p < 0.001$). There were no significant correlations between anti-MCV levels and age, disease duration, duration of morning stiffness, number of swollen and tender joints, HAQ or ESR in patients with RA, while serum levels correlates significantly with DAS28, VAS and CRP ($p < 0.05$). Anti-CCP2 correlates significantly with DAS28, VAS and CRP and ANA ($p < 0.05$). Serum anti-MCV and anti-CCP2 were significantly correlated with each other ($r = 0.483$; $p < 0.001$). The receiver operating characteristic (ROC) curve was drawn and it showed that anti-MCV had diagnostic specificity, sensitivity of 93.3%, 75.5%, respectively, while anti-CCP2 specificity, sensitivity of 98.1%, 85%, respectively. *Conclusion*: Serum anti-MCV as well as the anti-CCP-2 assay perform comparably well in the diagnosis of RA. In the high-specificity range, however, the anti-CCP2 assay appears to be superior to the anti-MCV test.

Keywords: Anti-Cyclic Citrullinated Peptide (Anti-CCP2); Anti-Citrullinated Vimentin Antibody (Anti-CMV) Rheumatoid Arthritis (RA)

1. Introduction

Rheumatoid arthritis (RA) is a chronic, inflammatory, autoimmune, systemic disease, in which various joints in the body are inflamed, leading to swelling, pain, stiffness, and the possible loss of function [1]. Early diagnosis and treatment may prevent joint destruction and suppress disease progression [2].

Several different autoantibodies with varying have been found in serum from patients with RA [3], but rheumatoid factor (RF) is at present the only autoantibody included in the 1987 American College of Rheumatology (ACR) classification criteria [4].

Highly specific and sensitive tests are necessary to diagnose early RA and initiate aggressive treatment regimens to prevent the irreversible joint damage. Testing for RF alone is not enough. It can be found in only 70% - 80% of RA patients. It is also present in other rheumatic disorders and healthy individuals [5].

Antibodies recognizing citrullinated proteins/peptides, especially the peptide mixture designated cyclic citrullinated peptides (CCP), have reasonable sensitivity and high specificity for RA and are incessantly used in the evaluation of patients with RA [6,7]. It is found to be highly specific for early diagnosis (97%) as well as prognosis of [8]. Vimentin is an intermediate filament that is widely expressed by mesenchymal cells and macrophages and easy to detect in the synovium. Modification of the protein occurs in macrophages undergoing apoptosis, and antibodies to citrullinated vimentin may emerge if the apoptotic material is inadequately cleared [9]. Recently, anti-mutated citrullinated vimentin (anti-MCV) antibodies have been recommended to be better diagnostic marker for early arthritis [10].

Some studies showed that anti-MCV antibody is more sensitive compared to other antibodies against citrulline-containing epitopes for RA diagnosis, and that anti-MCV antibody was present even earlier in the course of RA than anti-CCP, and therefore was a better marker of early RA [11]. Besides the higher sensitivity it has been shown that anti-MCV antibody is a better marker for early RA, and it correlates well with the disease activity score (DAS). The presence of anti-MCV antibodies at disease onset is associated with a more severe disease course, measured as higher level of inflammatory activity compared with anti-CCP [12].

Several studies demonstrated that anti-MCV antibodies have the same specificity as anti-CCP antibodies, but with better sensitivity [13,14]. Like anti-CCP antibodies, anti-MCV antibodies are also suitable for the early diagnosis of RA, with comparable sensitivity and specificity [15].

This work was aimed to evaluate the role of anti-mutated citrullinated vimentin antibodies (anti-MCV) and anti-CCP2 for the diagnosis of RA.

2. Patients and Methods

This case control study was conducted on RA patients attending the outpatient clinic of Rheumatology and Rehabilitation Department, Sohag University Hospital, in the period between May 2012 and September 2012. Forty patients (female/male = 26/14) fulfilling the 1987 American College of Rheumatology (ACR) criteria for a diagnosis of RA with a mean age of 46.95 ± 11.60 years were studied. Thirty healthy control subjects (female/male = 18/12). The mean age of the control subjects was 43.7 ± 9.9 years. Informed consent was obtained from patients and controls participating in the study. Age, sex, disease duration, Body Mass Index (BMI) (kg/m^2), swollen and tender joint counts of the RA patients were recorded. Duration of morning stiffness, Visual Analog Scale of pain (VAS) [16] disease activity index 28 (DAS28) [17], health assessment questionnaire (HAQ), erythrocyte sedimentation rate (ESR) and C-reactive protein (CRP) were used to assess disease activity. Disease Activity-Score 28 (DAS28) as a validated index of RA activity. It consists of four measures: 28 tender (TJC28) and swollen joint counts (SJC28), ESR, and patient global health assessment (VAS). Patients were grouped according to DAS28 scores as having high (DAS28 > 5.1) or mild to moderate (DAS28 < 5.1) disease activity.

3. Laboratory Methods

Six mL of peripheral venous blood were withdrawn asep-

tically from each patient and from each control subject. Two mL blood were left to clot for 15 minutes then centrifuged and sera were put into aliquots and stored at −20°C until assayed for anti-MCV and anti CCP2 antibodies for both patients and controls. The remaining 3 ml were used for other investigations done to patients:

1) Complete blood picture CBC was performed on The CELL-DYN 3700 automated hematology analyzer.

2) Renal and liver function tests were performed on Autoanalyzer Bechman Synchron cx5 system.

3) Measurement of ESR by the Westergren method.

4) Serum CRP concentrations were determined by immunonephelometry methods on a Turboxnephelometer (Orion Diagnostica, Finland). The titer of 6 mg/l was considered positive for CRP.

5) Rheumatoid factor IgMisotype was analyzed using the ELISA kit for RF IgM quantitation (Orgentec Diagnostika GmbH, Germany) according to the manufacturer's instructions. The titer of 20 IU/ml was regarded as positive [18].

6) Measurement of anti-nuclear antibody (ANA) was detected by the Fluro-kit supplied by DiaSorine Catalog No 1740 based on indirect immunoflorescent for the screening and titration ANA.

7) Anti-CCP2 antibodies were detected by enzyme-linked immunosorbent assay Kit supplies by INOVA Diagnostica Cat. NO 570139 is a semiquantitative enzyme-linked immunosorbent assay for the detection of IgG anti-CCP2 (Cyclic Citrullinated Peptide 2) antibodies in patient sera. The antigen is bound to the surface of a microwell plate, allowing any CCP2IgG antibodies present to bind to the immobilized antigen. A second incubation allows the enzyme labeled antihuman IgG to bind to any patient antibodies that have been attached to the microwells. After washing away any unbound enzyme labeled anti-human IgG, the remaining enzyme activity is measured by adding a chromogenic substrate and measuring the intensity of the color that develops spectrophotometrically. A titer above 20 units was considered as positive.

8) Determination of Anti-MCV antibodies were measured using ELISA kits (provided by ORGENTEC Diagnostica GmbH, Mainz, Germany) according to the manufacturer's instructions [19]. Serum samples were diluted 1:100 and incubated on MCV coated microtiter wells for 30 minutes at room temperature. Plates were washed three times and incubated with peroxidase-labeled anti-human IgG-conjugate for 15 minutes. Then substrate was incubated for 15 minutes after additional washing. Color development was stopped with 1 M HCl solution, and the optical density was measured. Results are expressed in U/ml using a simple point-to-point curve-fitting method. Values of 20.0 U/ml or greater were considered to be abnormal according to manufacturer's recommendations.

4. Statistics

The results were analyzed by IBM-SPSS (version 19). Results were given as means and standard deviation. Student's t-test for continuous variables was used to examine the significance of differences between RA and control groups. P-value less than 0.05 was regarded as significant. The correlation between anti -MCV, anti-CCP2 levels and age, disease duration, duration of morning stiffness, swollen and tender joint counts, VAS, DAS28, HAQ, ESR, CRP and BMI was analyzed by Pearson correlation analyses. Receiver operator characteristic curve (ROC) was drawn to find out the best cut-off value of anti-MCV in diagnosing RA. p value > 0.05 was considered insignificant, p < 0.05 was significant and p < 0.001 was highly significant.

5. Results

Age, sex and BMI did not show statistically significant differences between RA patients and control subjects (p > 0.05).Patients with RA had mild to moderate (DAS28 < 5.1) disease activity. The demographic and clinical characteristics of patients with RA and of control subjects are shown in **Table 1**. The mean serum Anti-CCP2 in patients with RA (89.2 ± 11.3 U/ml) was significantly higher (p < 0.001) than controls (14.8 ± 3.21 U/mL).

Table 1. Demographic and clinical characteristics of rheumatoid arthritis (RA) patients and control.

Characteristics (mean ± SD)	RA patients (40)	Control (30)	p value
Age (years)	46.95 ± 11.60	43.7 ± 9.9	0.542
Sex (F/M)	26/14	18/12	0.532
Disease duration (years)	4.57 ± 2.59	-	
Morning stiffness (min)	18.84 ± 9.04	-	
VAS (0 - 10)	4.62 ± 1.40	-	
Number of swollen joints	2.32 ± 1.18	-	
Number of tender joints	3.89 ± 2.08	-	
DAS28 score	3.79 ± 0.66	-	
HAQ score	11.49 ± 4.15	-	
ESR (mm/1st hr)	42.65 ± 8.59	-	
Rheumatoid factor (%)	46.0 ± 9.8	-	
CRP (mg/l)	18.65 ± 9.59	-	
Body mass index (BMI)	14.15 ± 11.48	27.85 ± 2.62	
Anti-CCP2 (U/ml)	89.2 ± 11.3	14.8 ± 3.21	<0.001**
Anti-MCV (U/mL)	114.45 ± 16.57	9.05 ± 3.67	<0.001**

RF: rheumatoid factor; MS: morning stiffness; VAS: visual analog scale of pain; DAS28: disease activity for 28 joint indices score; HAQ: health assessment questionnaire; ESR: erythrocyte sedimentation rate; CRP: C-reactive protein; BMI: body mass index. Anti-CCP2, antibodies against cyclic citrullinated peptide; MCV: Anti-MCV: antibodies against mutated citrullinated vimentin ** = Highly significant (**Figures 1** and **2**).

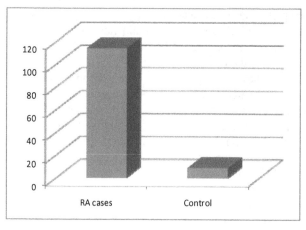

Figure 1. Serum anti-MCV levels in patients with RA and in controls.

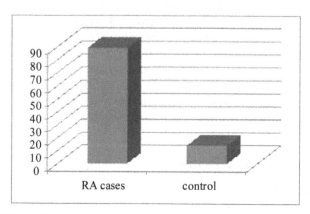

Figure 2. Serum anti-CCP2 levels in patients with RA and in controls.

Also, the anti-MCV levels (114.45 ± 16.57 U/ml) were higher (p < 0.001) in RA patients compared to healthy control subjects (9.05 ± 3.6 U/ml) **Table 1**.

Using Spearman's rank correlation coefficient, serum levels of anti-MCV correlated positively but insignificantly with age, onset of RA, duration of the disease, number of tender joints and ESR. (p > 0.05) and correlated negatively with the number of swollen joints (r = −0.053, p > 0.05) in RA patients. The anti-MCV level significantly correlated with CRP, VAS and DAS 28 (r.0.084, 0.747 and 0.802, p < 0.05). The level of anti-CCP2 correlated positively but insignificantly with age, onset of RA, duration of the disease, number of tender joints (p < 0.5) and significantly with VAS, DAS28, CRP, RF and ANA (p < 0.05). Anti-MCV and anti-CCP2 were significantly, correlated with each other (correlation coefficient = 0.483; p < 0.001) **Table 2**.

For direct comparison of the diagnostic values of the anti-MCV and the anti-CCP2 assays, we performed Receiver operator characteristic curve ROC analysis. The best cut-off value for the anti-MCV test was found at 21.5 U/mL (**Figure 3**). The area under the curve (AUC) was 0.893 at the 95% CI, Sensitivity was 75.6% and specificity was 93.3% indiagnosing RA patients, both positive and negative predictive values were (82.8% and 87.4%, respectively). At cut-off value 20 U/mL for the anti CCP2 test it was found that, the area under the curve was AUC 0.926 at the 95% CI, Sensitivity was 85.71% and specificity was 98.1% in diagnosing RA patients positive and negative predictive values were (86% and 93%, respectively) (**Table 3** and **Figure 4**).

The sensitivity of each test is plotted against one minus specificity for varying cutoffs (values lower than the cutoff were considered negative, and other values were considered positive) ($n = 40$).

6. Discussion

Therapeutic intervention early in the course of RA leads to more efficient disease control, less joint damage, and better prognosis of disease outcome [20]. So, it is of a particular importance to identify a sensitive diagnostic marker which permits early definitive diagnosis of RA. Several reports have demonstrated high diagnostic value of antibodies directed against citrullinated proteins in the

Table 2. Correlations between serums Anti CCP2, Anti-MCV and patients' characteristics.

Parameters	Anti-CCP2		Anti-MCV	
	r	p-value	r	p-value
Age	0.264	0.231	0.359	0.65
Onset of RA	0.658	0.455	0.236	0.742
Disease Duration	0.633	0.333	0.302	0.561
Number of tender joints	0.222	0.432	0.301	0.543
Number of swollen joints	0.651	0.652	-0.053	0.344
VAS	0.561	0.003**	0.747	0.005**
MS	0.233	0.645	-0.341	0.123
DAS28	0.351	0.001**	0.802	0.001**
HAQ	0.321	0.356	-0.29	0.06
ESR	0.452	0.442	0.029	0.367
CRP	0.568	0.031*	0.084	0.021*
RF	0.529	0.032*	0.560	0.312
ANA	0.333	0.051*	0.651	0.231
Anti-CCP2 (u/mL)	-	-	0.483	0.001**

Pearson correlation coefficients between Anti CCP2, Anti MCV R, RF in RA patients. RF: rheumatoid factor; MS: morning stiffness; VAS: visual analog scale of pain; DAS28: disease activity for 28 joint indices score; HAQ: health assessment questionnaire; ESR: erythrocyte sedimentation rate; CRP: C-reactive protein; BMI: body mass index. Anti-CCP2, antibodies against cyclic citrullinated peptide; MCV: Anti-MCV: antibodies against mutated citrullinated vimentin * = significant. ** = Highly significant.

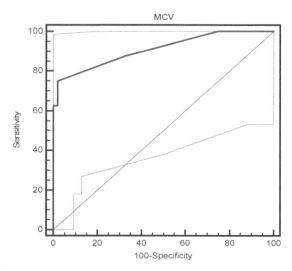

Figure 3. Receiver operator characteristic curve (ROC) assessing the validity of the anti-MCV test in diagnosing RA. The area under the curve was 0.893 at the 95% CI. The sensitivity of each test is plotted against one minus specificity for varying cutoffs (values lower than the cutoff were considered negative, and other values were considered positive) ($n = 40$).

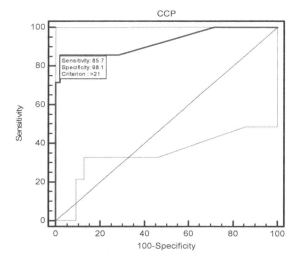

Figure 4. Receiver operator characteristic curve (ROC) assessing the validity of the anti-CCP2 test in diagnosing RA. The area under the curve was 0.923 at the 95% CI. The sensitivity of each test is plotted against one minus specificity for varying cutoffs (values lower than the cutoff were considered negative, and other values were considered positive) ($n = 40$).

diagnosis of RA. Although the specificity was more than 90% in most studies, the sensitivity of the same antibodies varied between 33% and 87.2%, possibly reflecting diverse genetic backgrounds and/or methodological differences in diverse antigen preparations and detection techniques applied [21].

In our study, we have shown that, the levels of anti-CCP2 were significantly increased in the serum of the

Table 3. Diagnostic effectiveness of the anti-MCV test and the anti-cyclic citrullinated peptide in RA patients.

	Cut off (U/ml)	Sensitivity % [95% CI]	Specificity % [95% CI]	Positive predictive values % [95% CI]	Negative predictive values % [95% CI]
Anti-MCV	21.5 (U/ml)	75.56 (60.5 - 87.1)	93.33 (68.1 - 99.8)	82.24 (78 - 96.22)	87.4 (69 - 81.42)
Anti-CCP2	21 (U/ml)	85.71 (42.1 - 99.6)	98.11 (89.9 - 100.0)	86 (62.1 - 89.6)	93 (89.7% - 99.6%)

patients with RA in comparison with the controls (p < 0.001). This results in agreement with other studies [22, 23].

The present study revealed a significantly higher serum anti-MCV antibody level in RA patients when compared to healthy controls (p < 0.001). This can be explained by the hypothesis that vimentin might trigger the initial immune response in RA [24]. It activates T lymphocytes by binding on HLA-DR4 on the surface of antigen presenting cells and may contribute to certain pathways in the pathogenesis of RA. Several studies demonstrated significant elevation in serum anti-MCV in RA-patients versus controls [25-27].

In contrast to this finding, Morbach *et al.*, [27], found no significant difference, a finding which can be explained by the fact that vimentin contains 43 arginine residues with 10 citrullination sites experimentally confirmed and anti-MCV antibodies are considered a heterogenous group of antibodies directed against different epitopes on the citrulline molecule [13].

In the present work, anti-MCV titer was significantly correlated with DAS-28, VAS and CRP (p < 0.05). Our finding is in consistent with the report of Innala *et al.*, [28] who concluded that anti-MCV titer was significantly correlated with DAS-28, VAS and ESR. Similarly, in a three-year follow-up study of 427 RA patients, Keskin *et al.*, [23] found that patients with active RA were found to have higher anti-MCV titers than patients with inactive disease, while, anti-CCP2 titer failed to show this correlation (a non-significant difference in anti-CCP2 titer between patients with active or inactive disease). Similarly he found that the mean serum anti-MCV levels were correlated with DAS 28, serum CRP levels, serum RF levels, swollen joints number and tender joints number (p = 0.001).

In a trial to assess the diagnostic performance of serum anti MCV antibodies in RA, the ROC curve was plotted. We found that at a cut off value of 21.5 u/ml serum anti MCV antibody had specificity and a sensitivity of 93.3% and 75.6% respectively and positive and negative predictive values were (82.8% and 87.4%, respectively). This is in consistent with the results of previous reports conducted by Damjanovska *et al.*, Soos *et al.*, and Mathsson *et al.*, [26,29,30]. So, detection of anti-MCV antibodies has been shown to provide a sensitivity of 62% - 84% and specificity of 83% - 95% for the diagnosis of RA. Poulsom and Charles [10] found a specificity and sensitivity

of 87% and 84% respectively, while Dejaco and associates [15] reported a result of 90.8% and 69.5% respectively. However, at a cut off value of 25 u/ml, Bang and colleagues [13] reported the specificity and sensitivity to be 88% and 82% respectively. Variation in the sensitivity and specificity can be attributed to the fact that some of the studies included patients with undifferentiated arthritis and psoriatic arthritis [31].

In the present study, out of 40 RA patients, 31 (77.5%) tested positive for anti-MCV. Anti-MCV sensitivity and specificity were 75.6% and 93.3%, respectively while anti-CCP2 was of sensitivity was 85.71% and specificity was 98.1% in diagnosing RA patients, similar to our finding a cutoff value of 20.0 U/ml (as recommended by the manufacturer), sensitivity and specificity of the anti-MCV ELISA were 69.5% and 90.8%, respectively, compared with 70.1% and 98.7% of the anti-CCP2 assay Dejaco *et al.*, [15].

While, Egerer *et al.*, [19] at cut-off value 20.5 found that anti-MCV antibodies in 1151 RA patients, have the same specificity as anti-CCP2 antibodies but with much better sensitivity (82% versus 72%). Similarly, Mathsson *et al.*, and Gross *et al.*, [20,26] who concluded that the anti-MCV assay extends the diagnostic spectrum for RA with higher sensitivity and prognostic value concerning radiological progression than anti-CCP2 antibodies (71% versus 58%, respectively).

7. Conclusion

In conclusion, Anti-MCV antibodies can be regarded as a promising diagnostic marker in RA patients with high sensitivity and specificity Autoantibodies to citrullinated proteins are specific for the diagnosis of RA. Antibodies directed against a modified citrullinated vimentin that demonstrates comparable overall diagnostic performance in relation to the anti-CCP2. In the high specificity range of both tests, which is clinically the most relevant, the anti-CCP2 appears to be superior to the anti-MCV assay. Serum anti-MCV antibody could be a promising tool in diagnosing RA, show a significant link with disease activity.

REFERENCES

[1]   J. H. Pedersen-Lane, R. B. Zurier and D. A. Lawrence, "Analysis of the Thiol Status of Peripheral Blood Leuko-

cytes in Rheumatoid Arthritis Patients," *Journal of Leukocyte Biology*, Vol. 81, No. 4, 2007, pp. 934-941. http://dx.doi.org/10.1189/jlb.0806533

[2] G. Serre, "Autoantibodies to Filaggrin/Deiminated Fibrin (AFA) Are Useful for the Diagnosis and Prognosis of Rheumatoid Arthritis, and Are Probably Involved in the Pathophysiology of the Disease," *Joint Bone Spine*, Vol. 68, No. 2, 2001, pp. 103-105. http://dx.doi.org/10.1016/S1297-319X(01)00259-7

[3] T. Mottonen, L. Paimela, M. Leirisalo-Repo, H. Kautiainen, J. Ilonen and P. Hannonen, "Only High Disease Activity and Positive Rheumatoid Factor Indicate Poor Prognosis in Patients with Early Rheumatoid Arthritis Treated with 'Sawtooth' Strategy," *Annals of the Rheumatic Diseases*, Vol. 57, No. 9, 1998, pp. 533-539. http://dx.doi.org/10.1136/ard.57.9.533

[4] F. C. Arnett, S. M. Edworthy, D. A. Bloch, *et al.*, "The American Rheumatism Association 1987 Revised Criteria for the Classification of Rheumatoid Arthritis," *Arthritis & Rheumatism*, Vol. 31, No. 3, 1988, pp. 315-324. http://dx.doi.org/10.1002/art.1780310302

[5] I. Vallbracht, J. Rieber, M. Oppermann, F. Forger, U. Siebert and K. Helmke, "Diagnostic and Clinical Value of Anti-Cyclic Citrullinated Peptide Antibodies Compared with Rheumatoid Factor Isotypes in Rheumatoid Arthritis," *Annals of the Rheumatic Diseases*, Vol. 63, No. 9, 2004, pp. 1079-1084. http://dx.doi.org/10.1136/ard.2003.019877

[6] G. A. Schellekens, B. A. de Jong, F. H. van den Hoogen, L. B. van de Putte and W. J. van Venrooij, "Citrulline Is an Essential Constituent of Antigenic Determinants Recognized by Rheumatoid Arthritis-Specific Autoantibodies," *The Journal of Clinical Investigation*, Vol. 101, No. 1, 1998, pp. 273-281. http://dx.doi.org/10.1172/JCI1316

[7] B. Harrison, W. Thomson, D. Symmons, *et al.*, "The Influence of HLA-DRB1 Alleles and Rheumatoid Factor on Disease Outcome in an Inception Cohort of Patients with Early Inflammatory Arthritis," *Arthritis & Rheumatism*, Vol. 42, No. 10, 1999, pp. 2174-2183. http://dx.doi.org/10.1002/1529-0131(199910)42:10<2174::AID-ANR19>3.0.CO;2-G

[8] E. Lindqvist, K. Eberhardt, K. Bendtzen, D. Heinegard and T. Saxne, "Prognostic Laboratory Markers of Joint Damage in Rheumatoid Arthritis," *Annals of the Rheumatic Diseases*, Vol. 64, No. 2, 2005, pp. 196-201. http://dx.doi.org/10.1136/ard.2003.019992

[9] E. R. Vossenaar, T. R. Radstake, A. van der Heijden, *et al.*, "Expression and Activity of Citrullinating Peptidylarginine Deiminase Enzymes in Monocytes and Macrophages," *Annals of the Rheumatic Diseases*, Vol. 63, No. 4, 2004, pp. 373-381. http://dx.doi.org/10.1136/ard.2003.012211

[10] H. Poulsom and P. J. Charles, "Antibodies to Citrullinated Vimentin Are a Specific and Sensitive Marker for the Diagnosis of Rheumatoid Arthritis," *Clinical Reviews in Allergy & Immunology*, Vol. 34, No. 1, 2008, pp. 4-10. http://dx.doi.org/10.1007/s12016-007-8016-3

[11] J. Ursum, M. M. Nielen, D. van Schaardenburg, *et al.*, "Antibodies to Mutated Citrullinated Vimentin and Disease Activity Score in Early Arthritis: A Cohort Study," *Arthritis Research & Therapy*, Vol. 10, No. 1, 2008, p. R12. http://dx.doi.org/10.1186/ar2362

[12] J. T. Cassidy, J. E. Levinson, J. C. Bass, *et al.*, "A Study of Classification Criteria for a Diagnosis of Juvenile Rheumatoid Arthritis," *Arthritis & Rheumatism*, Vol. 29, No. 2, 1986, pp. 274-281. http://dx.doi.org/10.1002/art.1780290216

[13] H. Bang, K. Egerer, A. Gauliard, *et al.*, "Mutation and Citrullination Modifies Vimentin to a Novel Autoantigen for Rheumatoid Arthritis," *Arthritis & Rheumatism*, Vol. 56, No. 8, 2007, pp. 2503-2511. http://dx.doi.org/10.1002/art.22817

[14] R. Sghiri, E. Bouajina, D. Bargaoui, *et al.*, "Value of Anti-Mutated Citrullinated Vimentin Antibodies in Diagnosing Rheumatoid Arthritis," *Rheumatology International*, Vol. 29, No. 1, 2008, pp. 59-62. http://dx.doi.org/10.1007/s00296-008-0614-8

[15] C. Dejaco, W. Klotz, H. Larcher, C. Duftner, M. Schirmer and M. Herold, "Diagnostic Value of Antibodies against a Modified Citrullinated Vimentin in Rheumatoid Arthritis," *Arthritis Research & Therapy*, Vol. 8, No. 4, 2006, p. R119. http://dx.doi.org/10.1186/ar2008

[16] R. K. Mallya and B. E. Mace, "The Assessment of Disease Activity in Rheumatoid Arthritis Using a Multivariate Analysis," *Rheumatology and Rehabilitation*, Vol. 20, No. 1, 1981, pp. 14-17. http://dx.doi.org/10.1093/rheumatology/20.1.14

[17] M. L. Prevoo, M. A. van 't Hof, H. H. Kuper, M. A. van Leeuwen, L. B. van de Putte and P. L. van Riel, "Modified Disease Activity Scores That Include Twenty-Eight-Joint Counts. Development and Validation in a Prospective Longitudinal Study of Patients with Rheumatoid Arthritis," *Arthritis & Rheumatism*, Vol. 38, No. 1, 1995, pp. 44-48. http://dx.doi.org/10.1002/art.1780380107

[18] G. Kleveland, T. Egeland and T. Lea, "Quantitation of Rheumatoid Factors (RF) of IgM, IgA and IgG Isotypes by a Simple and Sensitive ELISA. Discrimination between False and True IgG-RF," *Scandinavian Journal of Rheumatology*, Vol. 75, 1988, pp. 15-24.

[19] K. Egerer, E. Feist and G. R. Burmester, "The Serological Diagnosis of Rheumatoid Arthritis: Antibodies to Citrullinated Antigens," *Deutsches Ärzteblatt International*, Vol. 106, No. 10, 2009, pp. 159-163.

[20] W. L. Gross, F. Moosig and P. Lamprecht, "Anticitrullinated Protein/Peptide Antibodies in Rheumatoid Arthritis," *Deutsches Ärzteblatt International*, Vol. 106, No. 10, 2009, pp. 157-158.

[21] T. Mimori, "Clinical Significance of Anti-CCP Antibodies in Rheumatoid Arthritis," *Internal Medicine*, Vol. 44, No. 11, 2005, pp. 1122-1126. http://dx.doi.org/10.2169/internalmedicine.44.1122

[22] T. R. Mikuls, J. R. O'Dell, J. A. Stoner, *et al.*, "Association of Rheumatoid Arthritis Treatment Response and Disease Duration with Declines in Serum Levels of IgM Rheumatoid Factor and Anti-Cyclic Citrullinated Peptide Antibody," *Arthritis & Rheumatism*, Vol. 50, No. 12, 2004, pp. 3776-3782. http://dx.doi.org/10.1002/art.20659

[23] G. Keskin, A. Inal, D. Keskin, *et al.*, "Diagnostic Utility

of Anti-Cyclic Citrullinated Peptide and Anti-Modified Citrullinated Vimentin Antibodies in Rheumatoid Arthritis," *Protein & Peptide Letters*, Vol. 15, No. 3, 2008, pp. 314-317. http://dx.doi.org/10.2174/092986608783744153

[24] A. J. Zendman, W. J. van Venrooij and G. J. Pruijn, "Use and Significance of Anti-CCP Autoantibodies in Rheumatoid Arthritis," *Rheumatology (Oxford)*, Vol. 45, No. 1, 2006, pp. 20-25. http://dx.doi.org/10.1093/rheumatology/kei111

[25] X. Liu, R. Jia, J. Zhao and Z. Li, "The Role of Anti-Mutated Citrullinated Vimentin Antibodies in the Diagnosis of Early Rheumatoid Arthritis," *Journal of Rheumatology*, Vol. 36, No. 6, 2009, pp. 1136-1142. http://dx.doi.org/10.3899/jrheum.080796

[26] L. Mathsson, M. Mullazehi, M. C. Wick, *et al.*, "Antibodies against Citrullinated Vimentin in Rheumatoid Arthritis: Higher Sensitivity and Extended Prognostic Value Concerning Future Radiographic Progression as Compared with Antibodies against Cyclic Citrullinated Peptides," *Arthritis & Rheumatism*, Vol. 58, No. 1, 2008, pp. 36-45. http://dx.doi.org/10.1002/art.23188

[27] H. Morbach, H. Dannecker, T. Kerkau and H. J. Girschick, "Prevalence of Antibodies against Mutated Citrullinated Vimentin and Cyclic Citrullinated Peptide in Children with Juvenile Idiopathic Arthritis," *Clinical and Experimental Rheumatology*, Vol. 28, No. 5, 2010, p. 800.

[28] L. Innala, H. Kokkonen, C. Eriksson, E. Jidell, E. Berglin and S. R. Dahlqvst, "Antibodies against Mutated Citrullinated Vimentin Are a Better Predictor of Disease Activity at 24 Months in Early Rheumatoid Arthritis than Antibodies against Cyclic Citrullinated Peptides," *Journal of Rheumatology*, Vol. 35, No. 6, 2008, pp. 1002-1008.

[29] L. Damjanovska, M. M. Thabet, E. W. Levarth, *et al.*, "Diagnostic Value of Anti-MCV Antibodies in Differentiating Early Inflammatory Arthritis," *Annals of the Rheumatic Diseases*, Vol. 69, No. 4, 2010, pp. 730-732. http://dx.doi.org/10.1136/ard.2009.108456

[30] L. Soos, Z. Szekanecz, Z. Szabo, *et al.*, "Clinical Evaluation of Anti-Mutated Citrullinated Vimentin by ELISA in Rheumatoid Arthritis," *Journal of Rheumatology*, Vol. 34, No. 8, 2007, pp. 1658-1663.

[31] R. E. Petty, T. R. Southwood, P. Manners, *et al.*, "International League of Associations for Rheumatology Classification of sion, Edmonton, 2001," *Journal of Rheumatology*, Vol. 31, No. 2, 2004, pp. 390-392.

10

Effect of Anti-TNF Therapy on Resistance to Insulin in Patients with Rheumatoid Arthritis

Mario Pérez[1*], **Raul Ariza**[2], **Ruben Asencio**[1], **Adolfo Camargo**[1], **Heladia Garcia**[1], **Miguel Angel Vazquez**[1], **Leonor Barile-Fabris**[1]

[1]UMAE Specialty Hospital "Bernardo Sepulveda" CMNSXXI, IMSS, Mexico City, Mexico; [2]Hospital Angeles del Pedregal, Mexico City, Mexico.
Email: craulariza@yahoo.com.mx, axel190106@hotmail.com, lbarile@prodigy.net.mx, adolfo_camargo@yahoo.com, hely1802@yahoo.com.mx, vazza78@hotmail.com, *drmariopc@hotmail.com

ABSTRACT

Objective: To evaluate the effect of anti-TNF therapy on resistance to insulin in patients with rheumatoid arthritis (RA) compared with patients with RA being treated with non-biological DMARDs. **Methods:** Inactive patients diagnosed with RA (ACR 1987 criteria) (DAS 28 < 2.6) were included, being treated with anti-tumor necrosis factor inhibitors (anti-TNF) (cases) and non-biological disease-modifying anti-rheumatic drugs (DMARD) (controls), without risk factors for insulin resistance (administration of steroids, body mass index > 25 kg/m^2, diabetes mellitus or use of glucose lowering agents, systemic arterial hypertension or use of anti-hypertensive drugs, triglycerides > 150 mg/dl, hypercholesterolemia > 200 mg/dl, high-density lipoproteins < 40 mg/dl in men and < 50 mg/in women, or with lipids lowering agents, waist measurement > 88 cm in women and > 102 cm in men). We used HOMA (Homeostasis Model Assessment) to determine insulin resistance in both groups, HOMA being defined as >1 and sensitivity to insulin using QUICKI (Insulin Sensitivity Check Index), ≥0.38 being considered as normal. The Mann Whitney U was used for the statistical analysis. **Results:** A total of 28 patients, 15 being treated with non-biological DMARDs and 13 with anti-TNF therapy, were evaluated; 89.7%, of which were women. Average age: 43.5 (range 21 - 62); the average HOMA index of the non-biological DMARD group was 1.58 (range 0.7 - 5.4), compared with patients treated with anti-TNF therapy, 1.18 (range 0.2 - 4.3) (P = 0.5). The average QUICKI index was 0.36 (range 0.30 - 0.42) in patients treated with non-biological DMARD, compared with 0.37 in patients treated with anti-TNF therapy (range 0.30 - 0.51) (P = 0.8). **Conclusion:** Resistance to insulin manifested itself in both groups, although there was a greater trend of less insulin resistance and greater sensitivity in the anti-TNF group; this was probably not statistically significant due to the sample size.

Keywords: Anti-TNF; Resistance to Insulin; Rheumatoid Arthritis

1. Introduction

Rheumatoid arthritis (RA) is the most common form of chronic inflammatory joint disease that brings about osseous destruction. The inflammatory process causes thickening and hyperplasia of the synovium, which is infiltrated by numerous cells that produce pro-inflammatory cytokines, including IL-1, IL-6 and tumor necrosis factor (TNF) [1]. This inflammation plays an important part in the pathogenesis of atherosclerosis and contributes to the cardiovascular morbidity and mortality found in patients with RA [2]. Cardiovascular disease is twice

as common in patients with RA, in comparison with the general population [3].

The increase in insulin resistance is another major risk factor in the development of cardiovascular disease, several methods for evaluating insulin resistance have been developed, of these, homeostasis model assessment (HOMA) has been reported to be unable to evaluate insulin resistance. The quantitative insulin sensitivity check index (QUICKI) has been reported to be a useful marker of insulin resistance. [4]. An increase in insulin resistance has been reported in patients with auto-immune diseases, including patients with RA [5,6]. In a case-control study it was found that insulin resistance of patients with RA

*Corresponding author.

manifested itself in 88.9% of patients, compared with just 6.2% of the controls that consisted of patients with soft tissue disease. There was also a significant association with sub-clinical atherosclerosis evaluated by means of thickening of the intima-media layer of the carotid artery [7].

TNF is a pleiotropic cytokine that plays a pivotal role in the host's response against microorganisms. It is also an important component of the inflammatory path and is over-expressed in the synovial tissue and in serum of patients with RA and on the atherosclerotic plate [3,8]. It has been observed that it contributes to atherogenesis by means of a series of mechanisms: promoting the expression of adhesion molecules in endothelial cells and recruiting and activating inflammatory cells within the arterial wall [9]. Several studies have suggested that TNF may be an important mediator in insulin resistance in animal models [10,11]. There is also evidence that over-expression occurs in the adipose tissue and skeletal muscle of patients resistant to insulin [12,13]. Loss of weight in obese subjects with insulin resistant leads to a substantial reduction in the expression and secretion of the TNF in association with a decrease in levels of TNF, and the restoring of sensitivity to insulin [14].

Given the effects on inflammation and metabolism, it may be expected that neutralization of the TNF will decrease resistance to insulin and, in turn, decrease cardiovascular risk [15].

Kiortsis *et al.* did not show any major differences in patients with RA and ankylosing spondylitis treated with Infliximab for six months, in HOMA and QUICKI indices (methods of determining resistance to insulin and sensitivity to insulin, respectively) before and after treatment. Nevertheless, a considerable difference in pre- and post treatment values with anti-TNF [16] was found in patients with higher HOMA and QUICKI indices in basal determinations in a study carried out on 27 patients with RA (21 women and 6 men, with an average age of 57.1 and an average DAS 28 of 4.43) with reduction in serum levels of insulin and the HOMA index, after infusion of infliximab [17].

There is still some controversy concerning the role that the anti-TNF block has on resistance to insulin.

2. Design of the Study

Cases and controls.

3. Material and Methods

Cases included patients of the rheumatology service diagnosed with rheumatoid arthritis according to ACR classification criteria [18], being treated with anti-TNF therapy and with no details of activity (DAS 28 < 2.6).

Controls comprised inactive patients of the rheuma-

tology service diagnosed with rheumatoid arthritis according to ACR classification criteria, being treated with non-biological DMARD not being given anti-TNF therapy, who were paired with cases by gender and age.

The two groups studied did not show any signs of risk that would increase resistance to insulin. Insulin levels were determined using electrochemical luminescence and glucose by enzymatic colorimetric test during fasting, in serum, of both study groups.

The Homeostasis Model Assessment (HOMA) model was used to determine resistance to insulin and sensitivity to insulin using the Insulin Sensitivity Check Index (QUICKI) in both groups.

Statistical Analysis

The statistical analysis was carried out using a Mann Whitney U to compare differences in resistance to insulin among the two groups studied. The SPSS 15.0 program was used.

4. Results

Twenty-eight patients were included; 13 cases and 15 controls, treated as follows: Case 10 with Etanercept, 2 with Adalimumab and one with Infliximab Controls 86.6% under Methotrexate, 20% Leflunomide, 26.6% Sulfasalazine and 20% with anti-malariac drugs.

Out of the overall groups, only three were men, who belonged to the anti-TNF, the other 89.7% being women.

Table 1 shows the baseline demographic characteristics of both groups, age, body mass index (BMI) time evolution of RA in months, time inactivity of RA in months, disease activity score (DAS-28), rheumatoid factor in UI/ml, waist in cm, cholesterol in mg/dl, triglycerides in mg/dl and HDL-colesterol in mg/dl, in which there were no statistically significant differences.

The average serum glucose during fasting in the control group was 85 mg/dl (41 - 97), while it was 80 mg/dl (67 - 98) P = 0.628 for cases; the average level of serum insulin during fasting in the control group was 9.1 mIU/ml (4 - 25.6), compared with 6 mIU/ml (1.1 - 17.9) for cases, without there being a statistically significant difference (P = 0.387).

On an overall basis, an increase in insulin resistance was observed in both groups of patients, evidenced by an HOMA index greater than 1, in addition to a decrease in sensitivity to insulin to less than 0.38

In spite of there being a remission of the illness in the control group, most patients (66.6%) had an HOMA index of greater than 1 and 53% a QUICKI index less than 0.38. In the cases group, 53.8% of patients had an HOMA index greater than 1 and 61.5% a QUICKI index less than 0.38.

We did not find a statistically significant difference in

Table 1. Demographic characteristics of patients with and without anti-TNF therapy.

	DMARD N = 15	ANTI-TNF N = 13	P*
Age&, years (range)	44 (21 - 62)	43 (22 - 58)	0.695
Weight&, kg (range)	59 (44 - 68)	61 (48 - 70)	0.393
Size&, cm (range)	156 (149 - 163)	160 (147 - 168)	0.138
BMI&, kg/m² (range)	24.3 (16.9 - 25)	23.1 (20.7 - 24.8)	0.050
Time of evolution&, months (range)	6 (4 - 30)	6 (1 - 15)	0.432
Time of inactivity&, months (range)	5 (2 - 24)	4(1 - 48)	0.235
Rheumatoid factor&, UI/ml (range)	78.2 (9 - 553)	66.5 (5 - 632)	0.479
DAS 28& (range)	2.30 (2 - 2.5)	2.3 (1.1 - 2.5)	0.832
Waist&, cm (range)	85 (63 - 87)	83 (71 - 90)	0.745
Cholesterol&, mg/dl (range)	162 (110 - 199)	151 (116 - 194)	0.42
Triglycerides&, mg/dl (range)	92 (71 - 145)	95 (50 - 111)	0.419
HDL-colesterol&, mg/dl (rango)	57 (50 - 80)	55 (40 - 76)	0.196

*Mann-Whitney U; &Average values (range).

insulin resistance, the average HOMA index being 1.58 (0.7 - 5.4) in the control group, and 1.18 (0.2 - 4.3) on the case group (P = 0.534) (**Figure 1**).

Likewise, the average QUICKI index in the control group was 0.36 (0.30 - 0.42), compared with 0.37 (0.30 - 0.51) in the case group, without there being a statistically significant difference (**Figure 2**).

5. Conclusion

Resistance to insulin presented itself in both study groups, although there was less resistance to insulin and greater sensitivity in the group being treated with anti-TNF; this was probably not statistically significant due to the sample size.

6. Discussion

Two groups of patients with rheumatoid arthritis were selected for the study, who had no risk factor nor any predisposing factor concerning development of resistance to insulin, for example: activity of the disease, as a direct proportional relationship between activity of the disease and resistance to insulin [6] has been observed in some studies. The significant result was that in spite of the disease being in remission, the majority of patients of both groups showed an increase in resistance to insulin and a decrease in sensitivity to insulin.

Kiortsis *et al.* [16] studied the effect of anti-TNF therapy (Infliximab only) on 28 active patients with rheumatoid arthritis, in other words, they were refractory patients being treated with non-biological DMARDs and prednisone (5 mg a day). There were no substantial

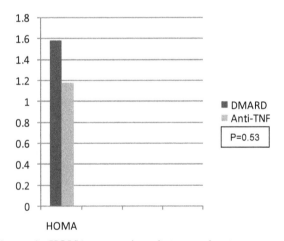

Figure 1. HOMA comparison between the two groups: DMARD vs anti-TNF.

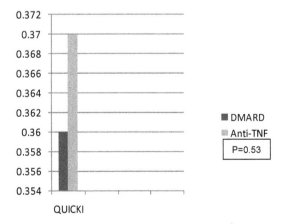

Figure 2. QUICKI comparison between the two groups: DMARD vs anti-TNF.

changes in their HOMA and QUICKI index, in spite of the anti-TNF therapy. We should point out the difference in our study as far as patient selection was concerned, as those with steroid and those that were active were excluded, but we found that there was no major difference in the HOMA and QUICKI of both treatment groups. Rosenvinge et al. [19] did also not observe any decrease in resistance to insulin, even though they used Adalimumab, unlike our study in which most patients of the anti-TNF therapy group were given Etanercept.

We have come across results that differ to ours. In a study carried out in Spain [17], 27 active patients with RA with an average DAS 28 of 4.43 were examined, whose seric insulin level and HOMA index were reduced after being administered Infliximab. A Turkish group headed by Oguz [20] included seven patients with RA who were treated with Infliximab, whose seric insulin level was reduced, as was their resistance to insulin by HOMA, with a statistically substantial difference. Results that favor a substantial decrease in resistance to insulin were also obtained in a group of patients with activity of the disease in China, with the use of Infliximab [21].

The particular aspect of our study was that we directly compared the effect of anti-TNF therapy with non-biological DMARDs, removing confusing factors that were definitely involved with resistance to insulin, unlike other studies that have examined this phenomenon, as they included patients who were obese, active, taking steroids, with dyslipidemia, etc., the only difference in our two groups of patients being the anti-TNF therapy.

There is no doubt that the limitation of our study is the size of the sample and this may explain the absence of substantial differences, so prospective, multi-centric and longitudinal studies need to be carried out to establish the actual impact of this type of treatment.

REFERENCES

[1] J. Zwerina, K. Redlich, G. Schett and J. S. Smolen, "Pathogenesis of Rheumatoid Arthritis: Targeting Cytokines," Annals of the New York Academy of Sciences, Vol. 1051, 2005, pp. 716-729. doi:10.1196/annals.1361.116

[2] S. Van Doornum, G. McColl and I. P. Wicks, "Accelerated Atherosclerosis: An Extraarticular Feature of Rheumatoid Arthritis?" Arthritis & Rheumatism, Vol. 46, No. 4, 2002, pp. 862-873. doi:10.1002/art.10089

[3] M. Boers, B. Dijkmans, S. Gabriel, H. Maradit-Kremers, J. O'Dell and T. Pincus, "Making an Impact on Mortality in Rheumatoid Arthritis: Targeting Cardiovascular Comorbidity," Arthritis & Rheumatism, Vol. 50, No. 6, 2004, pp. 1734-1739. doi:10.1002/art.20306

[4] G. Paolisso, G. Valentini, D. Guigliamo, G. Mavrazzo, R. Tirri, M. Gallo, et al., "Evidence for Peripheral Impaired Glucose Handling in Patients with Connective Tissue Diseases," Metabolism, Vol. 40, 1991, pp. 902-907. doi:10.1016/0026-0495(91)90064-4

[5] K. L. G. Svenson, T. Pollare, H. Lithell and R. Hallgren, "Impaired Glucose Handling in Active Rheumatoid Arthritis: Relationship to Peripheral Insulin Resistance," Metabolism, Vol. 37, 1998, pp. 125-130. doi:10.1016/S0026-0495(98)90005-1

[6] G. La Montagna, F. Cacciapuoti, R. Buono, D. Manzella, G. Mennillo, A. Arciello, G. Valentini and G. Paolisso, "Insulin Resistance Is and Independent Risk Factor for Atherosclerosis in Rheumatoid Arthritis," Diabetes and Vascular Disease Research, Vol. 4, No. 2, 2007, pp. 130-135. doi:10.3132/dvdr.2007.031

[7] J. P. Despres, B. Lamarche and P. Mauriege, "Hyperinsulinemia as an Independent Risk Factor for Ischemic Heart Disease," New England Journal of Medicine, Vol. 334, No. 15, 1996, pp. 952-957. doi:10.1056/NEJM199604113341504

[8] P. Libby, G. Sukhova, R. T. Lee and Z. S. Galis, "Cytokines Regulate Vascular Functions Related to Stability of the Atherosclerotic Plaque," Journal of Cardiovascular Pharmacology, Vol. 25, Suppl 2, 1995, pp. S9-S12. doi:10.1097/00005344-199500252-00003

[9] C. Book, T. Saxne and L. T. Jacobsson, "Prediction of Mortality in Rheumatoid Arthritis Based on Disease Activity Markers," Journal of Rheumatology, Vol. 32, No. 3, 2005, pp. 430-434.

[10] S. Wallberg-Jonsson, H. Johansson, M. L. Ohman and S. Rantapaa-Dahlqvist, "Extent of Inflammation Predicts Cardiovascular Disease and Overall Mortality in Seropositive Rheumatoid Arthritis. A Retrospective Cohort Study from Disease Onset," Journal of Rheumatology, Vol. 26, No. 12, 1999, pp. 2562-2571.

[11] G. S. Hotamisligil and B. M. Spiegelman, "Tumor Necrosis Factor Alpha: A Key Component of the Obesity-Diabetes Link," Diabetes, Vol. 43, No. 11, 1994, pp. 1271-1278. doi:10.2337/diabetes.43.11.1271

[12] G. S. Hotamisligil, P. Arner, J. F. Caro, R. L. Atkinson and B. M. Spiegelman, "Increased Adipose Tissue Expression of Tumor Necrosis Factor-Alpha in Human Obesity and Insulin Resistance," Journal of Clinical Investigation, Vol. 95, No. 5, 1995, pp. 2409-2415. doi:10.1172/JCI117936

[13] M. Saghizadeh, J. M. Ong, W. T. Garvey, R. R. Henry and P. A. Kern, "The Expression of TNF Alpha by Human Muscle. Relationship to Insulin Resistance," Journal of Clinical Investigation, Vol. 97, No. 4, 1996, pp. 1111-1116. doi:10.1172/JCI118504

[14] G. S. Hotamisligil, N. S. Shargill and B. M. Spiegelman, "Adipose Expression of Tumor Necrosis Factor Alpha: Direct Role in Obesity-Linked Insulin Resistance," Science, Vol. 259, No. 5091, 1993, pp. 87-91. doi:10.1126/science.7678183

[15] T. Saxne, M. A. Palladino Jr., D. Heinegard, N. Talal and F. A. Wollheim, "Detection of Tumor Necrosis Factor Alpha But Not Tumor Necrosis Factor Beta in Rheumatoid Arthritis Synovial Fluid and Serum," Arthritis & Rheumatism, Vol. 31, 1988, pp. 1041-1045. doi:10.1002/art.1780310816

[16] D. N. Kiortsis, A. K. Mavridis, S. Vasakos, S. N. Nikas and A. A. Drosos, "Effects of Infliximab Treatment on Insulin Resistance in Patients with Rheumatoid Arthritis and Ankylosing Spondylitis," *Annals of the Rheumatic Diseases*, Vol. 64, No. 5, 2005, pp. 765-766. doi:10.1136/ard.2004.026534

[17] M. A. Gonzalez-Gay, J. M. De Matias, C. Gonzalez-Juanatey, C. Garcia-Porrua, A. Sanchez-Andrade, J. Martin and J. Llorca, "Anti-Tumor Necrosis Factor-Alpha Blockade Improves Insulin Resistance in Patients with Rheumatoid Arthritis," *Clinical and Experimental Rheumatology*, Vol. 24, No. 1, 2006, pp. 83-86.

[18] F. C. Arnett, S. M. Edworthy, D. A. Bloch, D. J. McShane, J. F. Fries, N. S. Cooper, L. A. Healey, S. R. Kaplan, M. H. Liang, H. S. Luthra, *et al.*, "The American Rheumatism Association 1987 Revised Criteria for the Classification of Rheumatoid Arthritis," *Arthritis &*

Rheumatism, Vol. 31, No. 3, 1988, pp. 315-324. doi:10.1002/art.1780310302

[19] A. Rosenvinge, R. Krogh-Madsen, B. Baslund and B. K. Pedersen, "Insulin Resistance in Patient with Rheumatoid Arthritis: Effect of Anti-TNFalpha Therapy," *Scandinavian Journal of Rheumatology*, Vol. 36, No. 2, 2007, pp. 91-96. doi:10.1080/03009740601179605

[20] F. M. Oguz, A. Oguz and M. Uzunlulu, "The Effect of Infliximab Treatment on Insulin Resistance in Patients with Rheumatoid Arthritis," *Acta Clinica Belgica*, Vol. 62, No. 4, 2007, pp. 218-222.

[21] L. S. Tam, B. Tomlinson, T. T. Chu, T. K. Li and E. K. Li, "Impact of TNF Inhibition on Insulin Resistance and Lipids Levels in Patients with Rheumatoid Arthritis," *Clinical Rheumatology*, Vol. 26, No. 9, 2007, pp. 1495-1498. doi:10.1007/s10067-007-0539-8

List of Abbreviations

ACR—American college of rheumatology
RA—Rheumatoid arthritis
TNF—Tumor necrosis factor
DMARD—Disease-modifying anti-rheumatic drugs

HOMA—Homeostasis Model Assessment
QUICKI—Insulin Sensitivity Check Index
DAS 28—Disease activity score 28
BMI—Body mass index

11

Septic Arthritis: A Need to Strengthen the Referral Chain in a Developing Economy

Ikpeme A. Ikpeme[1], Ngim E. Ngim[1], Anthonia A. Ikpeme[2], Afiong O. Oku[3]

[1]Department of Surgery, University of Calabar Teaching Hospital, Calabar, Nigeria; [2]Department of Radiology, University of Calabar Teaching Hospital, Calabar, Nigeria; [3]Department of Community Medicine, University of Calabar Teaching Hospital, Calabar, Nigeria.
Email: iaikpeme@yahoo.com

ABSTRACT

Aim: This retrospective analysis documents the features and factors that potentially affect outcomes in septic arthritis in the Cross River Basin area of south-south Nigeria. Patients and Methods: A retrospective analysis of 43 patients who presented with septic arthritis in 45 joints between September 2007 and August 2010. All patients with pain, fever, joint swelling and non-weight bearing/refusal to move the limb and had a joint aspiration productive of a turbid and/or purulent aspirate were included in the analysis. Patients whose joint aspiration produced frank blood or a clear exudate were excluded. Results: There were 24 males and 19 females (M:F = 1.3:1). Forty patients were children while three were adults. Thirty-three patients were urban dwellers, 8 were semi-urban dwellers and 2 were rural dwellers. Twenty-five children were first seen by a Paediatrician. Only 5 patients were first seen by an Orthopaedic surgeon. Definitive treatment was conservative in 28 children and arthrotomy/washout in 12 children and 3 adults. *Staphylococcus aureus* was the commonest isolated pathogen in both age groups. Conclusion: Injudicious interventions in musculoskeletal conditions consist not only of traditional bone setting and other unorthodox practices, but also sub-optimal orthodox medical practices. Healthcare outcomes in Africa are a function of the skewed distribution of the healthcare workforce and a weak referral chain. The near absence of follow-up culture underscores the need for education on injudicious antibiotic therapy to be directed at patients and physicians. Judicious interventions in musculoskeletal sepsis at first contact and a strengthening of the referral chain are important.

Keywords: Septic Arthritis; Health Seeking Contact; Definitive Treatment; South-South Nigeria

1. Introduction

Pyogenic joint infections are surgical emergencies [1]. Being a commoner in children, the risk of rapid joint destruction, irreversible impairment of joint function and fatality, especially in neonates, underscores the need for prompt diagnosis and appropriate treatment. Permanent skeletal deformity can be a sequel of septic arthritis and in developing countries, septic arthritis can be a disabling and life threatening disease [1]. As with other orthopaedic conditions, late presentation, injudicious intervention by traditional bone setters and illiteracy are well documented factors that influence treatment outcomes for orthopaedic ailments in the developing world [2,3]. In the developed world, favorable long term outcomes are not uncommon in septic arthritis [1].

Previous Nigerian studies have documented the aetiology, presentation and outcome of this disease [1,4-6]. Studies also identify the paucity of African data in this condition [3,4,6]. The large joints including the hip, knee and shoulder are the most commonly affected and the disease is commoner in males. Although *Staphylococcus aureus* is the commonest identified organism [1,4-6], coliforms follow closely in a Nigerian local study [4]. Joint trauma has been identified as a possible predisposeing factor [1,3].

The burden of musculoskeletal sepsis in the developing world is enormous. The high incidence of complications because of late presentation and injudicious treatment of these conditions have also been documented [3]. These poor outcomes have been attributed to inadequate healthcare workforce distributions in Africa which ensure that these patients present first to general practitioners, paediatricians, herbalists, traditional bonesetters and surgeons without orthopaedic training [3]. Recent reports are now beginning to challenge the role of distance, poverty, lack of maternal education and care from traditional healers as the only significant underlying factors for late presentation and poor long term outcomes in Africa [3,7,8]. This is because in musculoskeletal septic conditions, inappropriate early antibiotic management or incorrect primary diagnoses are documented causes of late presentation with attendant poor long term outcomes in Africa [3]. The fact that orthopaedic surgeons or doctors with orthopaedic training are usually the last in the chain to see these patients may contribute significantly to late presentation and poor long term outcome.

Most episodes of acute septic arthritis result from haematogenous seeding of the vascular synovial membrane during a bacteraemia. Other routes of infection are direct inoculation and extension from a contiguous focus. *Staphylococcus aureus* is the most common cause of septic arthritis in Europe and all non-gonococcal septic arthritis in the United States [9]. Streptococcus species are the next most common isolates while Gram negative bacilli account for 10 - 20% cases. Patients with a history of intravenous drug abuse, immunocompromise or in the extremes of age have a higher prevalence of Gram negative infections. Polymicrobial infections occur in approximately 10% of patients with non gonococcal septic arthritis [9-11]. Historically, *Haemophilus influenzae*, *Staphylococcus aureus* and group A *Streptococci* were the commonest aetiologic organisms in children below the age of 2 years. However, the overall incidence of *Haemophilus influenzae* is decreasing because of the availability of *Haemophilus influenzae* type b (Hib) vaccine now being given to children [9].

The pathogenesis of septic arthritis is multifactorial and dependent on the interaction of the host immune response and bacterial adherence factors, toxins and immunoavoidance mechanisms. The synovial membrane is devoid of a limiting basement plate under the well vascularized synovium. This allows easy haemotogenous permeation of bacteria. Once bacteria are seeded in the joint space from any route of infection, low fluid shear properties encourage bacterial adherence and infection. In a joint that has undergone recent injury, the production of host derived extracellular matrix proteins like fibronectin which help in joint healing may promote bacterial adhesion and infection. *Staphylococcus aureus*, *Streptococcus spp* and *Neisseria gonorrhea* have a high selectivity for the synovium, probably as a result of adherence characteristics and toxin elaboration. The major determinants of establishing infection are the virulence and tropism of microorganisms combined with the resistance or susceptibility of the synovium.

An increasing body of evidence supports the importance of staphylococcal surface components as virulence determinants by mediating initial colonization. These receptors, termed microbial surface components recognizing adhesive matrix molecules (MSCRAMMs) adhere to host proteins in the joint extracellular matrix, and to implanted medical devices. Some of the host matrix proteins include fibronectin, laminin, elastin, collagen and hyaluronic acid. A number of studies show that mutations in bacterial surface receptors strongly reduce the ability of staphylococci to produce infection [12-15]. However, the role of collagen adhesion of staph aureus as a major virulence factor has been questioned since 30 - 60% of clinical isolates display neither collagen binding *in vitro* or the cna-encoded collagen adhesion [16]. Sequel to adherence, bacteria are internalized by host mechanisms involving membrane pseudopod formation or receptor-mediated endocytosis. These occur through the actions of host cytoskeletal rearrangements via microfilament activity. Once internalized, staphylococci may induce apoptosis via a host capase-dependent mechanism or survive intracellularly [17-20]. Induced apoptosis exacerbates the host cell damage in septic arthritis. Staphylococci may utilize invasion as an immunoavoidance technique and escape clearance by the immune system and antimicrobial therapy by persisting in host cells [9, 21,22].

The host immune response following colonization and proliferation of bacteria is an acute inflammatory response with elaboration of cytokines [interleukin 1-β (IL-1β) and interleukin-6(1L-6)] into the joint fluid by synovial cells. These cytokines activate the release of acute phase proteins like c-reactive protein from the liver which promote opsonization and complement activation. Bacterial phagocytosis by macrophages, synoviocytes and polymorphonuclear cells leads to the release of tumour alpha necrosis factor, interleukin-8 and granulocyte macrophage colony-stimulating factor. Nitric oxide is also required and 1L-1β and 1L-6 levels increase. T-cell mediated and humoral immune responses also play a role in bacterial clearance or pathogenesis of septic arthritis. When the host response fails to contain the infection quickly, the potent activation of the immune response leads to joint destruction mediated by high levels of cytokines and reactive oxygen species. Host matrix metalloproteinases, lysosomal enzymes and bacterial toxins damage the joint structures. Bacterial toxins include alpha-hemolysin, leukocyte-specific gamma toxin, *Staph aureus* leukocidin, bacterial superantigens and enterotoxins. Capsular polysaccharide also interferes with opsonization and phagocytosis [9].

The clinical manifestations of septic arthritis include fever and malaise, as well as pain, swelling, warmth and decreased range of movement in the involved joint. A detailed history is useful with attention to risk factors such as extremes of age, degenerative joint disease, rheumatoid arthritis, and corticosteroid therapy. Diabetes mellitus, intravenous drug abuse, immunosuppressive conditions like HIV, surgeries, renal disease, leukaemia and sepsis/infections in other sites are other risk factors. The Kocher diagnostic criteria for the paediatric septic hip is based on 4 parameters which help differentiate septic arthritis from transient synovitis in children. These are non-weight-bearing on affected side, erythrocyte sedimentation rate (ESR) greater than 40 mm/hr, fever > 38.5°C and a White Blood Cell (WBC) count greater than 12,000/mm³. The probability that the patient has septic arthritis is 99% when all 4 criteria are met, 93% when 3 criteria are present, 40% when 2 criteria are met and 3% when only one criteria is met. If none is met, the probability of septic arthritis is less than 0.2% [23-25]. To improve diagnostic accuracy, other researchers have added to Kocher's criteria a c-reactive protein > 200 mg/l or a history of a previous healthcare visit [26,27]. Ultimately, the diagnosis of septic arthritis is dependent on isolation of organism(s) from aspirated joint fluid.

Acute septic arthritis is a medical emergency with potential for significant morbidity and mortality. Prompt recognition coupled with rapid and appropriate treatments are pre-requisites for a good prognosis [28]. The treatment options include appropriate antimicrobial therapy and joint drainage. The initial antibiotic therapy is based on Gram Stain, joint fluid analysis, a good history and the mode of presentation. Generally, initial antimicrobials should be broad spectrum and are adjusted, if required based on the culture and sensitivity results. Few controlled studies assess the optimal duration, dose or route of administration of antibiotics [29]. Generally however, most antibiotics achieve excellent concentrations in joint fluid following the parenteral or oral routes, and the usual duration of therapy is 2 weeks for *Haemophillus influenza* and *Streptococcal* infections and 3 weeks for infections due to *Staphylococcus aureus* or the Gramnegative bacilli. The choice of antibiotic therapy in the elderly must be carefully made. These individuals have decreased organ reserve capacity, altered hepatic and renal capacity to handle medications, polypharmacy with associated drug-drug and drug-disease interactions [9]. Antibiotic loading and maintenance doses are estimated by measuring serum peak and trough concentrations after the 4th dose in the elderly.

Infection is a function of the interplay of such factors as host resistance, bacterial dose and virulence. In the developing world with the attendant malnutrition, more children are prone to infections [3]. A high index of suspicion is therefore required and it is important that clinicians bear the possibility in mind when evaluating the irritable or lethargic child. Ultrasonography is non-invasive and is becoming relatively common in urban and sub-urban areas of the developing world. In settings where this investigation is unavailable, arthrocentesis is simple to perform and the fluid sample can be easily assessed for colour, consistency, volume and Gram stain. These should make early diagnosis and appropriate therapy possible. In addition to early antibiotic display, the surgical options for treatment of septic arthritis include needle aspiration, tidal irrigation, arthroscopy and arthrotomy. These can be graded based on invasiveness, cost and effectiveness in the thoroughness of drainage [9]. The need for judicious intervention in this condition has to be understood by physicians especially in our setting where patients are easily lost to follow up and long term outcomes following sub-optimal interventions are difficult to document. Recurrent needle aspirations combined with antibiotics have been used to treat septic arthritis [9]. However, permanent joint damage is established after 5 days of infection [9,25] and there is insufficient evidence to recommend repeated aspirations as routine practice [25]. Tidal irrigation is as effective as Arthroscopy and may be useful when multiple joint aspiration yields fluid with different characteristics, an indication of loculation of pus in different pockets within the joint. Arthroscopic lavage has the advantage of offering extensive debridement with a small incision and is useful in deep joints like the hip. When less invasive options are unavailable or fail, when the patient presents after 3 - 4 days, in the presence of osteomyelitis, when the infective organism thrives in low oxygen tensions and require aminoglycosides for treatment, open arthrotomy is indicated [9]. Other indications are the need for urgent decompression because of neuropathy and compromised vascularization, pre-existing joint damage and when the affected joints are inaccessible by less invasive means. Open arthrotomy in all cases of hip and most cases of knee and shoulder sepsis remains a major therapeutic option among Orthopaedic surgeons [25].

This study will document the features and factors that can influence outcomes in this condition in the Cross River Basin area of South-South Nigeria. It will also document the eventual treatment offered patients even when they presented in the hospital first.

2. Patients & Methods

A retrospective analysis of forty-three (43) patients who presented to the University of Calabar Teaching Hospital, Nigeria, with septic arthritis in 45 joints between September, 2007 and August, 2010. Patients' case folders, radiological and microbiological laboratory records were retrieved and information obtained included age, sex, symptoms and duration before presentation, initial health facility used by the patient, and co-morbid factors.

Other information retrieved included place of abode of the patients, which health professional saw first, final treatment option, microbiological flora as well as the use of imaging studies in the diagnosis. Information obtained was analysed using SPSS version 16. Frequency tables and simple proportions were generated. This retrospective analysis was approved by the Ethics committee.

Inclusion Criteria

Patients who presented with joint pain, swelling, fever, non weight bearing or refusal to allow joint movement, and whose joint aspirates yielded cloudy or purulent material were included in this analysis. Those patients with the above clinical features but whose joint aspirate yield clear fluid or frank blood were excluded.

3. Results

There were forty-five (45) joints with septic arthritis in forty-three (43) patients during the period under review. There were 40 children (aged below 18 years) and 3 adults. Among the children, 24 (60%) were males and 16 (40%) were females giving a male: Female ratio of 1.5:1. All the adults in this series were females. The median age of the children was 22.5 months (interquartile range 22.5 months). Thirty-one (31) children (77.5%) and two (2) adults (66.6%) were urban-dwellers respectively, seven

children (17.5%) and one adult (33.3%) were semi-urban dwellers and two children (5%) were from rural communities (**Table 1**). Trauma, sickle cell anaemia and sepsis were significant co-morbid factors accounting for 15% each for trauma and sickle cell anaemia, and 12.5% for sepsis in children (**Table 2**). Fever, joint swelling, pain and non-weight bearing on the affected limb were the presenting clinical features with a median duration of 7 days in both age groups (**Figure 1**). The knee was the most commonly affected joint in children (60%) and adults (66.7%) with the left knee predominating in both age groups (37.5%, children and 66.7%, adults) (**Figure 2**). In terms of health seeking behavior, 22 children and one adult (62.5% and 33.3% respectively presented first to a hospital, 7 children (17.5%) and 2 adults (66.7%) tried self medication or a spiritual healer first before seeking hospital care and 3 children each (7.5% each) were first seen by either a Pharmacist or a traditional bone setter (**Table 3**). Twenty-five children (62.5%) were first seen by a Paediatrician, 3 (7.5%) by an Orthopaedic surgeon and 4 (10%) by a General duty doctor. Two of the adults were first seen by an Orthopaedic surgeon. The definitive treatment options were antibiotics alone in 28 children (70%) and arthrotomy and washout in 12 children (30%). All adults had arthrotomy and washout probably because they were all eventually seen by an Orthopaedic surgeon (**Table 4**). Nineteen (19) patients (44.2%) did not have a microbiological and sensitivity assay done owing to a

Table 1. Demographic characteristics of patients.

Characteristics	Children (n = 40) N (%)	Adults (n = 3)	N (%)
Age group (months)		Age (years)	
<12	12(30.0)		
12 - 24	10(25.0)	≤35	1(33.3)
25 - 36	2(5.0)	>35	2(66.7)
37 - 48	3(7.5)		
49 - 60	1(2.5)		
>60	12(30.0)		
Total	**40(100)**		**3(100)**
Sex		**Sex**	
Male	24(60.0)	Male	0(0)
Female	16(40.0)	Female	3(100)
Total	**40(100)**		**3(100)**
Habitation		**Habitation**	
Urban	31(77.5)	Urban	2(66.7)
Semi-urban	7(17.5)	Semi-urban	1(33.3)
Rural	2(5.0)	Rural	-
Total	**40(100)**		**3(100)**

The median age of children = 22.5 months (Interquartile range = 87).

Table 2. Co-morbid factors.

Co-morbid factors	Children (n = 40) n (%)	Adults (n = 3) n (%)
Trauma	6(15.0)	1(33.3)
Sickle cell anaemia	6(15.0)	-
Sepsis	5(12.5)	-
None	23(57.5)	2(66.7)
Total	**40(100.0)**	**3(100.0)**

Table 3. Health seeking behaviour.

	Children (n = 40) N (%)	Adults (n = 3) N (%)
First health seeking behavior		
Hospital	22(62.5)	1(33.3)
Self medication/spiritual healer	7(17.5)	2(66.7)
Chemist	5(12.5)	0(0)
Pharmacy	3(7.5)	0(0)
Traditional Bonesetter	3(7.5)	0(0)
Total	**40(100)**	**3(100)**

Table 4. Treatment Intervention.

	Children (n = 40) n (%)	Adults (n = 3) n (%)
Medical doctor who saw first		
Paediatrician	25(62.5)	0(0)
Orthopaedic surgeon	3(7.5)	2(66.7)
General duty doctor	4(10.0)	1(33.3)
Others[*]	8(20.0)	0(0.0)
Total	**40(100.0)**	**3(100.0)**
Definitive treatment option		
Conservative (Antibiotics alone)	28(70.0)	0(0)
Arthrotomy and washout	12(30.0)	3(100.0)
Total	**40(100)**	**3(100)**

[*]Others: Patent medicine vendors, Traditional bone setters, Spiritual healers.

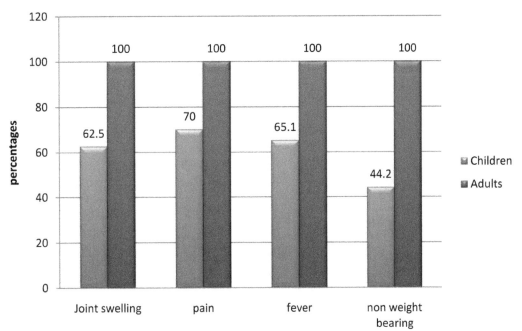

Median duration of joint swelling = 7 days (IQ range = 10); Median duration of fever = 7 days (IQ range = 8); Median duration of pain = 7 days (IQ range = 11); Median duration of loss of function = 7 days (IQ range = 11).

Figure 1. Clinical symptoms.

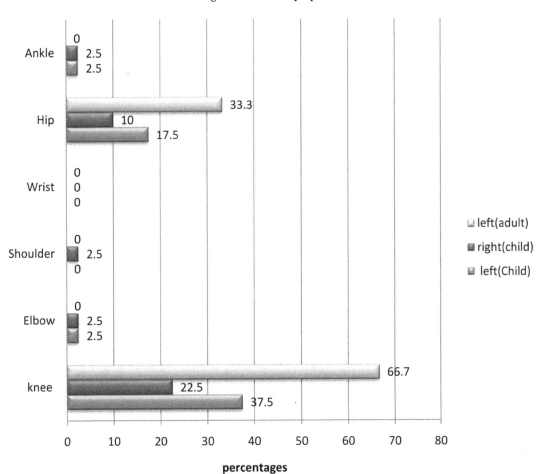

Figure 2. Sites of involvement.

variety of factors including poverty and faulty equipment. Among those who had a microbiological and sensitivity assay performed, *Staphylococcus aureus* was the most common pathogen (25%), followed by *Enterobacteriacae* and *Pseudomonas auroginosa* (5% each). Four specimens (10%) grew no isolates.

3. Discussion

Pyogenic arthritis is an emergency where prompt diagnosis, rapid and aggressive antimicrobial therapy, arthrotomy and washout are critical to ensuring good prognosis [1,9]. Whereas the pathogenesis is multifactorrial and diagnosis based on isolation of bacterial species from synovial fluid, there is a major role for clinical history, physical signs of inflammation, infection, laboratory features, and imaging studies [9]. The condition is managed in conjunction with an Orthopaedic surgeon [25].

The findings in this study agree with other studies that *Staphylococcus aureus* is the commonest causative organism [1,10,30,31], and the knee joint is the commonest affected joint [1,10,12]. Our findings also agree with other reports from Nigeria which identified trauma and sickle cell disease as significant co-morbid factors and a male preponderance [1,4,5], but differs from a South-Western Nigerian study which identified the upper limb joints as being the most commonly affected joints in children below the age of one year [1]. In our study, the knee joint remained the commonest affected joint in this age group (11 cases, 27.5%). Traditional massage practices may account for this difference.

The South-Western Nigerian study reported that inadequate antibiotic therapy occurred in 64.1% of their patients and concluded that patient education on early presentation, avoidance of improper use of antibiotics and regular follow up after acute pathology should be encouraged[1]. In our study, twenty-five children (62.5%) saw a Paediatrician first but only 12 (30%) out of 40 children had arthrotomy and washout combined with antibiotics. Education on the avoidance of improper antibiotic use may therefore need to be directed at patients and physicians as well. Considering the near absent tradition of follow-up in our setting [1,4,8], it will be difficult to assess the degree of disability that may attend a significant proportion of those patients who had conservative treatment without joint lavage. Antibiotic treatment alone is insufficient for established septic arthritis [32].

Studies from Africa commonly identify late presentation and injudicious health-seeking behavior as underlying factors in inappropriate treatment and potential poor outcomes [1,3,8,26,28]. This study however shows that a total of 23 patients (53.5%) sought healthcare in a hospital first. However, only 12 children and all 3 adults saw an orthopaedic surgeon either at their first visit or subsequently. Among those who were eventually referred to the orthopaedic surgeons the average interval between when the patients were seen by a paediatrician or general duty doctor and when they were referred was 4 days (96 hours). This may strengthen the argument that healthcare outcomes in Africa are a factor of the skewed distribution of the healthcare workforce and weak referral systems which may be significant determinants of poor outcomes in musculoskeletal disease in Africa [3].

Permanent destruction of intra-articular cartilage and sub-chondral bone loss begins within 24 hours and can be established by 3 days in septic arthritis [9,33]. A South African study has shown that patients with septic arthritis who had arthrotomy within 5 days of onset of symptoms had good long term prognosis while those who had arthrotomy after 5 days had poor long term prognosis [25,28]. Articular destruction results from a combination of high levels of cytokines, reactive oxygen species, release of lysosomal enzymes and bacterial toxins [33]. The early occurrence of cartilage and joint damage underscores the need for early and judicious intervention to reduce microbial load by joint lavage and reduce the potential risk for articular destruction. In this report, 30% of children had arthrotomy and joint lavage despite 62.5% seeking hospital care as the first health-seeking behavior. The remaining children received only antibiotics and were discharged. Although all the patients who had arthrotomy and joint washout combined with antibiotics in this study had a satisfactory outcome 12 weeks post operatively, a previous Nigerian study had reported poor outcomes in 47.1% of patients with septic arthritis of the hip [34]. Lack of adequate follow-up in our setting inhibits an objective evaluation of long-term outcomes, especially in the 70% of children who only received antibiotics without joint lavage. The combination of skewed healthcare workforce distributions, late presentation (median duration of symptoms of 7 days in this study) and a poor culture of follow-up strengthen the argument for judicious and often "radical" interventions in musculoskeletal septic diseases at first contact in the developing world [3,7,35]. This, and the strengthening of the referral chain must be the take home lesson for physicians working in these regions. A simple set of standard operating protocols that insist that all patients with septic arthritis must benefit from Orthopaedic review is an essential first step in these settings.

4. Conclusion

This study shows that despite a significant number of patients with septic arthritis presenting first to a hospital, the median duration of symptoms was prolonged and only a small proportion presented to an Orthopaedic surgeon. While patient education remains crucial, physicians also need to be targeted to address the issues of judicious interventions and strengthening of the referral chain. Continuing medical education must seek to draw attention to the issues of intra-professional communication and practices that promote poor outcomes in the developing world. This is especially critical in those regions where the patient's attitude to long term follow-up is poor. Simple practices like standard operating protocols that insist on minimum standards of care and referrals can have a dramatic impact on long term outcomes in this condition.

REFERENCES

[1] J. D. Ogunlusi, O. O. Ogunlusi, L. M. Oginni and J. A. Olowookere, "Septic Arthritis in a Nigerian Tertiary Hospital," *Iowa Orthopaedic Journal*, Vol. 26, 2006, pp. 45-47.

[2] I. A. Ikpeme, A. M. Udosen and I. Okereke-Okpa, "Patients' Perception of Traditional Bone Setting in Calabar," *Port Harcourt Medical Journal*, Vol. 1, No. 2, 2007, pp. 104-108.

[3] M. Segbefia and A. Howard, "Acute Septic Arthritis and Osteomyelitis in Children—An African Perspective," 2013. http://ptolemy.library.utoronto.ca/sites/default/files/review/2010/February-Acuteseptic Arthritis and Osteomyelitis.pdf

[4] G. O. Eyichukwu, "Outcome of Management of Non-Gonococcal Septic Arthritis at National Orthopaedic Hospital, Enugu, Nigeria," *Nigerian Medical Journal*, Vol. 19, No. 1, 2010, pp. 69-76.

[5] A. L. Akinyoola, P. O. Obiajunwa, L. M. Oginni, "Septic Arthritis in Children," *West African Journal of Medicine*, Vol. 25, No. 2, 2006, pp. 119-123.

[6] G. O. Onyemelukwe and R. D. Sturrock, "Septic Arthritis in Northern Nigeria," *Rheumatology*, Vol. 18, No. 1, 1979, pp. 13-17.

[7] M. Mijiyawa, O. Oniankitan, K. Attoh-Mensah, A. Tékou, E. K. Lawson, G. B. Priuli and J. K. Assimadi, "Musculoskeletal Conditions in Children Attending Two Togolese Hospitals," *Rheumatology*, Vol. 38 No. 10, 1999, pp. 1010-1013. doi:10.1093/rheumatology/38.10.1010

[8] N. Eke, "Late Presentation Begs for a Solution," *Port Harcourt Medical Journal*, Vol. 1, No. 2, 2007, p. 75.

[9] M. E. Shirtlift and J. T. Mader, "Acute Septic Arthritis," *Clinical Microbiology Reviews*, Vol. 15, No. 4, 2002, pp. 527-544.

[10] D. S. Morgan, D. Fisher, A. Merianos and B. J. Currie, "An 18-Year Clinical Review of Septic Arthritis from Tropical Australia," *Epidemiology & Infection*, Vol. 117, No. 3, 1996, pp. 423-428. doi:10.1017/S0950268800059070

[11] L. Le Dantec, F. Maury, R. M. Flipo, S. Laskri, B. Corlet, B. Duquesnoy and B. Delcambre, "Peripheral Septic Ar-

thritis. A Study of One Hundred and Seventy-Nine Cases," *Revue du rhumatisme (English Edition)*, Vol. 63, No. 2, 1996, pp. 103-110.

[12] I. M. Nilsson, J. M. Patti, T. Bremell, M. Hook and A. Tarwoski, "Vaccination with a Recombinant Fragment of Collagen Adhesin Provides Protection against Staphylococcus Aureus Mediated Septic Death," *Journal of Clinical Investigation*, Vol. 101, No. 12, 1998, pp. 2640-2649. doi:10.1172/JCI1823

[13] A. H. Patel, P. Nowlan, E. D. Weavers and T. Foster, "Virulence of Protein A-Deficient and alpha-Toxin-Deficient Mutants of *Staphylococcus aureus* Isolated by Allele Replacement," *Infection and Immunity*, Vol. 5, No. 12, 1987, pp. 3103-3110.

[14] S. J. Peacock, N. P. Day, M. G. Thomas, A. R. Berendt and T. J. Foster, "Clinical Isolates of *Staphylococcus aureus* Exhibit Diversity in Fnb Genes and Adhesion to Human Fibronectin," *Journal of Infection*, Vol. 41, No. 1, 2000, pp. 23-31. doi:10.1053/jinf.2000.0657

[15] L. M. Switalski, J. M. Patti, W. Butcher, A. G. Gristina, P. Speziale and M. Hook, "A Collagen Receptor on *Staphylococcus aureus* Strains Isolated from Patients with Septic Arthritis Mediates Adhesion to Cartilage," *Molecular Microbiology*, Vol. 7, No. 1, 1993. pp. 99-107. doi:10.1111/j.1365-2958.1993.tb01101.x

[16] M. G. Thomas, S. Peacock, S. Daenke and A. R. Berendt, "Adhesion of *Staphylococcus aureus* to Collagen Is Not a Major Virulence Determinant for Septic Arthritis, Osteomyelitis or Endocarditis," *The Journal of Infectious Diseases*, Vol. 179, No. 1, 1999, pp. 291-293. doi:10.1086/314576

[17] J. K. Ellington, S. S. Reilly, W. K. Ramp, M. S. Smeltzer, J. F. Kellam and M. C. Hudson, "Mechanisms of *Staphylococcus aureus* Invasion of Cultured Osteoblasts," *Microbial Pathogenesis*, Vol. 26, No. 6, 1999, pp. 317-323. doi:10.1006/mpat.1999.0272

[18] A. Lammers, P. J. Nuÿten and H. E. Smith, "The Fibronectin Binding Properties of *Staphylococcus aureus* Are Required for Adhesion to and Invasion of Bovine Mammary Gland Cells," *FEMS Microbiology Letters*, Vol. 180, No. 1, 1999, pp. 103-109. doi:10.1111/j.1574-6968.1999.tb08783.x

[19] B. E. Menzies and I. Kourteva, "Internalization of *Staphylococcus aureus* by Endothial Cells Induces Apoptosis," *Infection and Immunity*, Vol. 66, No. 12, 1998, pp. 5994-1998.

[20] C. A. Wesson, J. Deringer, L. E. Liou, K. W. Bayles, G. A. Bohach and W. R. Trumble, "Apoptosis Induced by *Staphylococcus aureus* in Epithelial Cells Utilizes a Mechanism Involving Caspases 8 and 3," *Infection and Immunity*, Vol. 68, No. 5, 2000, pp. 2998-3001. doi:10.1128/IAI.68.5.2998-3001.2000

[21] S. S. Reilly, M. C. Hudson, J. F. Kellam and W. K. Ramp, "*In Vivo* Internalization of *Staphylococcus aureus* by Embryonic Chick Osteoblasts," *Bone*, Vol. 26, No. 1, 2000, pp. 63-70. doi:10.1016/S8756-3282(99)00239-2

[22] H. D. Gresham, J. H. Lowrance, T. E. Caver, B. S. Wilson, A. L. Cleung and F. P. Lindberg, "Survival of Sta-

phylococcus aureus inside Neutrophils Contributes to Infection," *The Journal of Immunology*, Vol. 164, No. 7, 2000, pp. 3713-3722.

[23] M. S. Kocher, D. Zurakowski and J. R. KAsser, "Differentiating between Septic Arthritis and Transient Synovitis of the Hip in Children; an Evidence-Based Clinical Prediction Algorithm," *The Journal of Bone & Joint Surgery*, Vol. 81, No. 12, 1999, pp. 1662-1670.

[24] M. S. Kocher, R. Mandiga, D. Zurakowski, C. Barnwoh and J. R. Kasser, "Validation of a Clinical Prediction Rule for the Differentation between Septic Arthritis and Transient Synovitis of the Hip in Children," *The Journal of Bone & Joint Surgery*, Vol. 86, No. 8, 2004, pp. 1629-1635.

[25] A. Howard and M. Wilson, "Easily Missed? Septic Arthritis in Children," *BMJ*, Vol. 341, 2010, Article ID: c4407. doi:10.1136/bmj.c4407

[26] S. J. Luhmann, A. Jones, M. Schootman, J. E. Gordon, P. L. Schoeneker and J. D. Luhmann, "Differentiation between Septic Arthritis and Transient Synovitis of the Hip in Children with Clinical Prediction Algorithms," *The Journal of Bone & Joint Surgery*, Vol. 86, No. 5, 2004, pp. 956-962.

[27] M. S. Caird, J. M. Flynn, Y. L. Leung, J. E. Millman, J. G. D'Italia and J. P. Dormans, "Factors Distinguishing Septic Arthritis from Transient Synovitis of the Hip in Children. A Prospective Study," *The Journal of Bone & Joint Surgery*, Vol. 88, No. 6, 2006, pp. 1251-1257. doi:10.2106/JBJS.E.00216

[28] T. R. Nunn, W. Y. Cheung and P. D. Rollinson, "A Prospective Study of Pyogenic Sepsis of the Hip in Childhood," *The Journal of Bone & Joint Surgery*, Vol. 89, No.

1, 2007, pp. 100-106. doi:10.1302/0301-620X.89B1.17940

[29] J. Black, T. L. Hunt, P. J. Godley and E. Mathew, "Oral Antimicrobial Therapy for Adults with Osteomyelitis or Septic Arthritis," *The Journal of Infectious Diseases*, Vol. 155, No. 5, 1987, pp. 968-972. doi:10.1093/infdis/155.5.968

[30] M. Razak and J. Nasiruddin, "An Epidemiological Study of Septic Arthritis in Kuala Lumpur Hospital," *Medical Journal of Malaysia*, Vol. 53, Suppl. A, 1998, pp. 86-94.

[31] A. K. Shetty and A. Gedalia, "Management of Septic Arthritis," *Indian Journal of Pediatrics*, Vol. 71, No. 9, 2004, pp. 819-824. doi:10.1007/BF02730722

[32] P. Riegels-Nielsen, N. Frimodt-Moller, M. Sorensen and J. S. Jensen, "Antibiotic Treatment Insufficient for Established Septic Arthritis. *Staphylococcus aureus* Experiments in Rabbits," *Acta Orthopaedica Scandinavica*, Vol. 60, No. 1, 1989, pp. 113-115. doi:10.3109/17453678909150107

[33] S. Roy and J. Bhawan, "Ultrastructure of Articular Cartilage in Pyogenic Arthritis," *Archives of Pathology*, Vol. 99, No. 1, 1975, pp. 44-47.

[34] A. L. Akinyola, P. O. Obiajunwa, L. M. Oginni and S. I. I. Adeoye, "Septic Arthritis of the Hip in Nigerian Children," *African Journal of Paediatric Surgery*, Vol. 1, No. 2, 2005, pp. 56-61.

[35] I. A. Ikpeme, A. M. Udosen, A. A. Ikpeme, G. U. Inah and Q. N. Kalu, "Early Outcome of Treatment of Chronic Osteomyelitis Using the Improvised Irrigation and Drainage System for the Lautenbach Procedure," *International Journal of Tropical Surgery*, Vol. 3, No. 3, 2009, pp. 110-115.

12

Validation of Reference Genes for mRNA Quantification in Adjuvant Arthritis

Muhammad Ayaz Alam Qureshi[1], Aisha Siddiqah Ahmed[2], Jian Li[1], André Stark[3], Per Eriksson[4], Mahmood Ahmed[5*]

[1]Department of Molecular Medicine and Surgery, Karolinska University Hospital, Karolinska Institutet, Stockholm, Sweden; [2]Department of Clinical Neurosciences, Karolinska Institutet, Stockholm, Sweden; [3]Department of Clinical Sciences, Danderyd Hospital, Karolinska Institutet, Stockholm, Sweden; [4]Department of Medicine, Karolinska University Hospital, Karolinska Institutet, Stockholm, Sweden; [5]Department of Neurobiology, Care Sciences and Society, Karolinska Institutet, Stockholm, Sweden.
Email: *mahmood.ahmed@ki.se

ABSTRACT

Real time quantitative PCR (RT-qPCR) requires a method to normalize the expression of target genes against an endogenous reference gene. It is known that commonly used housekeeping genes (HKGs) vary tremendously in inflammatory conditions; however information about the stability and expression of HKGs in chronic inflammatory joint disease such as rheumatoid arthritis (RA) is scarce. The expressional stability of 10 commonly used HKGs was analyzed in the neuronal (spinal cord, dorsal root ganglia) and in the musculoskeletal tissues (tendon, muscle, epiphysis, capsule, periosteum and ankle joint) using RT-qPCR in the rat model of RA. In individual tissues, suitable HKGs were selected by $|\Delta Ct|$ ($|$ Ct control − Ct arthritis $|$) and further analyzed by using software programs; geNorm and normfinder. We found hypoxanthine-guanine phosphoribosyl tranferase (HPRT) as the most stable gene except ankle joint while glyceraldehyde-3-phosphate dehydrogenase (GAPDH) was found as the least stable gene in musculoskeletal tissues. In inflamed ankle joint where no reference gene was found to be stably expressed, an inflammatory cell marker CD3 was used to normalize peptidylprolyl isomerase B (PPIB), the most homogenous HKG identified among the 10 HKGs. The normalized PPIB was then used to analyze the gene expression of neurokinin 1 (NK1), receptor of substance P, a potent pro-inflammatory mediator. We observed a 3.5 fold increase (p = 0.009) in NK1 expression in inflamed ankle joint compared to control. Our results indicate that reference genes stability should be evaluated before using them as reference during inflammatory conditions. In tissues with intense inflammatory cell infiltration, an inflammatory cell marker should be used to normalize the selected reference gene to avoid erroneous results.

Keywords: Quantitative PCR; Adjuvant Arthritis; Housekeeping Gene

1. Introduction

Real time quantitative PCR (RT-qPCR) is a sensitive and reproducible method for the estimation and comparative analysis of mRNA expression [1]. However, it requires a method to normalize the expression of target genes against an endogenous reference or housekeeping gene (HKG) to see the difference in RNA concentration. A prerequisite for a gene to serve as endogenous reference is that its expression level should not vary in different tissue types and under various experimental conditions. Several structural and metabolic genes have been used as internal controls; however, none of them seems to be identified as universally accepted endogenous control. Previous studies indicate that most commonly used HKGs *i.e.*, glyceraldehyde-3-phosphate dehydrogenase

(*GAPDH*) and beta-actin (*ACTB*) show considerable variation between tissues as well as in different experimental conditions [2]. It has been reported that expression levels of both *GAPDH* and *ACTB* were unstable in pancreatic islet grafts [3], colonic cancerous tissues [4], asthmatic airways [5] and T-lymphocytes [6]. Little information is available about the expression of HKGs in chronic inflammatory joint diseases such as rheumatoid arthritis (RA). RA is a chronic immune-mediated disease marked by inflammation in synovium of joint and destruction of cartilage and bone. It seems reasonable to speculate that inflammatory cell infiltration can cause huge differences in the level of expression of HKGs genes leading to erroneous results. Thus, appropriate validation of HKGs is a crucial step in inflammatory conditions.

Currently many methods are used for the selection of stable and reliable HKGs [7,8]. One software-based ap-

*Corresponding author.

proach, developed by Vandesompele *et al.* [9] involves normalization of more than one housekeeping gene by using an algorithm based computer program, geNorm. GeNorm performs a pairwise comparison of candidate HKGs and ranks the potential reference genes according to their gene expression stability. Other software-based approaches include Excel-based BestKeeper [10], and normfinder [11]. Normfinder calculates a stability value based on the combined estimate of both intra- and inter-group values and further determines the optimal reference gene among the HKGs. For the selection of most stable HKGs during inflammatory conditions we used constant amount of RNA and HKGs were selected by comparing Ct values and further analyzed by using ge-Norm and normfinder software.

A number of animal models closely resembling the clinical and pathological picture of RA are being used to study the mechanisms of pain, inflammation and joint destruction as well as to identify better pharmacological tools to treat RA. Adjuvant arthritis (AA) is a commonly used animal model of RA with several clinical and pathological similarities regarding inflammation, pain, synovial hyperplasia, and joint destruction [12]. It has been implicated that the neuropeptide substance P (SP) is involved in the modulation of inflammation and pain through its receptor neurokinin 1 (NK1) in inflammatory joint disorders such as RA and AA [13]. However, to our knowledge, no study has evaluated HKGs for mRNA quantification in arthritic conditions. The aim of this study was to evaluate and to validate HKGs for a reliable mRNA quantification using RT-qPCR in AA.

2. Materials and Methods

The study included a total of 12 female Sprague Dawley rats (bw 230 - 250 g). The rats were housed 4/cage at 21°C in a 12-hour light/dark cycle with pellets and water ad lib according to the Karolinska Institute protocol. The study was approved by the Ethical Committee of Stockholm North.

2.1. Induction of Arthritis

Arthritis was induced in 6 rats by intradermal injections of a suspension (0.05 ml) of heat-killed *Mycobacterium-butyricum* in paraffin oil (10 mg/ml) into the base of the tail (day 0) under 3% - 5% isoflurane anaesthesia [14]. An additional 6 rats received 0.05 ml of paraffin oil and served as control group. In rats inoculated with *Mycobacterium butyrcium*, signs of inflammation including bilateral paw swelling, redness and warmth were observed on days 12 - 14 and sustained later on. Rats were sacrificed on day 15.

2.2. Tissue Collection and RNA Extraction

Rats were anaesthetised with sodium pentobarbitone (60 mg/kg, intraperitoneally) and decapitated. The lumbar

spinal cord, dorsal root ganglia (L2 - L6), ankle joint, achilles tendon, calf muscle, tibial epiphysis, knee joint capsule and periosteum were dissected and immediately frozen in liquid nitrogen. Frozen tissues were homogenized by Mikro-dismembrator S (B. Braun Biotech International), at 2600 rpm/min for 30 seconds and dissolved in 2 - 3 volumes of Trizol reagent (Invitrogen life technologies Inc., USA). RNA was then extracted and further purified using the RNeasy® MiniKit (Qiagen, USA) following the manufacturers protocol. Spectrophotometric analysis of the sample consistently showed absorption ratio (OD) $OD_{260 nm}/OD_{280 nm} = 1.8 - 2.2$ indicating excellent purity of the ribonucleic acids.

2.3. Real-Time Quantitative RT-PCR

Total RNA (1 μg) was reverse transcribed to cDNA with random hexamer primers using 1st strand cDNA Synthesis Kit for RT-PCR (Roche, Germany). For quantification cDNAs were diluted to 100 μl. A volume of 3 μl of individual cDNA for each HKG was used for real time RT-PCR with TaqMan 1X Universal PCR Master Mix (Applied Biosystems, Roche, Germany). Assay on Demand Kits containing corresponding primers and probes from Applied Biosystems were used. The 10 HKGs (**Table 1**) were evaluated as internal controls to normalize for RNA loading on ABI Prism 7700 Sequence Detection System. In addition, primers of NK1 (Rn00562004_m1) and CD3 (Rn00596773_m1) were run in the inflamed ankle joints. Data were collected in real-time during the elongation step of each cycle. Each cDNA sample was analyzed in duplicate. A standard curve was established using dilutions of cDNA from the spinal cord. Control with no template was included in each experiment. The standard curve was calculated by plotting the threshold cycle (Ct value) against the log nanograms of total RNA added to the reverse transcription reaction. The data acquired from each sample assayed was analysed for the stability of HKGs.

2.4. HKG Stability Analysis

Initially $|\Delta Ct| \pm$ SEM was calculated for each HKG in the spinal cord (SC), dorsal root ganglia (DRG), ankle joint, muscle, tendon, capsule, periosteum and epiphysis as the difference of Ct values obtained in the control and arthritic rats. The Ct is defined as the number of cycles needed for the fluorescence to reach a specific threshold level of detection and is inversely correlated with the amount of template present in the reaction. Ideally, a good reference gene should have ΔCt close to zero reflecting no change during pathological conditions. HKGs with $|\Delta Ct| > 1$ were excluded for further analysis considering unstable genes. The relative stability of selected reference genes was then calculated using geNorm [9] and Normfinder [11], two Excel-based software programs in each tissue. GeNorm ranked all HKGs according to their stability by average expression stability (M) which was derived by pairwise exclusion of unstable genes to find the best pair of HKGs and further calculates pair-wise variation value V for each HKG compared to all other HKGs. Normfinder ranked HKGs by calculating the stability values on the basis of inter-and intra-group variations. An arbitrary cut-off value of 0.4 for geNorm and normfinder was used. All HKGs with the stability values more than the cut-off values were considered unstable with both programs.

2.5. Statistics

All calculations were carried out using statview program. Differences in Ct values are shown as $|\Delta Ct| \pm$ SEM and RT-qPCR data is expressed as mean $\pm$ SD. The comparison between the groups was performed by using unpaired Student t-test. Significance level was set at $p \leq 0.01$.

3. Results

3.1. Analysis of HKG Stability

$|\Delta Ct| \pm$ SEM method. 10 HKGs were run in the neuronal (SC, DRG) and in the musculoskeletal tissues

(tendon, muscle, epiphysis, capsule, periosteum and ankle joint) from the control and arthritic rats (**Table 1**). A difference in Ct values ($|\Delta Ct|$) was calculated in the normal and arthritic tissues for all HKGs [15]. All HKGs with $|\Delta Ct| > 1$ were excluded for further analysis in the tissues analysed. Thus, 18S was excluded in DRG, *B2M* in muscle, *GAPDH* and *UCE* in capsule, *GAPDH* in epiphysis and *GUSB*, *PPIB*, *ACTB* and *ARBP* in periosteum (**Table 2**). No stable HKG was identified in the inflamed ankle joint according to the $|\Delta Ct|$ criteria. We observed minimal SEM in all tissues indicating a low biological and methodological variation.

GeNorm analysis. The HKGs selected on the basis of $|\Delta Ct|$ criteria were further analyzed by geNorm software program in the control and arthritic tissues. All HKGs with M value below the cut-off level of 0.4 were considered as stable while HKGs with M > 0.4 suggested unstable HKGs [16]. Based on the expressional stability (M), HKGs were ranked (**Table 3(a)**). Additionally, pairwise variation analysis (V) with default value 0.15 helped to choose the optimum number of HKGs for the calculation of normalization factor (NF) in each tissue. Using geNorm program, we identified *PPIB/GAPDH* as the most stable HKG pair in SC, *ARBP/GAPDH* in DRG, *ACTB/B2M* in tendon, *ACTB/PPIB* in muscle and capsule, *PPIB/ARBP* in epiphysis and *HPRT/B2M* in periosteum

Table 1. Housekeeping genes evaluated in the study.

Symbol	Name	Function	TaqMan Assay ID	Accession No.
ACTB	Beta-actin	Cytoskeletal structural protein	Rn00667869_ml	NM_031144.2
ACTG	Gama-actin	Cytoskeletal structural protein	Rn00563662_ml	NM_012893.1
B2M	Beta-2 microglubulin	Beta chain of major histocompatibility complex class 1 molecule	Rn00560865_ml	NM_012512.1
GAPDH	Glyceraldehyde-3-phosphate dehydrogenase	Oxidoreductase in glycolysis and gluconeogenesis	Rn99999916_sl	NM_017008.3
PPIB	Peptidylprolyl isomerase B (Cyclophilin B)	Immunosuppressant soluble cytosolic receptor	Rn00574762_ml	NM_022536.1
ARBP	Acidic ribosomal protein	Member of ribosomal protein	Rn00821065_gl	NM_022402.1
HPRT	Hypoxanthine-guanine phosphoribosyl tranferase	Purine synthesis in salvage pathway	Rn01527838_gl	NM_012583.2
GUSB	Glucoronidase beta	Lysosmal enzyme to degrade β-D-glucoronides	Rn00566655_ml	NM_017015.2
UCE	Ubiquitin conjugating enzyme	Enzyme in ubiquitin-proteasome pathway	Rn00732991_ml	NM_031138.2
18S	18s ribosomal RNA	Highly conserved RNA molecule in ribosome structure in eukaryote	Hs99999901_sl	X03205.1

Table 2. Difference in Ct values ($|\Delta Ct|$) in the spinal cord, dorsal root ganglia (DRG), tendon, muscle, epiphysis, capsule, periosteum and ankle joint of arthritis and control rats. HKGs are ranked from most stable to least stable. Values are expressed as $|\Delta Ct| \pm$ SEM. Boldface indicates genes removed for analysis by geNorm and normfinder. For details, see Materials and Results. n = 6 in each group.

Spinal cord	GUSB	GAPDH	18S	PPIB	B2M	ACTB	ARBP	UCE	HPRT	ACTG
	0.02 ± 0.07	0.02 ± 0.07	0.03 ± 0.09	0.15 ± 0.13	0.07 ± 0.06	0.11 ± 0.06	0.12 ± 0.07	0.36 ± 0.08	0.42 ± 0.11	0.47 ± 0.14
DRG	ARBP	HPRT	PPIB	UCE	GAPDH	GUSB	ACTG	B2M	ACTB	**18S**
	0.03 ± 0.11	0.07 ± 0.11	0.02 ± 0.06	0.17 ± 0.08	0.19 ± 0.07	0.21 ± 0.08	0.44 ± 0.26	0.58 ± 0.11	0.58 ± 0.12	1.04 ± 0.17
Tendon	ARBP	ACTB	HPRT	UCE	18S	B2M	ACTG	GAPDH	GUSB	PPIB
	0.26 ± 0.08	0.32 ± 0.13	0.36 ± 0.10	0.51 ± 0.16	0.55 ± 0.10	0.56 ± 0.12	0.78 ± 0.17	0.81 ± 0.23	0.86 ± 0.17	0.93 ± 0.17
Muscle	ACTG	18S	ARBP	ACTB	PPIB	GAPDH	HPRT	UCE	GUSB	**B2M**
	0.07 ± 0.14	0.08 ± 0.07	0.40 ± 0.09	0.51 ± 0.12	0.59 ± 0.13	0.60 ± 0.11	0.62 ± 0.11	0.76 ± 0.14	0.86 ± 0.25	1.40 ± 0.27
Epiphysis	B2M	UCE	HPRT	ACTG	ACTB	GUSB	18S	ARBP	PPIB	**GAPDH**
	0.00 ± 0.08	0.07 ± 0.13	0.09 ± 0.12	0.31 ± 0.20	0.32 ± 0.09	0.54 ± 0.10	0.56 ± 0.10	0.58 ± 0.12	0.59 ± 0.11	1.28 ± 0.20
Capsule	ARBP	B2M	18S	HPRT	GUSB	ACTB	PPIB	ACTG	UCE	**GAPDH**
	0.13 ± 0.10	0.13 ± 0.10	0.19 ± 0.09	0.19 ± 0.14	0.38 ± 0.11	0.53 ± 0.14	0.84 ± 0.17	0.90 ± 0.23	1.04 ± 0.23	1.23 ± 0.30
Periosteum	GAPDH	ACTG	HPRT	UCE	18S	B2M	**ARBP**	**ACTB**	**PPIB**	**GUSB**
	0.24 ± 0.15	0.28 ± 0.31	0.36 ± 0.10	0.37 ± 0.09	0.46 ± 0.10	0.77 ± 0.14	1.14 ± 0.18	1.21 ± 0.22	1.42 ± 0.25	1.77 ± 0.30
Ankle joint	**B2M**	**GUSB**	**18S**	**GAPDH**	**HPRT**	**UCE**	**ARBP**	**ACTB**	**ACTG**	**PPIB**
	1.27 ± 0.22	1.42 ± 0.26	1.79 ± 0.28	1.89 ± 0.33	2.00 ± 0.34	2.05 ± 0.34	2.39 ± 0.38	2.44 ± 0.39	2.46 ± 0.41	3.63 ± 0.58

Table 3. The expressional stability of housekeeping genes calculated by geNorm (a) and normfinder (b). Genes are ranked from most stable to least stable (top to bottom) in the spinal cord, dorsal root ganglia (DRG), tendon, muscle, epiphysis, capsule, periosteum and in ankle joint.

(a)

Spinal cord	M	DRG	M	Tendon	M	Muscle	M	Epiphysis	M	Capsule	M	Periosteum	M
HKG		HKG		HKGs		HKGs		HKG		HKG		HKG	
PPIB	0.11	ARBP	0.16	B2M	0.20	ACTB	0.15	PPIB	0.17	ACTB	0.16	HPRT	0.32
GAPDH	0.11	GAPDH	0.16	ACTB	0.20	PPIB	0.15	ARBP	0.17	PPIB	0.16	B2M	0.32
ARBP	0.14	HPRT	0.21	ARBP	0.26	ARBP	0.20	GUSB	0.19	GUSB	0.19	UCE	0.37
GUSB	0.16	PPIB	0.21	HPRT	0.27	HPRT	0.23	ACTB	0.21	B2M	0.26	18S	0.39
B2M	0.17	ACTB	0.23	PPIB	0.30	UCE	0.27	B2M	0.26	HPRT	0.30	GAPDH	0.44
ACTB	0.18	UCE	0.26	18S	0.31	18S	0.34	HPRT	0.29	ARBP	0.32	ACTG	0.67
UCE	0.20	GUSB	0.29	GUSB	0.34	GAPDH	0.44	UCE	0.32	18S	0.34		
18S	0.23	B2M	0.31	ACTG	0.40	ACTG	0.50	18S	0.34	ACTG	0.46		
HPRT	0.25	ACTG	0.48	UCE	0.49	GUSB	0.58	ACTG	0.39				
ACTG	0.28			GAPDH	0.60								

(b)

Spinal cord	M	DRG	M	Tendon	M	Muscle	M	Epiphysis	M	Capsule	M	Periosteum	M
HKG		HKG		HKGs		HKGs		HKG		HKG		HKG	
ARBP	0.00	HPRT	0.02	B2M	0.18	HPRT	0.05	PPIB	0.07	ACTB	0.04	HPRT	0.02
ACTB	0.01	PPIB	0.02	PPIB	0.19	ACTB	0.05	18S	0.09	PPIB	0.05	B2M	0.03
UCE	0.01	ACTB	0.03	18S	0.23	PPIB	0.06	ACTB	0.11	B2M	0.05	18S	0.04
HPRT	0.01	ARBP	0.03	ACTB	0.23	18S	0.11	ARBP	0.11	GUSB	0.08	UCE	0.06
GUSB	0.01	GAPDH	0.03	ARBP	0.24	ARBP	0.14	B2M	0.12	HPRT	0.09	ACTG	0.69
PPIB	0.01	UCE	0.03	HPRT	0.25	ACTG	0.18	UCE	0.13	18S	0.10	GAPDH	1.01
B2M	0.02	GUSB	0.04	GUSB	0.25	UCE	0.51	ACTG	0.13	ARBP	0.11		
ACTG	0.02	B2M	0.08	UCE	0.36	GUSB	0.53	HPRT	0.14	ACTG	0.32		
18S	0.04	ACTG	0.11	GAPDH	0.43	GAPDH	0.75	GUSB	0.34				
GAPDH	0.25			ACTG	1.89								

(**Table 4**). Pairwise variation analysis (Vn/n + 1) further indicated that inclusion of an additional gene in a selected pair of HKGs did not increase the stability of NF and accuracy of results in any of the tissues (**Figure 1**).

Normfinder analysis. The stability of HKGs in the control and arthritic tissues was further analyzed by Norm-Finder. Normfinder strengthened and further evaluated the best HKG in a group of HKGs selected by thege-Norm (**Table 3(b)**). When ranking the top candidate HKG previously selected by geNorm, the normfinder identified *ACTB* as more stable gene than *B2M* in tendon (stability value = 0.18 compared to 0.23), in epiphysis *PPIB* was selected over *ARBP* (stability value = 0.07 compared to 0.11), *ACTB* over *PPIB* in capsule (stability value = 0.04 compared to 0.05) and *HPRT* (stability value = 0.02) was selected as more reliable gene compared to *B2M* (stability value = 0.03) in periosteum. However, in the neuronal tissues (SC and DRG) as well as in muscle, normfinder selected different HKGs as selected by the geNorm although in the same stability range. Thus, in the SC, *ARBP* (stability value = 0.14) was selected as the most stable HKG. In DRG and muscle, *HPRT* was selected as the most stable HKG with stability value equal to 0.05 and 0.06 respectively. In muscle, the most stable pair of HKGs as selected by geNorm was *ACTB/PPIB*. Correspondingly, normfinder ranked *ACTB* as second and *PPIB* as third best gene with stability value equal to 0.05 for *ACTB* and 0.06 for *PPIB* compared to 0.05 for *HPRT* (**Table 4**).

3.2. Stability of HKG

Our results showed *HPRT* as the most stable HKG in all studied tissues except the inflamed ankle joint. GeNorm calculated the stability value (M) for *HPRT* ranging from 0.21 to 0.32 while normfinder showed stability value between 0.01 to 0.25, all below the arbitrary cut-off value of 0.4. On the other hand, by using all three analyses *GAPDH* was identified as the most unstable HKG in peripheral tissues in arthritic rats. Thus, Capsule, epiphysis and ankle joint had $|\Delta Ct| > 1$ and equal to 1.23, 1.28 and 1.89, respectively for *GAPDH* (**Table 2**). GeNorm calculated M for as 0.44 in muscle, 0.44 in periosteum and 0.60 in tendon. Furthermore, normfinder analyzed M equal to 0.43 in tendon, 0.75 in muscle and 1.01 in the periosteum, all above the arbitrary cut-off value of 0.4 (**Tables 3(a)** and **(b)**).

3.3. Selection of HKG in Ankle Joint

According to $|\Delta Ct|$ analysis (see Methods) all HKGs showed significant variations in the inflamed compared to normal ankle joint. Thus, $|\Delta Ct| > 1$ in the inflamed ankle joint for all the HKGs ranged from 1.27 for *B2M* to 3.63 for *PPIB* (**Table 2**). Considering the variability of

HKGs expression in the ankle joint as a result of severe inflammation, the expression of CD3, a T-lymphocyte marker was analyzed [17]. We observed an up-regulation of CD3 expression in the inflamed ankle joint with $|\Delta Ct| = 3.31 \pm 0.56$. Subsequent normalization of all HKGs with CD3 resulted in the differences in control and arthritis ankle joint ranging from 16.7% for *PPIB* to 79.4% for *B2M*. All the HKGs showed significant differences except *PPIB* and *ACTG* (**Figure 2**). The difference between the normal and inflamed ankle joints was 40.2% when *ACTG* normalized with CD was used but interestingly did not reach the level of significance (p = 0.07). The same difference for *PPIB* was 16.7% suggesting *PPIB* be the most homogenous HKG when normalized with CD3 (p = 0.6) (**Figure 2**). Therefore CD3-normalized *PPIB* (*PPIB*/CD3) was selected to analyse the gene expression of NK1 in inflamed ankle joint.

Table 4. Housekeeping genes selected by geNorm and Normfinder in the spinal cord, dorsal root ganglia (DRG), tendon, muscle, epiphysis, capsule and in periosteum of arthritis and control rats.

Tissue	geNorm	Normfinder
Spinal cord	*PPIB/GAPDH*	*ARBP*
DRG	*ARBP/GAPDH*	*HPRT*
Tendon	*ACTB/B2M*	*ACTB*
Muscle	*ACTB/PPIB*	*HPRT*
Epiphysis	*PPIB/ARBP*	*PPIB*
Capsule	*ACTB/PPIB*	*ACTB*
Periosteum	*HPRT/B2M*	*HPRT*

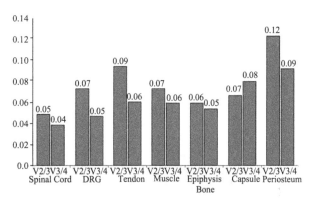

Figure 1. The optimum number of reference genes selected by the geNorm software. Variation analysis of the top four candidate HKGs in each tissue based on pairwise variation (Vn/n + 1) analysis. A value of V below the default value (V < 0.15) indicates no effect on increased stability by the inc- lusion of an additional HKG.

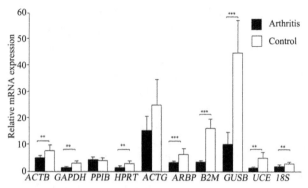

Figure 2. Variation in housekeeping genes expression in ankle joints of arthritis and control rats after CD3 normalization. Results are expressed as mean ± SD. $^{**}p \leq 0.005$ and $^{***}p \leq 0.0005$, comparison of arthritis and control groups (unpaired students t-test). n = 6 rats in each group.

3.4. Evaluation of CD3-Normalized HKG in Ankle Joint

Following the identification of *PPIB*/CD3 as the most stable HKG, it was tested as an internal control in inflamed ankle joint. Previous reports have shown increased expression of NK1 in inflamed tissues [13,18]. Consequently, we normalized NK1 expression in the control and inflamed ankle joints both with the non-normalized and CD3-normalized *PPIB* expression. We observed a down-regulation of NK1 expression by 3.2 fold (p = 0.06), when non-normalized *PPIB* was used, whereas an up-regulation of NK1 expression by 3.5 fold (p = 0.009) was demonstrated after normalizing *PPIB* with CD3 which was comparable with the results when NK1 data was analyzed without using any HKG (5.5 fold increase, p < 0.0001) (**Figure 3**).

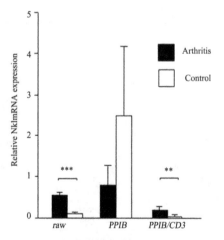

Figure 3. Non-normalized (raw), *PPIB* normalized and *PPIB*/CD3 normalized relative NK1 mRNA expression in the ankle joints of arthritis and control rats. Results are expressed as mean ± SD. $^{**}p \leq 0.005$ and $^{***}p \leq 0.0005$, comparison of arthritis and control groups (unpaired students t-test). n = 6 rats in each group.

4. Discussion

This study clearly highlights the importance of HKGs validation for analysis by RT-qPCR. Our results showed that the most stable HKG or the geometric mean of two most stable HKGs should be used as internal control to normalize genes of interest. We have demonstrated that most commonly used HKG, *GAPDH* is not stably expressed and therefore not suitable for normalization in peripheral tissues during inflammatory conditions. Moreover, our study indicates that in heavily inflamed tissues, normalization of HKGs, by an inflammatory cell marker, can be employed as an additional strategy.

To study the effects of inflammation on the expression of commonly used HKGs, we used adjuvant arthritis rat model which closely resemble the clinical, pathological and etiological picture of RA. Like RA, there is bilateral symmetrical involvement of peripheral joints where an intense inflammatory cell infiltration is identified in the hypertrophied synovium leading to cartilage and subchondral bone destruction. The pathological changes are not only confined to ankle joints but also observed in the draining lymph nodes, spleen, lever and the neuronal tissues like dorsal root ganglia and spinal cord.

It is known that for a reliable mRNA quantification, a stable internal control gene is a prerequisite which should express an inherent stability regardless of the experimental conditions. A number of studies have shown that the expression of commonly used HKGs vary not only between the different tissues in normal condition but also in pathological tissues [2-6]. Consistent with these observations, our present study reports that during peripheral inflammation, most of the commonly used reference genes are up-regulated in the peripheral and neuronal tissues. In the inflamed ankle joints with intense inflammatory cells infiltration, none of the ten HKGs used in this study was found to be expressed in a stable manner. It is known that inflammation not only change the phenotype of pro-inflammatory mediators like cytokines and neuropeptides but also trigger an increased expression of inflammatory mediators in the target organs. Thus, in adjuvant arthritis we have previously shown an increased expression of substance P and calcitonin gene-related peptide, the known pro-inflammatory neuropeptides, in the inflamed ankle joints as well as their increased synthesis in the corresponding dorsal root ganglia [19]. It is reasonable to speculate that the inflammatory reaction in the ankle joint and other tissues in adjuvant arthritis change the gene expression of neuropeptides but also the HKGs observed in this study.

Present study clearly demonstrates the importance of employing multiple approaches to select the reliable and stable HKG/s to detect the difference in target genes in conditions like adjuvant arthritis. A number of commonly used HKGs should be included and tested in individual tissues before a suitable HKG is selected for comparative analysis using RT-qPCR. Furthermore, the available methodologies like $|\Delta Ct|$, geNorm and norm-finders are recommended to utilize to further refine the selection of HKGs in order to avoid erroneous results. In the present study of adjuvant arthritis where inflammation affects all the analyzed tissues, application of $|\Delta Ct|$ method identifies and discards 8 out of 10 HKGs not suitable to be used as reference genes in DRG (*18S*), muscle (*B2M*), capsule (*GAPDH/UCE*), epiphysis (*GAPDH*) and periosteum (*GUSB/PPIB/ACTB/ARBP*). None of the 10 HKGs was found stable in inflamed ankle joints by this method. We then select the stable HKGs based on $|\Delta Ct|$ criteria in individual tissues and further analyzed by geNorm and normfinder. Using geNorm program, we identified 6 different pairs of HKGs suitable to be used as reference genes in spinal cord (*PPIB/GAPDH*), DRG (*ARBP/GAPDH*), tendon (*ACTB/B2M*), muscle/capsule (*ACTB/PPIB*), epiphysis (*PPIB/ARBP*) and periosteum (*HPRT/B2M*) but could not identify a common pair of HKGs to be used in all the tissues again highlighting the importance of testing a number of HKGs in individual pathological tissues. The results also indicate that adding a third HKG to a selected pain does not increase the stability and sensitivity of the pair. Also, geNorm program fails to identify a pair of stable HKGs in the inflamed ankle joints.

We then apply the normfinder program to further refine and select the best HKG in a pair of HKGs as selected by geNorm in individual tissues. Comparing the results of both programs, it is interesting to find that the top ranked HKGs more or less retain their positions in most of the peripheral tissues studied. It is safe to say that the reproducibility of the results obtained by the two methods reflects the inherent stability of the selected reference genes in a particular tissue. However, in spinal cord, DRG and muscle, minor differences were observed in the ranking of HKGs between the geNorm and normfinder methods, although the differences between the selected HKGs were in the acceptable range. Similar discrepancies have been reported earlier and our results are in line with previous reports [8,20]. It is assumed that minimal differences within the calculation algorithms of each applet may cause the observed differences in the ranking positions [8,20,21], probably due to the reason that the two programs use different methods for calculations. GeNorm calculates the stability value M on the basis of geometric mean expression levels. This program is not designed to choose a single gene rather it selects the best pair of HKG based on pairwise analysis. The principle is that the expression ratio of two ideal HKGs is identical in each experimental condition. Variations in expression ratio in tested HKGs can be due to the variation in one or both genes. Normfinder on the other hand,

is a more model-based program that calculates stability value based on inter-group and intra-group variations and chooses single best HKGs.

It has been reported that *GAPDH* is one of the most commonly used HKG even though several reports indicated that *GAPDH* is not stable in different tissues and during different experimental conditions [7,22,23]. Our results based on 3 different methods to select a stable HKG among 10 HKGs confirm that *GAPDH* is not suitable to be used as a reference gene to normalize the target gene expression in inflammatory tissues and can lead to totally misleading results. In our experiments, *HPRT* was the only HKG which was consistently ranked as a stable HKG in all the inflammatory tissues except ankle joint.

We were unable to identify any stable HKG among the ten commonly used HKGs in the inflamed ankle joint. We observed a significant up regulation of all HKGs in the ankle joint during inflammation compared to normal ankle joint. This change in the expression of HKGs is probably due to the reason that there is intense infiltration of various inflammatory cells in the ankle joint compared to other tissues in AA. The synovium of ankle joint in AA like RA transforms from relatively few cellular structure into a hyperplastic invasive tissue teeming with immunocompetent cells like lymphocytes, NK-cells, neutrophils and macrophages etc. T-lymphocyte is the most abundant and important cell present in the inflamed synovium which participate in the induction and maintenance of disease process. CD3 is a well known cell marker for T-lymphocyte.

In the present study, a significant up regulation of CD3 expression was demonstrated along with similar increased expression of HKGs in the inflamed ankle joint. It is clear that increased CD3 expression is due to intense inflammatory cell infiltration in inflamed ankle joint and we believe the same reason behind the increased expression of all the tested HKGs making them unstable to be used as reference genes. When all the HKGs were normalized with CD3 to remove the effects of inflammatory cells on HKGs, PPIB was found to be the least effected HKG. When normalized and non-normalized *PPIB* with CD3 was used to study the change in the expression of NK1, a receptor of pro inflammatory neuropeptide SP, opposite results were seen. A down regulation of NK1 expression was demonstrated when non-normalized *PPIB* was used and an expected significant up regulation of NK1 was observed with CD3 normalized. An increased expression of NK1 was also seen in the inflamed joint when no HKG (raw data) was used. Tricarico *et al.* encountered the similar problems when they could not identify appropriate HKGs in human breast tissue biopsies [23]. They suggested normalization of target genes with total RNA concentration as an acceptable method. Other suggested strategies are the measurements of sample volume, genomic DNA or incorporating alien molecules [24].

5. Conclusion

Thorough investigations of the expression pattern of HKGs should be performed before using them as internal control in inflammatory joint disorders. Furthermore, in tissues with intense inflammatory cell infiltration, an inflammatory cell marker should be used to normalize the selected HKG to avoid erroneous results.

6. Acknowledgements

This study was funded by a grant from Sven Noren Foundation to AS and a grant from Swedish research council (12660) to PE.

REFERENCES

[1] F. Ferre, "Quantitative or Semi-Quantitative PCR: Reality versus Myth," *PCR Methods and Applications*, Vol. 2, No. 1, 1992, pp. 1-9.

[2] T. J. Chang, C. C. Juan, P. H. Yin, C. W. Chi and H. J. Tsay, "Up-Regulation of Beta-Actin, Cyclophilin and GAPDH in N1S1 Rat Hepatoma," *Oncology Reports*, Vol. 5, No. 2, 1998, pp. 469-471.

[3] S. Rodriguez-Mulero and E. Montanya, "Selection of a Suitable Internal Control Gene for Expression Studies in Pancreatic Islet Grafts," *Transplantation*, Vol. 80, No. 5, 2005, pp. 650-652. doi:10.1097/01.tp.0000173790.12227.7b

[4] N. Tsuji, C. Kamagata, M. Furuya, D. Kobayashi, A. Yagihashi, T. Morita, S. Horita and N. Watanabe, "Selection of an Internal Control Gene for Quantitation of mRNA in Colonic Tissues," *Anticancer Research*, Vol. 22, No. 6C, 2002, pp. 4173-4178.

[5] E. M. Glare, M. Divjak, M. J. Bailey and E. H. Walters, "Beta-Actin and GAPDH Housekeeping Gene Expression in Asthmatic Airways Is Variable and Not Suitable for Normalising mRNA Levels," *Thorax*, Vol. 57, No. 9, 2002, pp. 765-770. doi:10.1136/thorax.57.9.765

[6] A. Bas, G. Forsberg, S. Hammarstrom and M. L. Hammarstrom, "Utility of the Housekeeping Genes 18S rRNA, Beta-Actin and Glyceraldehyde-3phosphate-dehydrogenase Fornormalization in Real-Time Quantitative Reverse Transcriptase-Polymerase Chain Reaction Analysis of Gene Expression in Human T lymphocytes," *Scandinavian Journal of Immunology*, Vol. 59, No. 6, 2004, pp. 566-573. doi:10.3171/jns.2004.100.3.0523

[7] M. D. Al-Bader and H. A. Al-Sarraf, "Housekeeping Gene Expression during Fetal Brain Development in the Rat-Validation by Semi-Quantitative RT-PCR," *Developmental Brain Research*, Vol. 156, No. 1, 2005, pp. 38-45. doi:10.1111/j.0300-9475.2004.01440.x

[8] N. Silver, E. Cotroneo, G. Proctor, S. Osailan, K. L. Paterson and G. H. Carpenter, "Selection of Housekeeping Genes for Gene Expression Studies in the Adult Rat Submandibular Gland under Normal, Inflamed, Atrophic and Regenerative States," *BMC Molecular Biology*, Vol. 9, 2008, p. 64. doi:10.1186/1471-2199-9-64

[9] J. Vandesompele, K. De Preter, F. Pattyn, B. Poppe, N. Van Roy, A. De Paepe and F. Speleman, "Accurate Normalization of Real-Time Quantitative RT-PCR Data by Geometric Averaging of Multiple Internal Control Genes," *Genome Biology*, Vol. 3, No. 7, 2002, pp. 1-21.

[10] M. W. Pfaffl, A. Tichopad and C. Prgomet, "Determination of Stable Housekeeping Genes, Differentially Regulated Target Genes and Sample Integrity: BestKeeper-Excel-Based Tool Using Pair-Wise Correlations," *Biotechnology Letters*, Vol. 26, No. 6, 2004, pp. 509-515.

[11] C. L. Andersen, J. L. Jensen and T. F. Orntoft, "Normalization of Real-Time Quantitative Reverse Transcription-PCR Data: A Model-Based Variance Estimation Approach to Identify Genes Suited for Normalization, Applied to Bladder and Colon Cancer Data Sets," *Cancer Research*, Vol. 64, No. 15, 2004, pp. 5245-5250.

[12] P. H. Wooley, "Animal Models of Rheumatoid Arthritis," *Current Opinion in Rheumatology*, Vol. 3, No. 3, 1991, pp. 407-420. doi:10.1097/00002281-199106000-00013

[13] S. M. Carlton and R. E. Coggeshall, "Inflammation-Induced Up-Regulation of Neurokinin 1 Receptors in Rat Glabrous Skin," *Neuroscience Letters*, Vol. 326, No. 1, 2002, pp. 29-32. doi:10.1016/S0304-3940(02)00299-9

[14] C. M. Pearson and F. D. Wood, "Studies of Arthritis and Other Lesions Induced in Rats by the Injection of Mycobacterial Adjuvant. VII. Pathologic Details of the Arthritis and Spondylitis," *American Journal of Pathology*, Vol. 42, No. 1, 1963, pp. 73-95.

[15] A. T. McCurley and G. V. Callard, "Characterization of Housekeeping Genes in Zebrafish: Male-Female Differences and Effects of Tissue Type, Developmental Stage and Chemical Treatment," *BMC Molecular Biology*, Vol. 9, 2008, p. 102. doi:10.1186/1471-2199-9-102

[16] L. J Maccoux, D. N. Clements, F. Salway and P. J. Day, "Identification of New Reference Genes for the Normalisation of Canine Osteoarthritic Joint Tissue Transcripts from Microarray Data," *BMC Molecular Biology*, Vol. 8, 2007, p. 62. doi:10.1186/1471-2199-8-62

[17] Y. Yoshikai, G. Matsuzaki, T. Inoue and K. Nomoto, "An Increase in Number of T-Cell Receptor Gamma/Delta-Bearing T Cells in Athymic Nude Mice Treated with Complete Freund's Adjuvants," *Immunology*, Vol. 70, 1990, pp. 61-65.

[18] M. K. Schafer, D. Nohr, J. E. Krause and E. Weihe, "Inflammation-Induced Upregulation of NK1 Receptor mRNA in Dorsal Horn Neurones," *Neuroreport*, Vol. 4, No. 8, 1993, pp. 1007-1010. doi:10.1097/00001756-199308000-00003

[19] M. Ahmed, A. Bjurholm, M. Schultzberg, E. Theodorsson and A. Kreicbergs, "Increased Levels of Substance P and Calcitonin Gene-Related Peptide in Rat Adjuvant Arthritis. A Combined Immunohistochemical and Radioimmunoassay Analysis," *Arthritis & Rheumatism*, Vol. 38, No. 5, 1995, pp. 699-709.

[20] V. R. Cicinnati, Q. Shen, G. C. Sotiropoulos, A. Radtke,

G. Gerken and S. Beckebaum, "Validation of Putative Reference Genes for Gene Expression Studies in Human Hepatocellular Carcinoma Using Real-Time Quantitative RT-PCR," *BMC Cancer*, Vol. 8, 2008, p. 350. doi:10.1186/1471-2407-8-350

[21] H. Schmid, C. D. Cohen, A. Henger, S. Irrgang, D. Schlondorff and M. Kretzler, "Validation of Endogenous Controls for Gene Expression Analysis in Microdissected Human Renal Biopsies," *Kidney International*, Vol. 64, No. 1, 2003, pp. 356-360. doi:10.1046/j.1523-1755.2003.00074.x

[22] R. D. Barber, D. W. Harmer, R. A. Coleman and B. J. Clark, "GAPDH as a Housekeeping Gene: Analysis of GAPDH mRNA Expression in a Panel of 72 Human Tis-

sues," *Physiological Genomics*, Vol. 21, No. 3, 2005, pp. 389-395. doi:10.1152/physiolgenomics.00025.2005

[23] C. Tricarico, P. Pinzani, S. Bianchi, M. Paglierani, V. Distante, M. Pazzagli, S. A. Bustin and C. Orlando, "Quantitative Real-Time Reverse Transcription Polymerase Chain Reaction: Normalization to rRNA or Single Housekeeping Genes Is Inappropriate for Human Tissue Biopsies," *Analytical Biochemistry*, Vol. 309, No. 2, 2002, pp. 293-300. doi:10.1016/S0003-2697(02)00311-1

[24] J. Huggett, K. Dheda, S. Bustin and A. Zumla, "Real-Time RT-PCR Normalisation; Strategies and Considerations," *Genes and Immunity*, Vol. 6, No. 4, 2005, pp. 279-284. doi:10.1038/sj.gene.6364190

13

Open-Label, Pilot Study of the Safety and Clinical Effects of Rituximab in Patients with Rheumatoid Arthritis-Associated Interstitial Pneumonia

Eric L. Matteson[1,2], Tim Bongartz[1], Jay H. Ryu[3], Cynthia S. Crowson[2], Thomas E. Hartman[4], Paul F. Dellaripa[5]

[1]Division of Rheumatology, Rochester, USA; [2]Department of Health Sciences Research, Rochester, USA; [3]Division of Pulmonary and Critical Care Medicine, Rochester, USA; [4]Department of Radiology, Mayo Clinic College of Medicine, Rochester, USA; [5]Division of Rheumatology, Brigham and Womens Hospital, Boston, USA.
Email: matteson.eric@mayo.edu

ABSTRACT

Objective: To investigate the clinical effect of rituximab (RTX) in the management of progressive rheumatoid arthritis related interstitial lung disease (RA-ILD). **Methods:** A total of 10 patients with progressive RA-ILD were enrolled into this 48-week, open-label treatment study. Treatment was with RTX at 1000 mg at day 1, day 15, and again at weeks 24 and 26, with concomitant methotrexate therapy. **Results:** The study included 4 men and 6 women. Of 7 evaluable patients at week 48, the diffusing capacity to carbon monoxide had worsened by at least 15% in 1 patient, and was stable in 4 patients, and increased by >15% of baseline value in 2 patients. The forced vital capacity declined by at least 10% in 1 patient, was stable in 4 patients, and increased by at least 10% in 2 patients. High resolution computed tomography of the chest showed improvement in 1 patient, and was unchanged in 5. Three patients were withdrawn, one who had an infusion reaction at week 0, one at week 5 who was hospitalized for congestive heart failure at week 5 and who later died at week 32 of complications following a traumatic hip fracture, and one died at week 6 of possible pneumonia. **Conclusions:** In this pilot study of 10 patients with RA-ILD treated with RTX, measures of lung disease remained stable in the majority of study completers. Further research is needed to clarify whether this treatment has a role in management of RA-ILD.

Keywords: Rheumatoid Arthritis; Interstitial Pneumonitis; Rituximab

1. Introduction

Pulmonary involvement is common in patients with rheumatoid arthritis (RA), and clinically overt interstitial lung disease (ILD) is prevalent in about 8% of patients with early RA and 19% of patients with a longer disease duration [1-3]. The 10 year incidence rate of symptomatic pulmonary fibrosis has been described as high as 6% in patients with RA [2,3]. The presence of ILD in RA has a significant adverse impact on mortality [2,4].

To date, no clinical trial has assessed the efficacy of any therapy in RA-ILD. Therapeutic strategies are entirely based on therapeutic recommendations in idiopathic interstitial pneumonias (IIP) [5-7]. In view of some histologic differences between IIPs and their counterparts in RA, there might be important features which could impact on treatment efficacy and prognosis [3]. At the same time, assumptions about effectiveness of diease modifying drugs (DMARDs) on pulmonary disease de-

rived from their impact on joint disease should be treated with caution.

The pathogenesis of RA-ILD is unknown. Other disease related features and smoking are risk factors, and a number of immunologic, cellular and humoral abnormalities have been described in RA-ILD [2,8-10]. Formation of B-cell follicles and germinal centers and the presence of circulating antibodies to lung proteins have been detected in IIP [8]. There may be a significant increase in B-cell numbers in RA-ILD compared to normal lung tissue and IIPs, and there are dense B-cell follicles in the two most common histologic subtypes of RA-ILD, nonspecific interstitial pneumonia (NSIP) and usual interstitial pneumonia (UIP) [9].

These observations provide a rationale for a potential efficacy of B-cell ablative therapies in RA-ILD. The use of a monoclonal antibody directed against CD20, a B-cell surface marker, has already proven effectiveness in the treatment of RA joint disease, but the effect on lung disease has not been evaluated [11]. This study was performed to gain a preliminary assessment of the safety and clinical effect of rituximab, an established therapy for RA, in patients with moderate to severe clinically overt and progressive RA-ILD.

2. Methods

2.1. Patients

The study population consisted of 4 male and 6 female outpatients with RA associated UIP or NSIP, ages 43 to 80 years. All patients met the revised 1987 American College of Rheumatology classification criteria for RA [12]. The study was approved by the Institutional Review Boards of the Mayo Clinic and the Brigham and Women's Hospital, and registered with Clinicaltrials gov. as NCT00578565.

Diagnosis of progressive RA-ILD of UIP or NSIP subtype was based on the following criteria: 1) Clinical symptoms consistent with ILD with onset between 3 months and 36 months prior to screening; 2) Progressive ILD as demonstrated by any one of the following within the past year: >10% decrease in forced vital capacity (FVC), increasing infiltrates on chest radiograph or high resolution computed tomography (HRCT), or worsening dyspnea at rest or on exertion; 3) Diagnosis of UIP or NSIP by either surgical lung biopsy or HRCT showing definite or probable UIP or NSIP; 4) Abnormal pulmonary function results (reduced FVC or decreased diffusing capacity to carbon monoxide (DLco) or impaired gas exchange at rest or with exercise and 5) Insidious onset of otherwise unexplained dyspnea or exertion and bibasilar, inspiratory crackles on auscultation. Only patients with an FVC > 50% of predicted value at screening and DLco > 30% of predicted value at screening were enrolled. No patient had lung biopsy.

Patients were excluded who had clinical features suggesting infection, neoplasm, sarcoidosis, ILD other than UIP or NSIP, other collagen vascular disease, or exposure to known fibrogenic drugs or environmental factors. Other exclusions included FEV1/FVC ratio <0.6 at screening (pre or post-bronchodilator), residual volume > 120% predicted at screening, history of unstable or deteriorating cardiac or neurologic disease, abnormal neurologic examination, history of tuberculosis or test positive for human immunodeficiency virus or hepatitis B or C, pregnancy or lactation, creatinine > 1.5x upper limit of normal, and IgG and IgM levels below lower limit of normal. Treatment exclusions included previous exposure to cyclophosphamide, cyclosporine, interferon gamma or beta, anti-tumor necrosis factor therapy, anti-IL1 therapy or with endothelin receptor blockers within the last 8 weeks. Patients who had previously received rituximab or experimental therapy for RA were also ex-

cluded. No change of DMARD treatment within the last 3 months prior to trial enrollment was allowed.

2.2. Treatment

Rituximab 1000 mg was administered by intravenous (i.v.) infusion on days 1 and 15 with repeat dosing at weeks 24 and 26. All subjects received 100 mg of i.v. methylprednisolone as premedication. Continuation of DMARD treatment and oral prednisone established at least 3 months prior to inclusion at a stable dose was allowed. The use of systemic corticosteroid therapy was permitted up to a dose of 15 mg/day during the study. Administration of higher doses of corticosteroids at the discretion of the patient's primary physician was permitted for a period not to exceed two weeks in the event of a rapid clinical deterioration in clinical status.

2.3. Clinical Assessments

Measures of pulmonary efficacy and function including the FVC, DLco and St. George's respiratory questionnaire were obtained at screening and at weeks 12, 24 and 48 [13]. HRCT was performed at screening and weeks 24 and 48. The HRCTs were independently assessed by a radiologist expert in pulmonary radiology for ILD related changes using a standard scoring system for ground glass attenuation, reticulation, honeycombing, decreased attenuation, centrilobular nodules, other nodules, emphysema and consolidation on a 0 to 4 scale: 0 = no involvement, 1 = 1% - 25% involvement, 2 = 26% - 50% involvement, 3 = 51% - 75% involvement, 4 = 76% - 100% involvement [8]. Health-related quality of life and function were assessed with patient questionnaires, including the Medical Outcomes Study Short Form 36 item instrument (SF-36), the Health Assessment Questionnaire (HAQ), Clinical Disease Activity Index (CDAI) and the 28 joint disease activity score (DAS28).

2.4. Biomarkers

CD19 counts were measured at baseline and 12, 24, 36, and 48 weeks.

2.5. Analytic Approach

The primary endpoint of the study was the safety of rituximab therapy in RA-ILD as assessed through patient history, physical exams and laboratory parameters at 48 weeks. Secondary endpoints were assessment of progression-free survival at 48 weeks. Based on consensus recommendations, progression was defined as: decrease of baseline FVC ≥ 10% (and at least ≥200-ml change), 15% decrease in single-breath DLco or death from progressive lung [7]. Other outcome parameters included radiographic progression over 48 weeks on HRCT, the St. George respiratory questionnaire, quality of life measures Medical Outcomes Study SF-36, HAQ, DAS28 and CDAI.

3. Results

The study included 4 men and 6 women with mean age 64.7 years (range 43 to 80) who had RA (mean duration 13.8 years; range 0.4 to 44) and ILD (mean duration 3.2 years; range 0.0 to 7.5). Rheumatoid factor and/or anti CCP antibody was present in 7/10 patients (pts). UIP was present in 4 patients, and NSIP in 6. Medications at enrollment included prednisone (8 pts), methotrexate (4 pts), and sulfasalazine (1 pt).

Function and activity measures over the course of the study are contained in **Table 1**. Baseline pulmonary function included mean FVC 68% (min: 47%, max: 89%), mean DLco 47.6% (min: 28%, max: 73%), mean FEV1/FVC ratio 86.5 (min: 68.8, max: 101), mean St. George's score 54.7 (min: 4.0, max 92.5; 0 = best, and

100 = worst), Mean SF-36 physical component score was 23.2 (min: 11.4, max: 43.5), and the mean mental component score was 47.8 (min: 32.4, max: 57.3).

Changes in the function and activity measures are contained in **Table 1**. By week 48, the DLco had worsened by at least 15% (at least ≥3 ml/min/mm Hg) in 1 patient, was stable in 4 patients, and increased by >15% of baseline in 2 patients. The FVC declined by at least 10% (and at least ≥200 ml) in 1 patient, was stable in 4 patients, and increased by at least 10% in 2 patients. There was no clinically meaningful change in the St. George's respiratory score. Serial HRCT examinations revealed improvement in 1 patient, and worsening in another patient, with no changes noted on HRCT for the other 5 patients assessed at week 48 (**Table 2**).

Among the 7 patients who reached week 48, 4 had NSIP and 3 had UIP. Of the 3 UIP patents, 1 improved by FVC and DLco and the other 2 remained stable by DLco, FVC and HRCT. Of the 4 NSIP patients, 1 worsened

Table 1. Function and activity measures in patients with rheumatoid arthritis related intersitial pneumonia treated with rituximab.

Measure	Baseline N = 10	Week 12 N = 7	Week 12 change from baseline	Week 24 N = 7	Week 24 change from baseline	Week 48 N = 7	Week 48 change from baseline
FVC, %	68 (47, 89)	80.5 (67, 100)	6.5% (0%, 15%)	76.3 (51, 104)	1.5% (−11%, 20%)	75.3 (50, 102)	2.4% (−12%, 17%)
DLco, %	47.6 (28, 73)	52.4 (35, 70)	−0.5% (−18%, 13%)	53.2 (33, 63)	15.3% (−7%, 54%)	52.0 (30, 75)	11.6% (−22%, 47%)
FEV1/FVC	86.5 (68.8, 101)	88.4 (79.1, 109)	2.4% (−5%, 8%)	91.5 (75.9, 115)	3.4% (−4%, 14%)	88.1 (77, 109)	0% (−10%, 8%)
St. George's score	54.7 (4.0, 92.5)	50.6 (2.3, 85.5)	4.9% (−43%, 62%)	49.5 (5.0, 81.9)	14.4% (−17%, 107%)	51.5 (23.3, 68.5)	81.1% (−33%, 478%)
SF-36 physical component score	23.2 (11.4, 43.5)	26.7 (13.4, 42.7)	8.1% (−33%, 48%)	23.9 (17.5, 40.6)	21.0% (−1%, 54%)	28.0 (19.6, 34.4)	37.0% (−31%, 116%)
SF-36 mental component score	47.8 (32.4, 57.3)	56.9 (47.7, 62.6)	7.3% (−2%, 20%)	50.0 (43.1, 64.3)	−4.3% (−21%, 13%)	54.5 (39.0, 65.1)	9.9% (−10%, 62%)
DAS28 ESR	5.5 (2.2, 7.3)	-	-	4.6 (3.2, 6.8)	−21.3% (−42%, 9%)	3.3 (2.5, 4.4)	−31.8% (−62%, 24%)
CDAI	32.5 (2.9, 54.7)	−9.3, N = 1	−66%, N = 1	18.5 (2.1, 59.4)	−12.4% (−80%, 121%)	10.4 (2.5, 24.6)	−38.5% (−92%, 59%)
HAQ	1.2 (0.25, 2.375)	0.8 (0.125, 1.625)	50.7% (−67%, 200%)	1.0 (0.375, 1.5)	49.1% (−21%, 250%)	1.0 (0.25, 1.5)	85.9% (−80%, 300%)

Values in table are means (minimum, maximum); N = Number, FVC = Forced vital capacity; DLco = Diffusing capacity of carbon monoxide; SF-36 = Medical Outcomes Study Short Form 36; DAS = Disease activity score; ESR = Erythrocyte sedimentation rate; CDAI = Clinical disease activity index; HAQ = Health assessment questionnaire.

Table 2. Finding on high resolution computed tomography of the lungs.

	Prior to base-line (N = 8)	Baseline (N = 10)	Week 24 (N = 7)	Week 48 (N = 7)
Nodular opacities	4	3	1	1
Size ≤ 5 mm	3	1	1	1
6 - 10 mm	0	1	0	0
>10 mm	1	1	0	0
Extent < 10%	3	2	0	0
10% - 40%	1	0	0	0
>40%	0	1	1	1
Irregular linear opacities	7	9	7	7
Extent < 10%	4	4	2	2
10% - 40%	3	5	5	5
>40%	0	0	0	0
Interlobular septa thickening	0	1	1	0
Ground glass infiltrates	5	9	7	6
Extent away from fibrosis 0%	1	5	4	4
<10%	2	2	2	1
10% - 40%	2	2	1	1
>40%	0	0	0	0
Extent in areas of fibrosis 0%	0	3	2	1
<10%	4	3	3	3
10% - 40%	1	3	2	2
>40%	0	0	0	0
Consolidation	0	1	2	1
Emphysema	2	3	2	3
Extent < 10%	2	2	1	2
10% - 40%	0	1	1	1
>40%	0	0	0	0
Honeycombing	2	5	3	3
Extent < 10%	2	5	3	3
10% - 40%	0	0	0	0
>40%	0	0	0	0

Table 3. Individual patient pulmonary data at week 48 for 10 patients with rheumatoid arthritis related interstitial pneumonia disease treated with rituximab.

Parameter	Pt 1 NSIP	Pt 2 NSIP	Pt 3 UIP	Pt 4 UIP	Pt 5 UIP	Pt 6 NSIP	Pt 7 NSIP	Pt 8 NSIP	Pt 9 NSIP	Pt 10 UIP
DLco	S	WD	S	S	D	D	S	W	I	I
FVC	S	WD	S	S	D	D	I	S	W	I
HRCT	S	WD	S	S	D	D	S	I	W	S

I = Improved; S = Stable; W = Worsened; D = Death, and WD = Withdrew from study. For DLco, worsening was defined as decrease of at least 15% and improvement was defined as increase of at least 15%. For FVC, worsening was defined as decrease of at least 10% and improvement was defined as increase of at least 10%. Pt = Patient; FVC = Forced vital capacity; DLco = Diffusing capacity of carbon monoxide; NSIP = Nonspecific interstitial pneumonitis; UIP = Usual interstitial pneumonitis.

by FVC and HRCT but improved by DLco and another worsened by DLco, 1 improved by FVC and 1 remained stable by DLco, FVC and HRCT (**Table 3**).

Although not formally assessed, clinical joint disease activity parameters including the mean DAS28 and CDAI were improved in surviving patients by weeks 24 and 48. Mean Medical Outcomes Study Short Form 36 and Health Assessment Questionnaire scores were globally unchanged by weeks 24 and 48. As expected, CD19 counts dropped dramatically, from normal to zero or near 0 in most patients by week 24, and continued to be low at week 48 (data not shown).

Three patients did not complete the 48 weeks study. One patient had an infusion reaction with the first infusion, and withdrew from the study. One patient was hospitalized for congestive heart failure at week 5, unlikely to be related to study drug, and later died at week 32 of complications following a traumatic hip fracture. Another patient died at week 6 of possible pneumonia and adult respiratory distress syndrome; a causative organism was not recovered.

4. Discussion

The overall research objective of this study was to examine the course of patients with progressive RA-ILD treated with rituximab by evaluation of safety and progression-free survival at 48 weeks following initial treatment. Facing the current lack of clinical trial data in RA-ILD, we expected also to gain important information on the usefulness of potential study endpoints, the magnitude of response that can be expected in a clinical trial of RA-ILD, and potential difficulties that can be associated with a certain trial design and the overall feasibility of a full-scale randomized controlled trial.

In this pilot study of 10 patients with progressive RA-ILD who were treated with conventional doses of rituximab used in the management of RA, there were significant adverse events including two deaths. Given the small number of patients, the relationship of these events to treatment vs. underlying disease is unclear. Of the 7 patients who reached week 48, only 1 could be said to have improved, while 1 worsened and 5 were stable. Although the numbers of patients in the study was small, it could not be determined whether patients with NSIP or UIP were more likely to respond.

As an aim of the study was to determine if use of this therapy would result in improvement, it could be concluded that there was not a signal for clinical efficacy of this treatment for RA IP. However, 5 patients remained stable, which may be of significance since worsening of parameters of lung disease was a requirement for enrollment into the trial. Nevertheless, it cannot be disregarded that three patients did not complete the study, including

two patients who died. Of these noncompleters, the death following the hip fracture was unlikely related to the study drug, and it is uncertain whether the death at week 6 due to possible pneumonia and respiratory distress syndrome was related to the study drug. Pulmonary toxicity to rituximab has been reported principally in patients receiving it for malignancy indications, with isolated cases reported in rheumatoid arthritis [14,15]. In general, the most common presentation is acute/subacute hypoxemic organizing pneumonia starting 2 weeks after the last infusion (often around the 4th cycle when given weekly). Adult respiratory distress syndrome has also been reported, usually within hours after the first infusion [16]. In one survey of 45 patients with presumed rituximab pulmonary injury, 8 patients died [16].

Clearly, further research is needed to clarify whether this treatment has a role in management of RA-ILD in less advanced disease, or in specific histopathologic patterns of disease. This research will necessarily include the development of improved sets of outcomes for evaluation of patients with RA-ILD [14].

5. Author Contributions

All authors were involved in drafting the article or revising it critically for important intellectual content, and all authors approved the final version to be published. Dr. Matteson had full access to all of the data in the study and takes responsibility for the integrity of the data and the accuracy of the data analysis. Study conception and design: Bongartz, Matteson, Ryu. Acquisition of data: Matteson, Bongartz, Dellarippa. Analysis and interpretation of data: Matteson, Bongartz, Dellaripa, Hartman, Ryu, Crowson.

6. Funding

Funding for this project was provided by the Mayo Clinic Foundation, and was supported by NIH/NCRR CTSA Grant Number UL1 RR024150. Its contents are solely the responsibility of the authors and do not necessarily represent the official views of the NIH. The study drug was provided without cost by Genentech, Inc.

7. Acknowledgements

We would like to especially thank our study coordinators Ms. Jane Jaquith and Jade Cumberbatch as well as the staff of the Mayo Clinic Clinical and the Brigham and Women's Hospital Research Units for their time and dedication in facilitating the conduct of this study.

REFERENCES

[1]   C. Turesson, W. M. O'Fallon, C. S. Crowson, S. E.

Gabriel and E. L. Matteson, "Extra-Articular Disease Manifestations in Rheumatoid Arthritis: Incidence Trends and Risk Factors over 46 Years," *Annals of the Rheumatic Diseases*, Vol. 62, No. 8, 2003, pp. 722-727. doi:10.1136/ard.62.8.722

[2] T. Bongartz, C. Nannini, Y. F. Medina-Velasquez, S. J. Achenbach, C. S. Crowson, J. H. Ryu, R. Vassallo, S. E. Gabriel and E. L. Matteson, "Incidence and Mortality of Interstitial Lung Disease in Rheumatoid Arthritis," *Arthritis & Rheumatism*, Vol. 62, No. 5, 2010, pp. 1583-1591. doi:10.1002/art.27405

[3] C. Nannini, J. H. Ryu and E. L. Matteson, "Lung Disease in Rheumatoid Arthritis," *Current Opinion in Rheumatology*, Vol. 20, No. 3, 2008, pp. 340-346.

[4] S. V. Kocheril, B. E. Appleton, E. C. Somers, E. A. Kazerooni, K. R. Flaherty, F. J. Martinez, et al., "Comparison of Disease Progression and Mortality of Connective Tissue Disease-Related Interstitial Lung Disease and Idiopathic Interstitial Pneumonia," *Arthritis & Rheumatism*, Vol. 53, No. 2, 2005, pp. 549-557.

[5] K. Phillips, K. R. Flaherty, E. L. Matteson, T. Bongartz, J. Bathon, K. K. Brown and P. F. Dellaripa, "Interstitial Lung Disease in Rheumatoid Arthritis," *Current Rheumatology Reviews*, Vol. 6, No. 2, 2010, pp. 120-126.

[6] C. Turesson and E. L. Matteson, "Extraarticular Features of Rheumatoid Arthritis and Systemic Involvement," In: M. C. Hochberg, A. J. Silman, J. S. Smolen, M. E. Weinblatt and M. H. Weisman, Eds., *Rheumatology*, 5th Edition, Mosby, Philadelphia, 2011, pp. 839-847.

[7] G. Raghu, H. R. Collard, J. J. Egan, F. J. Martinez, J. Behr, K. K. Brown, et al., "An Official ATS/ERS/JRS/ALAT Statement: Idiopathic Pulmonary Fibrosis: Evidence-Based Guidelines For Diagnosis and Management," *American Journal of Respiratory and Critical Care Medicine*, Vol. 183, No. 7, 2011, pp. 788-782.

[8] W. A. Wallace, S. E. Howie, A. S. Krajewski and D. Lamb, "The Immunological Architecture of B-Lymphocyte Aggregates in Cryptogenic Fibrosing Alveolitis," *Journal of Pathology*, Vol. 178, No. 3, 1996, pp. 323-329.

[9] S. R. Atkins, C. Turesson, J. L. Myers, H. D. Tazelaar, J. H. Ryu, E. L. Matteson, et al., "Morphologic and Quantitative Assessment of CD20+ B Cell Infiltrates in Rheumatoid Arthritis-Associated Nonspecific Interstitial Pneumonia and Usual Interstitial Pneumonia," *Arthritis &*

Rheumatism, Vol. 54, No. 2, 2006, pp. 6635-6641.

[10] C. Turesson, E. L. Matteson, T. V. Colby, Z. Vuk-Pavlovic, R. Vassallo, C. M. Weyand, et al., "Increased CD4+ T cell Infiltrates in Rheumatoid Arthritis-Associated Interstitial Pneumonitis Compared with Idiopathic Interstitial Pneumonitis," *Arthritis & Rheumatism*, Vol. 52, No. 1, 2005, pp. 73-79.

[11] P. Emery, R.Fleischmann, A. Filiowicz-Sosnowska, J. Schechtman, L. Szczepanski, A. Kavanaugh, et al., "The Efficacy and Safety of Rituximab in Patients with Active Rheumatoid Arthritis Despite Methotrexate Treatment: Results of a Phase IIB Randomized, Double-Blind, Placebo-Controlled, Dose-Ranging Trial," *Arthritis & Rheumatism*, Vol. 54, No. 5, 2006, pp. 1390-1400. doi:10.1002/art.21778

[12] F. C. Arnett, S. M. Edworthy, D. A. Bloch, D. J. McShane, J. F. Fries, N. S. Cooper, et al., "The American Rheumatism Association 1987 Revised Criteria for the Classification of Rheumatoid Arthritis," *Arthritis & Rheumatism*, Vol. 31, No. 3, 1988, pp. 315-324. doi:10.1002/art.1780310302

[13] P. W. Jones, "The St George's Respiratory Questionnaire," *Respiratory Medicine*, Vol. 85, No. B, 1991, pp. 25-31.

[14] L. A. Saketkoo, E. L. Matteson, K. K. Brown, J. R. Seibold, V. Strand, P. Dellaripa, K. Flaherty, D. Huscher, D. Khanna, C. V. Oddis, K. Phillips, D. Pittrow, A. Wells, C. Denton, O. Distler, A. Fischer, O. Kowal-Bielecka, S. Mittoo and J. Swigris, "Developing Disease Activity and Response Criteria in Connective Tissue Disease-Related Interstitial Lung Disease," *The Journal of Rheumatology*, Vol. 38, No. 7, 2011, pp. 1514-1518. doi:10.3899/jrheum.110281

[15] A. V. Hadjinicolaou, M. K. Nisar, H. Parfrey, E. R. Chilvers and A. J. K. Östör, "Non-Infectious Pulmonary Toxicity of Rituximab: A Systematic Review," *Rheumatology*, Vol. 51, No. 4, 2012, pp. 653-662. doi:10.1093/rheumatology/ker290

[16] H. Liote, F. Liote, B. Seroussi, C. Mayaud and J. Cadranel, "Rituximab-Induced Lung Disease: A Systematic Literature Review," *European Respiratory Journal*, Vol. 35, No. 3, 2010, pp. 681-687. doi:10.1183/09031936.00080209

14

Low-to-Moderate Alcohol Consumption May Be Safe When Taking Methotrexate for Rheumatoid Arthritis or Psoriasis

Bernard Ng[1,2]

[1]Houston Veterans Affairs HSR&D Center of Excellence, Michael E. DeBakey Veterans Affairs Medical Center, Houston, USA;
[2]Department of Medicine, Baylor College of Medicine, Houston, USA.
Email: Bernard.Ng@va.gov

ABSTRACT

It is unclear if consumption of small to moderate amounts of alcohol is safe while taking methotrexate. We set out to determine whether there is an association between liver enzyme abnormalities and alcohol consumption in subjects taking methotrexate. The study sample was identified from the database of the South Central Veteran Affairs Healthcare Network, consisting of 10 hospitals in Texas, Oklahoma, Mississippi and Louisiana. From a cohort of 2443 eligible Veterans with rheumatoid arthritis and/or psoriasis taking methotrexate from 10/1/2007 to 9/30/2009, 120 cases with abnormal liver-enzyme elevation were randomly selected to compare with 120 controls. Data were collected from mailed survey forms that inquired about alcohol consumption habits, physicians' advice on alcohol, and methotrexate compliance. There was no significant difference in the number of non-drinkers and low-to-moderate alcohol drinkers between cases and controls ($p = 0.217$). Few persons identified themselves as heavy drinkers. Our data suggest that it is likely safe for patients with rheumatoid arthritis and psoriasis to consume low-to-moderate amounts of alcohol while taking methotrexate. However, alternative methods to improve capturing alcohol consumption in heavy drinkers are needed for more comprehensive results.

Keywords: Methotrexate; Alcohol; Liver Enzymes; Rheumatoid Arthritis; Psoriasis

1. Introduction

In 2000, the National Household Survey on Drug Abuse estimated that 1.9 million Veterans reported heavy alcohol use [1]. The rate of past-month alcohol use was estimated to be similar in male Veterans and non-Veterans. In another report from the same source, men were twice as likely as women to be dependent on alcohol (10.5% versus 5.1%) [2]. With a 94% preponderance of men in the US Veteran population, the issue of alcohol use influencing compliance with a methotrexate (MTX) regimen and increasing risk of adverse effects is of greater importance for Veterans than it is for the general US population.

Rheumatoid arthritis (RA) and psoriasis are common conditions that afflict over 1.3 million and 4.5 million Americans, respectively [3,4]. The economic burden associated with such inflammatory conditions, with an average age of onset between 30 and 50, is exceptionally high because they affect working-age adults. Work disability accounts for much of the economic burden associated with RA and psoriatic arthritis. Therefore, early treatment of these chronic diseases is important to reduce the associated morbidity and mortality [4].

MTX has been used extensively in the treatment of RA and psoriasis since the early 1980s. It is a drug with a high benefit-to-risk ratio compared with other traditional disease-modifying, anti-rheumatic drugs (DMARDs). It has been estimated that about 20% - 25% of psoriasis patients have been treated with MTX [5] and all new biological agents for RA rely on concomitant use of MTX for synergistic effects. Optimal dosing and patient compliance with the drug are important factors for successful treatment.

It is usually recommended that an individual abstain from or consume minimal amounts of alcohol while taking MTX because of potential liver toxicities [6]. This is a conservative recommendation that is based solely on expert opinion because there are no clinical data about the quantity of alcohol that can be safely consumed with MTX [6]. A review of 27 prospective studies estimated that, in subjects taking MTX, 20.2% had at least one episode of elevated liver enzymes but that only 3.7% had to discontinue MTX because of liver toxicity [6]. Elevation of liver enzymes is often transient and reverts to normal when alcohol or other hepatotoxic drugs (for example, non-steroidal anti-inflammatory drugs, statins, etc.) are stopped. Subsequently, MTX can be resumed at the same or a lower dose.

In the case of leflunomide, a DMARD that requires total abstinence from alcohol, one study reported that patients refused to take it when told that they needed to abstain from alcohol [8]. Unlike the treatment of HIV and diabetes, for which alcohol dependence has been shown to reduce medication compliance, there is little evidence that MTX compliance is affected by alcohol dependence [9,10].

The purpose of this study was to examine whether there is an association between low-to-moderate alcohol consumption in patients taking MTX and elevated liver enzymes. The lack of an association would provide preliminary evidence that it might be safe for patients taking MTX to consume low-to-moderate amounts of alcohol.

2. Methodology

This study was approved by the Baylor College of Medicine Institutional Review Board and the Michael E. DeBakey Veterans Affairs Medical Center Research and Development Committee. In addition, because the study involved questions related to alcohol consumption, we also received a National Institutes of Health certificate of confidentiality.

2.1. Study Setting

The research was carried out with RA and psoriasis patients from the South Central Veteran Affairs Healthcare Network (SCVHCN), consisting of 10 VA hospitals in Texas, Oklahoma, Mississippi, and Louisiana.

Using an administrative database from the SCVHCN that contained patient demographics, diagnosis codes, drug prescriptions and laboratory results, we identified our incipient cohort as patients with RA and/or psoriasis who had been prescribed MTX for at least 6 months. Patients were eligible for inclusion if they met the following criteria: 1) had one ICD-9 code of 714.xx for RA or 696.xx for psoriasis between 10/1/2007 to 9/30/2009 and 2) had been taking MTX for at least 6 months. To ensure that we captured everyone who was prescribed at least 6 months of MTX, we searched drug prescriptions back to 4/1/2007. Exclusion criteria included having 1) abnormal liver enzymes prior to 10/1/2007 and 2) a known history of chronic viral hepatitis, autoimmune hepatitis or Sjögren's syndrome. A total of 2443 patients met these criteria.

2.2. Study Population

We used a case-control study design because of the small

number of liver enzyme abnormalities in our cohort of RA and psoriasis patients on MTX. We defined cases as patients who had elevated liver enzymes (having at least one reading of high serum alanine aminotransferase (ALT) (i.e., greater than 80 U/L) and/or high serum aspartate aminotransferase (AST) (i.e., greater than 120 U/L) while they were taking MTX within the study period. Controls had normal levels of ALT and AST while taking MTX.

From the incipient cohort of 2443 identified patients, we randomly selected 120 cases and 120 controls to whom a survey questionnaire, "Alcohol Use in Patients on Methotrexate" was mailed. This sample size was chosen based on the results of an earlier study for which the questionnaire was developed [11].

2.3. Survey Questionnaire

The "Alcohol Use in Patients on Methotrexate" survey for our study consisted of seven questions designed to estimate weekly alcohol consumption and to inquire about MTX compliance (see Appendix). The survey questions have been validated by a study in Norfolk, United Kingdom [11]. With permission from the author (Dr. Chris Deighton), we adapted the survey questions to be applicable to the US Veteran population.

Under the supervision of a psychometrician, we first conducted cognitive testing of the survey questions to ensure that the items were understandable and able to be answered by our Veteran population. In this part of the study, patients were not asked to answer the actual survey questions but asked to provide comments about the wording and meaning of the questions. In view of this brief survey, the psychometrician ascertained that four subjects would suffice for the cognitive testing process if there were a general consensus that the questions were clear and easy to understand. We enrolled four consecutive patients on MTX (with RA and/or psoriasis) from our rheumatology outpatient clinics.

For each of the seven questions in the survey, the subjects participating in the cognitive testing were asked to comment on the followings:

1) How important do you feel this question is?

2) Describe what comes to mind when you hear this question.

3) Do you get a clear picture in your mind right away of what your answer would be?

    a) If so, what makes this question clear?

    b) If not, what makes this question unclear?

4) How would you ask this question to make it clearer?

5) How hard would it be to answer this question?

    a) If you think it would be hard, what makes it hard?

    b) What would make it easier to answer?

6) How comfortable would you feel answering this

question?

    a) If comfortable, what makes you feel comfortable about answering this question?

    b) If uncomfortable, what makes you feel uncomfortable about answering this question?

2.4. Survey Administration

The survey and a consent form were mailed to study subjects. Subjects were instructed in the consent form to sign the consent form, complete the survey, and return the documents to us in a self-addressed, stamped envelope. One week after mailing out the surveys, we contacted subjects by telephone to ask if they had questions about the survey. Phone interviews to obtain survey answers or verbal consents were not allowed by our IRB.

2.5. Data Analysis

Using the Chi-square test, we examined whether the percentage of patients with abnormal liver enzymes in our eligible study population differed among patients with RA only, psoriasis only, and those with both RA and psoriasis. We also conducted a multivariable logistic regression analysis in which the dependent variable was whether or not the patient had abnormal liver enzymes. Gender and disease diagnoses were used as independent variables.

We next compared the cases and controls to whom surveys were sent on their mortality rates, survey response rates, demographic characteristics and medication use. For continuous variables such as age, we used the nonparametric Wilcoxon two-sample test to compare cases and controls. For categorical variables, we used the Chi-square test. For survey questions with low response rates, we did not conduct formal statistical tests but instead reported only the numbers and percentages of patients responding to the survey items. When examining questions related to MTX compliance and doctor's advice, we categorized patients into three categories: nondrinkers, low-to-moderate drinkers, and heavy drinkers. From the many possible definitions of moderate alcohol consumption, we selected the widely accepted—National Institute on Alcohol Abuse and Alcoholism (NIAAA) definition of 7 - 14 standard drinks per week for men and up to 1 - 7 standard drinks per week for women. We use the definition of *standard drink* as any drink that contains about 14 g pure alcohol (12 oz. of beer/8 - 9 oz. of malt liquor/5 oz. of table wine/1.5 oz. of hard liquor or spirits) [12,13]. We tabulated the responses of the cases and controls as to whether they were drinkers, what their level of alcohol consumption was, and what their views of alcohol consumption and use of MTX were.

3. Results

3.1. Characteristics of Study Population Taken from the SCVHCN Administrative Database

Within our regional VA administrative database, there were 2443 RA and psoriasis patients meeting our study criteria. Among these, there were 179 subjects (7.3%) with at least one abnormal liver function test during the study period. **Table 1** shows significant differences among patients with RA only, those with psoriasis only, and those with both conditions as to whether they had abnormal liver enzymes (p < 0.001). In terms of patients with RA only, 6.3% had abnormal levels, compared with 10.8% of those with psoriasis only and 13.6% of those with both diseases.

In the multivariable logistic regression model, we found that psoriasis only patients and patients with both diseases were more likely than RA only patients to have abnormal liver enzymes (odds ratio for psoriasis only patients = 1.76, 95% CI: 1.21 - 2.55 and odds ratio for patients with both diseases = 2.31, 95% CI: 1.28 - 4.18). Males were more likely to have abnormal liver enzymes than females, but this did not reach statistical significance (odds ratio = 2.21, 95% CI: 0.89 - 5.48).

3.2. Cognitive Testing Phase of the Survey

Four consecutive patients (two men and two women) participated in the cognitive testing of the survey questions. All four patients felt that all seven questions were important and clearly worded. They also reported that they felt comfortable answering these questions.

Table 1. Summary of our study population taken from the SCVHCN administrative database.

Disease	Abnormal liver enzymes (%)	Normal liver enzymes (%)
RA only (n = 1959)	6.3	93.7
Males (n = 1833)	6.6	93.4
Females (n = 126)	3.2	96.8
Psoriasis only (n = 381)	10.8	89.2
Males (n = 366)	10.9	89.1
Females (n = 15)	6.7	93.3
Both diseases (n = 103)	13.6	86.4
Males (n = 98)	14.3	85.7
Females (n = 5)	0.0	100.0

Overall: x_2^2 = 15.4 (p < 0.001); Males: x_2^2 = 15.0 (p = 0.001); Females: Fisher's exact test (p = 0.53).

3.3. Survey Results

At the time of the survey, 14 patients in the case group and four patients in the control group were unreachable. **Table 2** compares the patients' demographics. There were no significant differences in the distribution of age, gender and diagnoses between cases and controls. The use of related drugs such as folic acid and other oral DMARDs was similar in both groups. The average daily prednisone dose was significantly higher in the cases. Although the percentage of patients ever using 10 mg or more of prednisone daily was higher amongst the cases, this did not reach statistical significance. We would expect MTX to be a confounding factor for abnormal raised liver enzymes if average MTX dose is higher amongst the cases. However, average MTX dose was significantly higher in the control group. This could be due to MTX dose being reduced when abnormal levels of liver enzymes were found.

With regard to the differences in patients' compliance with MTX and physicians' advice on alcohol consumption, 70.3% of non-drinkers reported to have never missed a dose of MTX compared to 24.3% of low-to-moderate drinkers and 5.4% of heavy drinkers. Most of the non-drinkers remembered being advised by their physicians to avoid alcohol completely (60%) while only 10% of heavy drinkers remembered hearing this advice. Among those who were told that they could consume small amounts of alcohol (up to 2 drinks per day for men and 1 drink per day for women) while on MTX, 67% were low-to-moderate drinkers and 33% were heavy drinkers. None of the non-drinkers remembered hearing the advice that low-to-moderate alcohol consumption was acceptable.

Table 2. Comparison of cases and controls to whom surveys were sent on their response rate, demographic characteristics and use of related medicines.

	Cases (n = 106)	Controls (n = 116)	p-value
Response rate (%)	24.5	23.3	0.88[¶]
Average age (as of 6/1/2010)	64.0	65.1	0.37[*]
Sex (% male)	91.5	92.2	0.85§
RA only (%)	68.9	76.7	
Psoriasis only (%)	24.5	14.7	0.17§
RA and psoriasis (%)	6.6	8.6	
Average methotrexate dose (per week)	13.4	14.7	0.03[*]
% on folic acid	91.5	91.4	0.97§
Concomitant use of other DMARDS (% of patients on the following drugs):	14.2	12.9	0.79§
a) Leflunomide	16.0	11.2	0.29§
b) Sulfasalazine	31.1	37.9	0.29§
c) Hydroxychloroquine			
% who had been on 10 mg or more of prednisone during study	46.3	34.5	0.07§
Average prednisone dose daily (mg)	15.4	11.8	<0.01[*]
% with concomitant use of statins	60.4	56.0	0.51[§]
% with concomitant use of retinols	3.8	5.2	0.75[¶]

[¶] Fischer's exact test; [*] Wilcoxon two sample test; [§]Chi-square.

The amount of alcohol consumed between the cases and controls were not significantly different (p = 0.17). There was also no significant difference when we compared the distribution among cases and controls of non-drinkers with light-to-moderate drinkers and heavy drinkers (p = 0.37, Fisher's exact).

All heavy alcohol drinkers reported that knowing low-to-moderate alcohol consumption is acceptable when taking MTX would not change their methotrexate compliance. The heavy alcohol drinkers also reported no reduction in the amount of alcohol consumed since they started MTX. However, some of those who consume low-to-moderate amounts of alcohol did report that they might improve MTX compliance if they knew that low-to-moderate alcohol consumption is acceptable when taking MTX.

4. Discussion

There is a lack of information about the amount of alcohol that can be safely consumed by patients with RA or psoriasis while taking MTX. Due to concerns for increased risk of hepatotoxicity, many physicians prefer that patients adhere to strict alcohol abstinence. However, despite the high rates of alcohol use in a predominantly male VA population, elevated liver enzymes among patients with RA or psoriasis while on MTX are lower (7.3%) compared with studies done on the general population (9.3% and 17.0%) [11,14]. Our study used a case-control design because of the low rate of elevated liver enzymes while on MTX among our study population of patients with RA or psoriasis.

Elevations of liver enzymes in patients taking MTX are typically more frequently observed in patients with psoriasis than in patients with RA. This is consistent with previous findings that MTX-associated hepatotoxicity is more often observed in patients with psoriasis than in patients with RA [15]. Such observations had been attributed to the greater preponderance of men with psoriasis compared with RA and higher alcohol consumption by men. However, in our study population which has a low number of females, there is a no difference in the proportion of males and females between the two diagnoses. Yet we still have significantly higher abnormal liver enzyme occurrences among psoriatic patients. In addition, when we looked only at males, the occurrence of abnormal liver enzymes was still significantly higher in psoriasis only patients compared with RA only patients. This point is supported by our logistic regression model where we found increased odds of having abnormal liver enzymes in patients with psoriasis only and with both diseases compared with RA only. The increased odds remained significant even when corrected for gender. Therefore, there could be other possible rea-

sons (e.g., genetic factors) because gender differences between the two diagnoses cannot fully explain these observations.

Studies using a large database have the advantages of being cost effective, convenient and able to provide a larger study population which would be difficult to achieve with other study methods [16-22]. The VA database is the largest healthcare administrative database in the United States and is a useful resource for epidemiologic studies [23]. However, epidemiologic studies using databases rely heavily on the accuracy of diagnostic coding, and their reliability depends on the physicians' ability to make an accurate diagnosis. Singh et al. have pointed out that using only diagnosis code 714.xx to define a prevalent sample of RA patients has a low specificity of 55% ,with an unacceptably high false-positive rate of 34% [24]. However, we have further added the criterion of being on MTX for at least 2 years. This criterion, according to Singh et al., would increase the specificity to an acceptable level of 83% - 97% and increase the positive predictive value from 81% - 97%. In a report of another study, Singh et al. indicated that using the ICD-9 diagnosis code to screen for psoriatic arthritis is both sensitive (57% - 100%) and specific (98% - 100%) [25]. However, adding the DMARD criterion to define the cohort could result in lowering the sensitivity. Our study design omitted patients who had discontinued MTX within 6 months for various adverse effects, such as abnormal liver function tests or drug hypersensitivity. We excluded cases with less than 6 months of MTX use because of the following:

1) It could indicate that MTX was discontinued upon the physician's realization of a misdiagnosis of RA or psoriasis;

2) Elevated liver enzymes for other reasons could have preceded initiation of MTX, and the prescribing physician would have discontinued MTX when he/she realized this.

A limitation resulting from the exclusion of such cases is that true cases may have been omitted, such as those of patients who consumed alcohol and developed elevated liver enzymes because they were unable to reduce alcohol intake, and so the prescribing physician discontinued MTX within the first 6 months. Another limitation includes our inability to capture drug prescription information when patients obtained drugs from outside the VA system—for example, aspirin and other non-steroidal anti-inflammatory drugs which may be cheaper to purchase from a retail pharmacy. In addition, we have a predominantly male Veteran population which reduces the ability to extrapolate our findings to the general population.

Our data suggest that liver enzyme elevations in subjects with RA or psoriasis taking MTX are unlikely to be affected by low-to-moderate amounts of alcohol consumption.

5. Acknowledgments

This work was supported by a local grant from the Houston Center for Quality of Care and Utilization Studies (CF.HQU.LFP.0110.000-00.B_N) and also partly supported by the Houston Veterans Affairs Health Services Research and Development Center of Excellence (HFP 90-020). The views expressed are those of the authors and do not necessarily represent those of the Department of Veterans Affairs/Baylor College of Medicine.

The authors would like to thank Sonora Hudson for editing the manuscript, Crystal Booker for helping to contact the survey participants and tabulation of results, Dr. Fawad Aslam for helping with initial study design and pre-testing phase of the survey, and the Veterans Affairs South Central Mental Illness Research, Education and Clinical Center for providing help from Dr. Adam Kelly with the psychometrics of the survey form and from Annette Walder with data organization.

REFERENCES

[1] Office of Applied Studies, "Alcohol Use among Veterans," Office of Applied Studies, Rockville, 2001.

[2] Office of Applied Studies, "Gender Differences in Alcohol Use and Alcohol Dependence or Abuse: 2004 and 2005," Office of Applied Studies, Rockville, 2007.

[3] R. S. Stern, T. Nijsten, S. R. Feldman, et al., "Psoriasis Is Common, Carries a Substantial Burden Even When Not Extensive, and Is Associated with Widespread Treatment Dissatisfaction," Journal of Investigative Dermatology Symposium, Vol. 9, No. 2, 2004, pp. 136-139. doi:10.1046/j.1087-0024.2003.09102.x

[4] C. G. Helmick, D. T. Felson, R. C. Lawrence, et al., "Estimates of the Prevalence of Arthritis and Other Rheumatic Conditions in the United States. Part I," Arthritis & Rheumatism, Vol. 58, No. 1, 2008, pp. 15-25. doi:10.1002/art.23177

[5] T. Nijsten, D. J. Margolis, S. R. Feldman, et al., "Traditional Systemic Treatments Have Not Fully Met the Needs of Psoriasis Patients: Results from a National Survey," Journal of the American Academy of Dermatology, Vol. 52, No. 3, 2005, pp. 434-444.

[6] J. M. Kremer, G. S. Alarcon, R. W. Lightfoot Jr., et al., "Methotrexate for Rheumatoid Arthritis. Suggested Guidelines for Monitoring Liver Toxicity. American College of Rheumatology," Arthritis & Rheumatism, Vol. 37, No. 3, 1994, pp. 316-328. doi:10.1002/art.1780370304

[7] C. Salliot and D. van der Heijde, "Long Term Safety of Methotrexate Monotherapy in Rheumatoid Arthritis Patients: A Systematic Literature Research," Annals of the Rheumatic Diseases, Vol. 68, No. 7, 2008, pp. 1100-1104.

[8] S. Rajakulendran and C. Deighton, "Do Guidelines for the Prescribing and Monitoring of Leflunomide Need to Be Modified?" Rheumatology, Vol. 43, No. 11, 2004, pp. 1447-1448. doi:10.1093/rheumatology/keh348

[9] C. L. Bryson, D. H. Au, H. Sun, et al., "Alcohol Screening Scores and Medication Nonadherence," Annals of Internal Medicine, Vol. 149, No. 11, 2008, pp. 795-804.

[10] J. Dunbar-Jacob, J. L. Holmes, S. Sereika, et al., "Factors Associated with Attrition of African Americans during the Recruitment Phase of a Clinical Trial Examining Adherence among Individuals with Rheumatoid Arthritis," Arthritis & Rheumatism, Vol. 51, No. 3, 2004, pp. 422-428. doi:10.1002/art.20411

[11] S. Rajakulendran, K. Gadsby and C. Deighton, "Rheumatoid Arthritis, Alcohol, Leflunomide and Methotrexate. Can Changes to the BSR Guidelines for Leflunomide and Methotrexate on Alcohol Consumption Be Justified?" Musculoskeletal Care, Vol. 6, No. 4, 2008, pp. 233-245. doi:10.1002/msc.135

[12] US Department of Health and Human Services, "Helping Patients Who Drink Too Much: A Clinician's Guide," NIAAA Publications Distribution Center, Rockville, 2005, p. 24.

[13] M. C. Dufour, "What Is Moderate Drinking? Defining 'Drinks' and Drinking Levels," Alcohol Research & Health, Vol. 23, No. 1, 1999, pp. 5-14.

[14] K. Visser and D. M. Van der Heidje, "Incidence of Liver Enzyme Elevations and Liver Biopsy Abnormalities during Methotrexate Treatment in Rheumatoid Arthritis: A Systematic Review of the Literature," Arthritis & Rheumatism, Vol. 58, 2008, p. S557.

[15] R. E. Kalb, B. Strober, G. Weinstein, et al., "Methotrexate and Psoriasis: 2009 National Psoriasis Foundation Consensus Conference," Journal of the American Academy of Dermatology, Vol. 60, No. 5, 2009, pp. 824-837. doi:10.1016/j.jaad.2008.11.906

[16] R. A. Bright, J. Avorn and D. E. Everitt, "Medicaid Data as a Resource for Epidemiologic Studies: Strengths and Limitations," Journal of Clinical Epidemiology, Vol. 42, No. 10, 1989, pp. 937-945. doi:10.1016/0895-4356(89)90158-3

[17] J. P. Burke, H. H. Tilson and R. Platt, "Expanding Roles of Hospital Epidemiology: Pharmacoepidemiology," Infection Control and Hospital Epidemiology, Vol. 10, No. 6, 1989, pp. 253-254. doi:10.1086/646016

[18] I. K. Crombie, "The Role of Record Linkage in Post-Marketing Drug Surveillance," British Journal of Clinical Pharmacology, Vol. 22, No. 1, 1986, pp. 77S-82S. doi:10.1111/j.1365-2125.1986.tb02987.x

[19] G. A. Faich, "Record Linkage for Postmarketing Surveillance," Clinical Pharmacology and Therapeutics, Vol. 46, No. 4, 1989, pp. 479-480. doi:10.1038/clpt.1989.169

[20] W. A. Ray and M. R. Griffin, "Use of Medicaid Data for Pharmacoepidemiology," American Journal of Epidemiology, Vol. 129, No. 4, 1989, pp. 837-849.

[21] S. Shapiro, "The Role of Automated Record Linkage in the Postmarketing Surveillance of Drug Safety: A Critique," Clinical Pharmacology and Therapeutics, Vol. 46,

No. 4, 1989, pp. 371-386. doi:10.1038/clpt.1989.154

[22] H. H. Tilson, "Pharmacoepidemiology: The Lessons Learned; the Challenges Ahead," *Clinical Pharmacology and Therapeutics*, Vol. 46, No. 4, 1989, p. 480. doi:10.1038/clpt.1989.170

[23] E. J. Boyko, T. D. Koepsell, J. M. Gaziano, *et al.*, "US Department of Veterans Affairs Medical Care System as a Resource to Epidemiologists," *American Journal of Epidemiology*, Vol. 151, No. 3, 2000, pp. 307-314. doi:10.1093/oxfordjournals.aje.a010207

[24] J. A. Singh, A. R. Holmgren and S. Noorbaloochi, "Accuracy of Veterans Administration Databases for a Diagnosis of Rheumatoid Arthritis," *Arthritis Care & Research*, Vol. 51, No. 6, 2004, pp. 952-957. doi:10.1002/art.20827

[25] J. A. Singh, A. R. Holmgren, H. Krug, *et al.*, "Accuracy of the Diagnoses of Spondylarthritides in Veterans Affairs Medical Center Databases," *Arthritis Care & Research*, Vol. 57, No. 4, 2007, pp. 648-655. doi:10.1002/art.22682

APPENDIX: Questions in Alcohol Use in Patients on Methotrexate Survey

Adapted from a study in Norfolk, United Kingdom with permission from the author (Dr. Chris Deighton) [11].

1) How often do you miss your Methotrexate dose?
a) In ever miss a dose.
b) On average, I miss a dose once in six months.
c) On average, I miss a dose once in four months.
d) On average, I miss a dose once in two months.
e) On average, I miss a dose every month.
f) I am not sure about this.

2) What did your doctor tell you about drinking alcohol when you were started on Methotrexate?
a) Avoid alcohol completely.
b) Drink as you like.
c) No advice was given.
d) Cannot remember.
e) Not applicable to me since I do not drink alcohol.

3) Were you told that drinking alcohol up to 2 standard drinks per day for men and 1 standard drink per day for women is ok?
a) Yes.
b) No.
c) Cannot remember.

4) Do you drink any alcohol? (Please include social drinking as well)
a) Yes.
b) No.
If you answer no, then you need not answer any further questions.

5) Please average your alcohol intake over the last 6 months. Please include episodes, if any, of binge drinking as well. You may choose as many answers as they apply to you.
a) If you drink beer, please state the average number of drinks:

i) Number of 12 oz. drinks consumed in one week:
_____
ii) Number of 16 oz. drinks consumed in one week:
_____
iii) Number of 22 oz. drinks consumed in one week:
_____
iv) Number of 40 oz. drinks consumed in one week:
_____
v) Other: _____
b) If you drink malt liquor (example: Forty, Colt 45, Private Stock, Camo 40, King Cobra and others) please state the average number:
i) Number of 12 oz. drinks consumed in one week:
_____
ii) Number of 16 oz. drinks consumed in one week:
_____
iii) Number of 20 oz. drinks consumed in one week:
_____
iv) Number of 40 oz. drinks consumed in one week:
_____
v) Other: _____
c) If you drink hard liquor/spirits (80-proof drinks) (example: brandy, gin, vodka, whiskey) please state the average number:
i) Number of shots (1.5 oz.) consumed in one week:
_____
ii) Number of Pint (16 oz.) drinks consumed in one week: _____
iii) Number of Fifth (25 oz.) drinks consumed in one week: _____
iv) Number of 1.75 liters (59 oz.) drinks consumed in one week: _____
v) Number of Mixed drink (please specify):
_____

If you drink table wine, fortified wine, Cordial, Liqueurs (example Sherry, Port) please state the average number:
i) Number of servings/single bottle/glasses (5 oz.)

glasses consumed in one week: _____

    ii) Number of standard 750ml (25oz.) bottle consumed in one week: _____

    iii) Other: _____

6) The current recommendation is to avoid alcohol while taking Methotrexate. If the recommendation were changed such that alcohol drinking was allowed while taking Methotrexate, how would that affect your Methotrexate intake?

a) I would use my medicine more regularly.

b) I would use my medicine less regularly.

c) It would not make a difference.

7) How has your alcohol drinking changed since you have been on Methotrexate?

a) I have been drinking more alcohol.

b) I have been drinking less alcohol.

c) I have completely stopped drinking alcohol.

d) There has been no change in my drinking habits.

15

Rheumatoid Arthritis of the Temporomandibular Joint; Comparison of Digital Panoramic Radiographs Taken Using the Joint Limitation Program [JLA View] and CT Scans

Antigone Delantoni

Department of Dentoalveolar Surgery, Implant Surgery and Radiology, Faculty of Dentistry, Aristotle University of Thessaloniki, Thessaloniki, Greece.
Email: adelantoni@yahoo.com

ABSTRACT

Objective: The aim of this study was to evaluate the efficacy of digital panoramic radiographs using the JLA view program in cases of rheumatoid arthritis and compare them to CT scans of the patients. **Methods:** 40 patients with known condition of RA and clinical symptoms in the TMJ were selected for the study. Radiological evaluation included a panoramic radiograph of the TMJs that was taken and a computer tomography of the joints. In the panoramic radiographs taken, isolation of the TMJs was done using the JLA view program, while in the CT scans of the patients, all scans were taken with closed mouth, with a distance of 0.5 mm per slice. The parameters examined were: 1) bony changes of the condyle; 2) the position of the condyle in the mandibular fossa; 3) the joint space; 4) bony changes of mandibular fossa. **Results:** There were no statistically significant differences found between the two observers or between the two joints of the same patient [right and left] on the panoramic radiographs. For the case of CT scans there were significant differences between the joint space of right and left joints, while in the ANOVA performed differences were found for the evaluation of the bony changes of the condyle. **Conclusion:** There were no significant differences between the two radiographic methods selected and therefore when a proper simple radiograph is taken and well evaluated, the conclusions drawn from it are well based and there is no need for further examinations.

Keywords: Rheumatoid Arthritis; Imaging; Temporomandibular Joint; Panoramic Radiography

1. Introduction

The temporomandibular joint [TMJ] is one the most frequently involved small joints of the skeleton in the case of inflammatory diseases, the most frequent of which is rheumatoid arthritis [1]. The radiographic involvement of the TMJ in inflammatory conditions has been studied and reported by many laboratories [1-5].

The lately introduced digital panoramic radiographs have not however been studied for the condition, though the efficacy of digital radiographs in other joints involved in the disease is not doubted anymore. The low radiation dose and the increased details of the radiographs plus the ability to manipulate the radiograph taken are the major advantages of digital radiographs.

Since the beginning of the description and classification of the TMJ syndrome by Costen in 1934 there has been no full clinical description of the condition until the 80's where Weinberg [3] first mentions the etiology and

the need for a thorough and complete knowledge of the TMJ. Similar reports have been made by Laskin [1] where the author mentions the difficulty in classifying the condition since it has numerous causes but one clinical expression. In more recent studies the TMJ syndrome is always mentioned with the cause of the condition.

One can therefore state that though the temporomandibular joint is a frequently involved joint in rheumatoid arthritis, there has been little research on whether the conventional radiographic techniques are adequate for the joint's evaluation. In this paper an attempt to compare conventional imaging techniques to CT scans is made.

2. Materials and Methods

40 patients of known rheumatoid arthritis have been included in the study. The patients were of ages 19 - 57 and had no other condition that could cause TMJ dysfunction

(e.g. dentures, missing teeth, trismus, malocclusion etc.). They were selected among a number of 85 patients of rheumatoid arthritis and were carefully examined so that the disease would be active at the TMJ upon the examination (trigger points to muscles, clicking sounds etc.). Therefore the 40 patients selected were patients with RA that presented TMJ dysfunction syndrome. They were asked to take a digital panoramic radiograph of the TMJ (Joint Limitation Program) (**Figure 1**) and then a CT scan of the joint (**Figure 2**).

The panoramic radiographs were taken using the PM 2002 CC Proline orthopantomogram by Planmeka (PM 2002 CC Proline Panoramic X-Ray Unit, Planmeca Co. Helsinki, Finland) where the JLA program was applied (Joint limitation program). The CT scans were also performed the same way. All exams were performed with the patients mouth closed. Sections of 0, 5 or 1 mm were selected to have homogeneity in all the exams and the viewing of the radiographs were performed. The radiographs taken were viewed by two expert Oral Surgeons and one Dentomaxillofacial Radiology expert who supervised the procedure prior to the analysis of the results.

The observers viewed the radiographs in random order and under identical conditions [dark room with ambient background light]. They were then asked to evaluate the condition of the joint based on points that could be

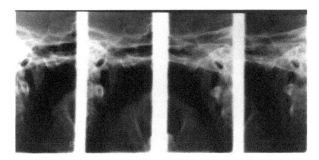

Figure 1. Panoramic radiograph using the Joint Limitation Program with open and closed mouth. They cystic lesions are prominent and easily identified.

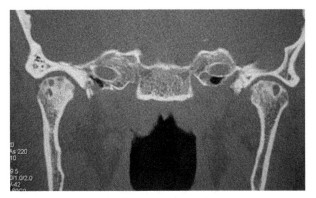

Figure 2. CT section of the same patient showing the cyst shaped erosions on the condylar head.

viewed on the radiographs. Both right and left joint were viewed separately since the involvement of one joint does not necessarily mean involvement of the other joint.

The observers were asked to evaluate: 1) Bony changes of the condyle (flattening, erosion, osteophytes, sclerosis, resorption); 2) The position of the condyle in the mandibular fossa (anterior, concentric, posterior); 3) The joint space (increased, normal, reduced); 4) Bony changes of mandibular fossa [erosion, sclerosis, resorption, normal]. All images, both panoramic radiographs and the CT scans of the patients were examined for the above parameters by the observers.

3. Results

There was comparison made between the right and left joints of the patients and no statistically significant differences were found for the cases of panoramic radiographs (p value: 0.3836). For the case of CT scans there were significant differences between the joint space of right and left joints (p value: 0.1794), while in the ANOVA performed differences were found for the evaluation of the bony changes of the condyle (p value: 0.0153).

No statistical differences were found between right and left joints of the same patients for the case of panoramic radiographs while statistical significant differences were found between right and left joints for the case of the articular space and its size estimate (p value: 0.3026) which is partly expected since the articular space depends on the joints' elements and the two joints are completely independent.

Besides the initial descriptive statistics ANOVA was performed for each of the four areas of interest on the radiographs and the following results were obtained.

Statistical significant differences were measured between CT scans and panoramic radiographs for the 1st feature of the joint, meaning the condylar head and the lesions that appear on it. No statistical significant differences were found for the other three parts of the joint measured articular space, condylar head's position and temporal articular surface. The differences found for the condylar head between the two radiographic techniques measured are observed in **Table 1**.

Table 1. ANOVA table for A.

	P value	Power
Type	0.0003	0.971
Position	0.4143	0.123
Type + Position	0.6829	0.069

Due to the difference of the measurements for the condylar head evaluation there were differences found in the overall estimate of the joint as is observed in **Table 2**.

Due to the differences in the numbers given by the observers in order to evaluate the four different parts of the joint involved in RA Principal Component Analysis was performed. The PCA is a statistical technique that bears into account the gravity of each of the variables selected in the total result thus giving us more accurate results considering that each joint segment is of equal significance [as is assumed]. The results for the PCA was 0.882 (**Table 3**), proving that when each feature of the joint is equally valued there are no statistical significant differences between the two radiographic techniques selected.

Therefore the results obtained could be summarized to the following. There were no statistical significant differences between the two observers since a consensus decision was reached. There were differences between the two imaging modalities for the first of the four viewed features of the TMJ, the condylar head and its lesions. However the PCA which considers the importance of each independent variable, no statistical significant differences were measured between the two methods.

4. Discussion

The purpose of the current study was to subjectively study the radiographic findings in patient with TMJ syndrome that had a known history of rheumatoid arthritis. More specifically an attempt to correlate the radiographic findings according to the radiographic technique used and to measure the efficacy of conventional plain radiographs [panoramic] when compared to high specificity CT.

Table 2. ANOVA table for total.

	P value	Power
Type	0.0351	0.556
Position	0.1028	0.354
Type + Position	0.5190	0.098

Table 3. Wilcoxon Signed Rank Test for condylar position between panoramic and CT scans.

#0 Differences	0
#Ties	1
Z value	−0.148
P value	0.8825

The first thorough radiographic analysis of the TMJ in cases of rheumatoid arthritis has been made by Worth in 1963 [4] though initial mention of the condition was in 1951 by Steinhardt [5] and Fiumicelli [6]. Since then there have been numerous studies involving the TMJ and rheumatoid arthritis. Tabeling and Dolwick 1985 [7] mention that 50% of the RA patients studied had TMJ problems. In 1987 a more thorough description of the clinical symptoms of the TMJ in patients with RA was made by Braunwald, Isselbacher και Petersdorf [8] where the radiological symptoms are well described.

In the present study a clinical examination protocol used by the Dental Faculty [altered Helkimo] was used to determine the patients to be included in the study. Patients with a known RA history showed a higher TMJ syndrome condition (40 out of 85) than the patients not included in the study (45 of the initial 85). Similar results have been presented in numerous studies [9-16].

In previous studies the frequency of TMJ involvement in RA varies from 2% to 98% [17]. In the majority of reports though 40% to 50% of all RA patients presents some clinical involvement of the TMJ [18-20]. This result is in agreement with the results from the present study since from the initial number of patients 40 fulfilled all the criteria to be included in the study.

For the radiographic implications of the condition most authors agree to a percentage of about 60% involvement for CT scans in the case of known RA of the patients ranging from 50% to 80% [7,21]. There is agreement that the radiographic findings of the patients are not as visible in the initial stages of the condition while the primary lesions are the erosions the anterior and inner condylar surface. The initial lesions are not as visible in panoramic radiographs [22,23]. However in the present study in the cases of involvement of the TMJ for lesions that are not extended [erosions and osteophytes, there were no significant statistical differences between the two methods This is in agreement with the number of authors that claim that the Joint Limitation Program [JLA view] is more useful in the patients classification and as markers for the joints inflammatory condition [24,25]. What should be noted here is that in the present study a large number of patients with active RA of the TMJ were not included in the study for other reasons such as occlusal problems, trismus and other conditions. If all active RA patients were included, the percentile of patients having radiographic findings could be significantly higher.

Regarding the comparison of the two different techniques, though there were differences between the isolated findings of both techniques [condylar head] there were no statistical significant differences overall in the joints. The reason for this is that the condylar head imaging is significantly different in imaging between the two methods [panoramic and CT] due to the large number of anatomical elements that superimpose it in panoramic radiographs [26,27]. Also CT scans are known to have a larger specificity in small size lesions [28-31]. However it is of great value that overall there were no differences between the two techniques which could partly prove the importance of a detailed initial radiographic examination that could not mean large radiation doses as is the case of CT.

Conclusively we can say that there is increased involvement of the TMJ in the patients with RA. The involvement is visible in simple radiographs such as digital panoramic radiographs if they are properly taken though CT scans do tend to have a higher specificity and detail in the case of initial lesions. In the present study there were no significant differences found between the two radiographic methods selected for both joints, and therefore when a proper simple radiograph is taken and well evaluated, the conclusions drawn from it are well based and there is no need for further examinations.

REFERENCES

[1]　D. M. Laskin, "Diagnosis of Pathology of the Temporomandibular Joint, Clinical and Imaging Perspectives," *Radiologic Clinics of North America*, Vol. 31, No. 1, 1993, pp. 135-147.

[2]　H. H. Yilmaz, D. Yildirim, Y. Ugan, S. E. Tunc, A. Yesildag, H. Orhan and C. Akdag, "Clinical and Magnetic Resonance Imaging Findings of the Temporomandibular Joint and Masticatory Muscles in Patients with Rheumatoid Arthritis," *Rheumatology International*, Vol. 32, No. 5, 2011, pp. 1171-1178.

[3]　L. A. Weinberg, "The Etiology, Diagnosis, and Treatment of TMJ Dysfunction-Pain Syndrome. Part I: Etiology," *Journal of Prosthetic Dentistry*, Vol. 42, No. 6, 1979, pp. 654-664. doi:10.1016/0022-3913(79)90197-5

[4]　H. M. Worth, "Principles and Practice of Oral Radiographic Interpretation," Year Book Medical Publishers, Chicago,1963.

[5]　G. Steinhardt, "Rheumatoid Arthritis of the Temporomaxillary Joint," *Zeitschrift fur Laryngologie, Rhinologie, Otologie und Ihre Grenzgebiete*, Vol. 30, No. 11, 1951, pp. 475-485.

[6]　A. Fiumicelli, "Involvement of the Temporo-Mandibular Joint in Rheumatoid Arthritis," *Nova Acta Stomatol*, Vol. 3, No. 1, 1951, pp. 1-10.

[7]　H. J. Tabeling and M. F. Dolwick, "Rheumatoid Arthritis: Diagnosis and Treatment," *Florida Dental Journal*, Vol. 56, No. 1, 1985, pp. 16-18.

[8]　E. Braunwald and R. G. Petersdorf, "Harrison's Principles of Internal Medicine," McGraw-Hill, New York, 1987.

[9]　B. Wenneberg, L. Hollender and S. Kopp, "Radiographic Changes in the Temporomandibular Joint in Ankylosing Spondylitis," *Dentomaxillofacial Radiology*, Vol. 12, No. 1, 1983, pp. 25-30.

[10]　B. Wenneberg, S. Kopp and L. Hollender, "The Temporomandibular Joint in Ankylosing Spondylitis. Correlations between Subjective, Clinical, and Radiographic Features in the Stomatognathic System and Effects of Treatment," *Acta Odontologica Scandinavica*, Vol. 42, No. 3, 1984, pp. 165-173. doi:10.3109/00016358408993868

[11]　P. L. Westesson, "Temporomandibular Joint and Dental Imaging," *Neuroimaging Clinics of North America*, Vol. 6, No. 2,1996, pp. 333-355.

[12]　K. Marton, "Oral Symptoms of Immunologic Disorders. Part I. Systemic Autoimmune Diseases," *Fogorvosi Szemle*, Vol. 96, No. 1, 2003, pp. 9-15.

[13]　A. G. Pullinger, D. A. Seligman and W. K. Solberg, "Temporomandibular Disorders. Part I: Functional Status, Dentomorphologic Features, and Sex Differences in a Nonpatient Population," *Journal of Prosthetic Dentistry*, Vol. 59, No. 2, 1988, pp. 228-235. doi:10.1016/0022-3913(88)90019-4

[14]　A. G. Pullinger, D. A. Seligman and W. K. Solberg, "Temporomandibular Disorders. Part II: Occlusal Factors Associated with Temporomandibular Joint Tenderness and Dysfunction," *Journal of Prosthetic Dentistry*, Vol. 59, No. 3, 1988, pp. 363-367. doi:10.1016/0022-3913(88)90191-6

[15]　D. E. Ryan, "Temporomandibular Disorders," *Current Opinion in Rheumatology*, Vol. 5, No. 2, 1993, pp. 209-218. doi:10.1097/00002281-199305020-00014

[16]　P. N. Scutellari, C. Orzincolo and S. Ceruti, "The Temporo-Mandibular Joint in Pathologic Conditions: Rheumatoid Arthritis and Seronegative Spondyloarthritis," *Radiologia Medica*, Vol. 86, No. 4, 1993, pp. 456-466.

[17]　M. Kononen, B. Wenneberg and A. Kallenberg, "Craniomandibular Disorders in Rheumatoid Arthritis, Psoriatic Arthritis, and Ankylosing Spondylitis: A Clinical Study," *Acta Odontologica Scandinavica*, Vol. 50, No. 5, 1992, pp. 281-287. doi:10.3109/00016359209012774

[18]　I. M. Chalmers and G. S. Blair, "Rheumatoid Arthritis of the Temporomandibular Joint. A Clinical and Radiological Study Using Circular Tomography," *Quarterly Journal of Medicine*, Vol. 42, No. 166, 1973, pp. 369-386.

[19]　J. E. Chenitz, "Rheumatoid Arthritis and Its Implications in Temporomandibular Disorders," *Cranio*, Vol. 10, No. 1, 1992, pp. 59-69.

[20]　T. A. Larheim, H. J. Smith and F. Aspestrand, "Rheumatic Disease of the Temporomandibular Joint: MR Imaging and Tomographic Manifestations," *Radiology*, Vol. 175, No. 2, 1990, pp. 527-531.

[21]　N. Bayar, S. A. Kara, I. Keles, M. C. Koc, D. Altinok and S. Orkun, "Temporomandibular Joint Involvement in Rheumatoid Arthritis: A Radiological and Clinical Study," *Cranio*, Vol. 20, No. 2, 2002, pp. 105-110.

[22]　E. T. Koh, A. U. Yap, C. K. Koh, T. S. Chee, S. P. Chan and I. C. Boudville, "Temporomandibular Disorders in Rheumatoid Arthritis," *Journal of Rheumatology*, Vol. 26,

No. 9, 1999, pp. 1918-1922.

[23] L. Z. Arvidsson, B. Flatø and T. A. Larheim, "Radiographic TMJ Abnormalities in Patients with Juvenile Idiopathic Arthritis Followed for 27 Years," *Oral Surgery, Oral Medicine, Oral Pathology, Oral Radiology and Endodontics*, Vol. 108, No. 1, 2009, pp. 114-123.

[24] L. M. Helenius, D. Hallikainen, I. Helenius, J. H. Meurman, M. Kononen, M. Leirisalo-Repo and C. Lindqvist, "Clinical and Radiographic Findings of the Temporomandibular Joint in Patients with Various Rheumatic Diseases. A Case-Control Study," *Oral Surgery, Oral Medicine, Oral Pathology, Oral Radiology, and Endodontics*, Vol. 99, No. 4, 2005, pp. 455-463. doi:10.1016/j.tripleo.2004.06.079

[25] P. L. Westesson, "Temporomandibular Joint and Dental Imaging," *Neuroimaging Clinics of North America*, Vol. 6, No. 2, 1996, pp. 333-355.

[26] J. V. Manzione, R. W. Katzberg and T. J. Manzione, "Internal Derangements of the Temporomandibular Joint. II. Diagnosis by Arthrography and Computed Tomography," *International Journal of Periodontics & Restorative Dentistry*, Vol. 4, No. 4, 1984, pp. 16-27.

[27] T. A. Larheim, "Comparative Imaging of the Temporomandibular Joint," *Current Opinion in Dentistry*, Vol. 2, 1992, pp. 163-169.

[28] T. A. Larheim, "Comparison between Three Radiographic Techniques for Examination of the Temporomandibular Joints in Juvenile Rheumatoid Arthritis," *Acta Radiologica Diagnosis*, Vol. 22, No. 2, 1981, pp. 195-201.

[29] T. A. Larheim, "Imaging of the Temporomandibular Joint in Rheumatic Disease," *Cranio Clinics International*, Vol. 1, No. 1, 1991, pp. 133-153.

[30] T. A. Larheim, T. Bjornland, H. J. Smith, F. Aspestrand and A. Kolbenstvedt, "Imaging Temporomandibular Joint Abnormalities in Patients with Rheumatic Disease. Comparison with Surgical Observations," *Oral Surgery, Oral Medicine, Oral Pathology*, Vol. 73, No. 4, 1992, pp. 494-501. doi:10.1016/0030-4220(92)90333-L

[31] T. A. Larheim, H. J. Smith and F. Aspestrand, "Rheumatic Disease of the Temporomandibular Joint: MR Imaging and Tomographic Manifestations," *Radiology*, Vol. 175, No. 2, 1990, pp. 527-531.

16

A Focus on the Diagnosis of Early Rheumatoid Arthritis

Marta Olivieri*, Maria Chiara Gerardi, Francesca Romana Spinelli, Manuela Di Franco

Rheumatology Unit, Department of Internal Medicine and Medical Specialities, Sapienza University of Rome, Rome, Italy.
Email: *marta.olivieri11@gmail.com

ABSTRACT

Nowadays it is worldwide accepted that early diagnosis and early treatment of Rheumatoid Arthritis (RA) can improve the prognosis in most of patients. In this way, the 2010 ACR/EULAR Rheumatoid Arthritis classification criteria have shown to be more sensitive than the ACR 1987 criteria and include better patients with early RA. Other important point to focus on is to identify predictive factors for outcome, in order to propose a more aggressive treatment for early RA patients who could develop a persistent and/or erosive disease. The presence of Rheumatoid Factors (RF) and Anti-citrullinated peptides antibobies (ACPA), as well as the duration of the disease at the time of diagnosis, are independent risk factors for the development of erosive RA. As for imaging, both traditional X-ray and Magnetic Resonance Imaging (MRI) highlight respectively the Rapid Radiological Progression (RRP) and the presence of bone edema which are associated to a more aggressive disease. In the last years, the musculoskeletal ultrasonography (MSUS) has emerged as a useful imaging technique since it allows to identify synovitis and bone alteration earlier than the radiological examination. Interating clinical, serological and imaging data the clinician can define the effective disease activity of each patient.

Keywords: Early Rheumatoid Arthritis; Diagnosis

1. Introduction

Rheumatoid arthritis (RA) is a chronic systemic inflammatory disease affecting 1% of the population. It is associated with significant morbidity, mortality, and high burden for the National Health Service (NHS). The disease is characterized by inflammation of the synovium, most frequently occurring in the small joints of the hands and feet, but also large joints can be involved; the inflammatory process frequently leads to loss of cartilage and bone erosions. The joint destruction is correlated with the severity of inflammation [1]. If patients are no treated, work disability, comorbidity and mortality can generally occur within ten years. In the last years, development of new biological drugs directed against molecular targets known as key pathogenetic factors (cytokynes such as TNF alfa, interleukin-6), has improved the prognosis of the disease with significant reduction of radiological erosive damage and disability.

2. Classification Criteria

In the recent past, 1987 Classificative Criteria of American College of Rheumatology (ACR) have been used for the diagnosis of RA [2]; however, these criteria are un-

able to identify the disease at its onset [3]. Moreover, these criteria do not include laboratory findings, such as anti-citrullinated peptide antibodies (ACPA) that are more specific for RA than Rheumatoid Factor (RF). New classification criteria has been validated in 2010 by ACR and European League Against Rheumatism (EULAR) [4] and include 4 items: joint involvement (number of joints with definite synovitis), presence and titre of RF and ACPA, evaluation of acute-phase reactants such as Cre-active protein (CRP) and erithrocyte sedimentation rate (ESR), and duration of symptoms (more or less than 6 weeks). Patients can be classified as RA if a score of ≥6 out of 10 is obtained. Thus, RA can be diagnosed using a combination of clinical and serological parameters.

Even if they are classificative and not diagnostic, ACR 2010 criteria and 1987 criteria have different specificity and sensitivity to identify early RA patients [3]. Indeed some studies have compared the specificity and sensitivity of both classification criteria showed better sensitivity in 2010 criteria (73.5%), and a better specificity in those of 1987 (92.9%) [5].

Better performance of the 2010 criteria in term of sensitivity but not of specificity has been confirmed in a recent work carried out on polyarthritis patients with less than 6 weeks disease duration: in this cohort, only 71.5% of patients with a score of ≥6 points at the first evaluation has been later classified as having RA [6].

3. Pathogenesis and Antibodies

The pathogenesis of RA implies an interaction between environmental factors and genetic background: in genetically predisposed individuals, an arthritogenic peptide may trigger the innate immune response which is followed by an upregulation of adaptive immunity. The earliest, preclinical phase of the disease, in which asymptomatic subjects develop ACPA and IgM-RF has been clearly demonstrated in recent studies on healthy blood donors who later have developed RA [7]. RF are antibodies (IgM, IgG, IgA) directed against Fc region of IgG; RF (usually IgM) is not specific for RA, as it is also detected in other connective tissue diseases, infections, and autoimmune disorders, as well as in 1% - 5% of healthy people. The presence of RF represent an independent risk factor for bone erosion and seems to predict radiographic progression [8]. The autoantibodies directed against citrullinated cyclic pepetides belong to a group of antibodies able to react with several citrullinated peptides on multiple proteins (filaggrin, vimentin, fibrin, alpha-enolase), and for this reason, indicated as ACPA [9]. These autoantibodies are found in 70% of RA patients and are highly specific; APCA also represent early predictors identifying patients at risk for more aggressive and erosive disease [10].

4. Early Diagnosis

Early diagnosis, as early as the symptoms of disease begin, is mandatory since early treatment is known to improve prognosis in most of patients. It is necessary to identify as soon as possible those subjects who might develop an aggressive disease and carry out all possible strategies to slow the disease progression [11]. Most important questions in the last years are: when does RA start? Can it be stopped [11]? In the preclinical phase, the adaptive immune response impairs the synovial membrane, leading to an influx of immune and inflammatory cells and increased vascularity of the joints followed by a destructive synovitis. In the asymptomatic phase, it is not feasible to identify the beginning of the disease from a biological point of view. An early diagnosis can be made as soon as the first clinical symptoms of arthritis start. The concept of a "window-of-opportunity" suggests that there is a period, early in the course of the disease, between biological changes and clinical evidence. In this period the disease process can be altered or maybe even reversed with a complete return to normality. Therapy during this period may have a much greater effect than treatment at a later stage in terms of halting disease progression and achieving remission [12]. "Early arthritis" is defined as symptomatic arthritis appeared from less than 24 weeks and "very early arthritis" from no more than 12

weeks. This range of time results from the evidence that 70% of patients reveal an irreversible joint damage after 2 years of disease, but 28% of RA patients already shows erosions at disease onset [13]. On the other hand, though the diagnosis of RA should be made as soon as possible, the differential diagnosis, particularly at an early stage, can be difficult and should include other arthritis such as spondyloarthritis, reactive arthritis, connective tissue disease and microcrystalline arthritis. As clinical evidence strongly supports the observations that structural damage occurs early and permanently in RA and intervention slows the progression of damage, a rapid referral to a rheumatologist when RA is suspected is recommended. In order to identify early disease, referral recommendation has been developed to help primary care physicians. Patients with any of the following criteria should be referred to the rheumatologist [14]:

- $\geq$3 swollen joints;
- metatarsophalangeal/metacarpophalangeal involvement;
- morning stiffness $\geq$ 30 min.

If the first key point is an early diagnosis, the second one is to identify the predictive factors of disease outcomes [15]. In the last years, different predictive models have been developed to identify in a very early stage of inflammatory arthritis those patients that will develop a persistent and/or erosive RA [16] and will need a more aggressive treatment.

In these models the presence of ACPA and the disease duration at the time of diagnosis have been identified as independent risk factors for the development of erosive RA and of persistent synovitis; particularly, the ACPA positivity is significantly linked to RA diagnosis [17].

As recommended by the ACR, a periodic measurement of disease activity with validated indices to evaluate disease activity and response to the therapy is mandatory [18]. The composite disease activity indices such as DAS28 (Disease Activity Score 28 joints), SDAI (Simplified Disease Activity Index 28 joints) and CDAI (Clinical Disease Activity Index 28 joints), allow the rheumatologist to define the arthritis activity discriminating between low, moderate and high disease activity [19] (**Tables 1** and **2**).

The earlier inflammatory arthritis is detected and treated, better the long-term outcome in terms of damage and function is obtained. Further benefit is shown with regular monitoring of disease activity and rapid therapeutic escalation to gain disease control. Sensitive measures are therefore required for the assessment and monitoring of treatment in early arthritis.

As for imaging, the X-ray examination is still the first choice in the evaluation of erosive damage; however, even though it is highly specific, its sensitivity is low.

Patients that showed bone erosions in early stage of

Table 1. Clinimetric index in RA.

Elements	SDAI	CDAI	DAS28
Number of swollen joints	Simple count (0 - 28)	Simple count (0 - 28)	Simple count, square root Transformed
Number of tender joints	Simple count (0 - 28)	Simple count (0 - 28)	Simple count, square root Transformed
Acute phase reactants	CRP in mg/dL (0.1 - 10.0)	-	ESR, log transformed
Patient global health	-	-	VAS in mm
Patient global disease activity	VAS in cm (0 - 10.0)	VAS in cm (0 - 10.0)	-
Evaluator global disease activity	VAS in cm (0 - 10.0)	VAS in cm (0 - 10.0)	-
Total index	No immediate scoring due to CRP; simple possible	Immediate scoring possible; simple calculation possible	No immediate scoring due to ESR; calculator required

Legend: CRP (creactive protein), ESR (erithrocyte sedimentation rate), VAS (visual analogue scale), DAS28 (disease activity score 28 joints), SDAI (simplified disease activity index 28 joints), and CDAI (clinical disease activity index 28 joints).

Table 2. Instruments to measure rheumatoid arthritis disease activity and to define remission.

Instruments	Thresholds of disease activity levels
Disease activity score in 28 joints (DAS 28) (range 0 - 9.4)	Remission: <2.6 Low activity: ≥2.6 to <3.2 Moderate activity: ≥3.2 to ≤5.1 High activity: >5.1
Clinical disease activity index (CDAI) (range 0 - 76.0)	Remission: ≤2.8 Low activity: >2.8 to 10.0 Moderate activity: >10.0 to 22.0 High activity: >22
Simplified disease activity index (SDAI) (range 0 - 86.0)	Remission: ≤3.3 Low activity: >3.3 to ≤11.0 Moderate activity: >11.0 to ≤26 High activity: >26

disease detected by X-ray (Rapid Radiological Progression-PRP) have a worst outcome and need of early and aggressive treatment.

It has been demonstrated that RRP, defined as an increase of 5 or more points in radiological scores such as Sharp/van der Heijde score (SHS) in the first year of treatment, is associated with worst functional ability in later and more radiological damage progression in long term follow-up. Thus, RRP in the first year of treatment is an independent predictor of later functional disability, and represents not only a radiologically but also a clinically relevant early outcome helpful to define the initial choice of treatment [20].

This may mean that, as earlier studies have shown, patients with a low risk of RRP require less intensive initial therapy to prevent radiological damage progression than patients with a high risk [21,22].

Magneting Resonance Imaging (MRI) is shown to perform better than conventional radiology to identify articular alterations in RA patients, particularly bone edema, precursor of erosions, as early as after 4 weeks from the

onset of symptoms [23] and gives 65% of sensitivity and 82.5% of specificity [24].

Muscoloskeletal ultrasound (MSUS) is cheaper and more accessible even if it is dependent on examiner and the reproducibility should be improved. It allows to identify the presence of synovitis, structural abnormalities of tendons, ligaments, entheses and bone alteration such as erosions before they can be detected by conventional X-ray examination [25]. Moreover through power Doppler (PD) it is possible to visualize the vascularity of the synovium that is linked to the presence of an active synovitis [26, 27]. It has been recently shown a bigger sensitivity of MSUS compared with clinical examination in identifying articular inflammation in "early undifferentiated arthritis" (earlyUA) patients with evidence of sub-clinical disease in 64% of patients [28]. Although further studies are required to assess the value of MRI and MSUS in the differential diagnosis of early arthritis, the findings of erosions and synovitis are useful in clinical practice to confirm suspected cases of RA. Furthermore, the detection of erosions and synovitis/PD signal on MSUS have a prognostic value and may be used to guide the choice of treatment strategies. Whilst MRI has been used as a monitoring tool in early arthritis, further research is ongoing for the standardisation of US as an outcome measure in response to treatment.

The importance of early diagnosis in RA patients is linked to the evidence of a better prognosis in patients treated in the early stage of the disease.

It has also been demonstrated that steroids therapy, started within the first 12 weeks shows clinical remission in a significant number of patients within 6 months [29] and that the therapy with Disease modifying anti-rheumatic drugs (DMARDs) is efficacy in 50% of patients if started within 12 weeks compared with 15% of patients if started after 20 weeks from the beginning of disease [30].

A recent meta-analysis carried out in 1133 RA patients with disease duration of less than 2 years, has shown that an average delay of 9 months in the treatment with DMARDs is associated with an increase of radiological progression [31].

5. Conclusions

As highlighted in this review, a key point of RA diagnosis is today represented by an early detection of patients at risk of a severe disease progression. Due to the complexity of disease, only the contemporary assessment of clinical features, laboratory tests and imaging findings can suggest the prognosis of each patient and drive the therapeutic approach. Early referral to rheumatologist is required when physicians suspect an inflammatory arthritis. Nowadays we have a diagnostic tool to diagnose early RA, even if it is can be improved.

The risk stratification allows to select patients who may need a more aggressive therapy since the earlier stage of the disease. Aim of the targeted therapy is to achieve a complete remission or, at least, a low disease activity as defined by clinimetric indices, early in the course of the disease and to warrant a clinical improvement at short and long term and a better quality of life.

REFERENCES

[1] M. C. Wick, S. Lindblad, L. Klareskog and R. F. van Vollenhoven, "Relationship between Inflammation and Joint Destruction in Early Rheumatoid Arthritis: A Mathematical Description," *Annals of the Rheumatic Diseases*, Vol. 63, No. 7, 2004, pp. 848-852. doi:10.1136/ard.2003.015172

[2] A. J. MacGregor, "Classification Criteria for Rheumatoid Arthritis," *Bailliere's Clinical Rheumatology*, Vol. 9, No. 2, 1995, pp. 287-304. doi:10.1016/S0950-3579(05)80191-8

[3] M. P. van der Linden, R. Knevel, T. W. Huizinga and A. H. M. van der Helm-van, "Classification of Rheumatoid Arthritis: Comparison of the 1987 American College of Rheumatology Criteria and the 2010 American College of Rheumatology/European League against Rheumatism Criteria," *Arthritis & Rheumatism*, Vol. 63, No. 1, 2011, pp. 37-42. doi:10.1002/art.30100

[4] D. Aletaha, T. Neogi, A. J. Silman, *et al.*, "2010 Rheumatoid Arthritis Classification Criteria: An American College of Rheumatology/European League against Rheumatism Collaborative Initiative," *Annals of the Rheumatic Diseases*, Vol. 69, No. 9, 2010, pp. 1580-1588. doi:10.1136/ard.2010.138461

[5] Y. Kaneko, M. Kuwana, H. Kameda and T. Takeuchi, "Sensitivity and Specificity of 2010 Rheumatoid Arthritis Classification Criteria," *Rheumatology*, Vol. 50, No. 7, 2011, pp. 1268-1274. doi:10.1093/rheumatology/keq442

[6] A. F. Mourão, *et al.*, "Markers of Progression to Rheumatoid Arthritis: Discriminative Value of the New ACR/EULAR Rheumatoid Arthritis Criteria in a Portuguese Population with Early Polyarthritis," *Acta Reumatologica Portuguesa*, Vol. 36, No. 4, 2011, pp. 370-376.

[7] H. Kokkonen, *et al.*, "Antibodies of IgG, IgA and IgM Isotypes against Cyclic Citrullinated Peptide Precede the Development of Rheumatoid Arthritis," *Arthritis Research & Therapy*, Vol. 13, No. 1, 2011, p. R13. doi:10.1186/ar3237

[8] D. Aletaha, F. Alasti and J. S. Smolen, "Rheumatoid Factor Determines Structural Progression of Rheumatoid Arthritis Dependent and Independent of Disease Activity," *Annals of Rheumatic Diseases*, 2012.

[9] C. Alessandri, R. Priori, M. Modesti, R. Mancini and G. Valesini, "The Role of Anti-Cyclic Cytrullinate Antibodies Testing in Rheumatoid Arthritis," *Clinic Reviews in Allergy & Immunology*, Vol. 34, No. 1, 2008, pp. 45-49. doi:10.1007/s12016-007-8023-4

[10] L. A. van de Stadt, M. H. de Koning, R. J. van de Stadt, G. Wolbink, B. A. Dijkmans, *et al.*, "Development of the Anti-Citrullinated Protein Antibody Repertoire Prior to the Onset of Rheumatoid Arthritis," *Arthritis & Rheumatism*, Vol. 63, No. 11, 2011, pp. 3226-3233. doi:10.1002/art.30537

[11] V. P. Bykerk and J. M. Hazes, "When Does Rheumatoid Arthritis Start and Can It Be Stopped before It Does?" *Annals of the Rheumatic Diseases*, Vol. 69, No. 3, 2010, pp. 473-475. doi:10.1136/ard.2009.116020

[12] J. Nam, B. Combe and P. Emery, "Early Arthiritis: Diagnosis and Management," *Eular On-Line Course on Rheumatic Diseases*, Module 13-2007-2009 EULAR.

[13] S. Bosello, A. L. Fedele, G. Peluso, E. Gremese, B. Tolusso and G. Ferraccioli, "Very Early Rheumatoid Arthritis Is the Major Predictor of Major Outcomes: Clinical ACR Remissionand Radiographic Non-Progression," *Annals of the Rheumatic Diseases*, Vol. 70, No. 7, 2011, pp. 1292-1295. doi:10.1136/ard.2010.142729

[14] P. Emerty, "Evidence Supporting the Benefit of Early Interventionin Rheumatoid Arthritis," *Journal of Rheumatology*, Vol. 66, 2002, pp. 3-8.

[15] P. G. Conaghan, "Predicting Outcomes in Rheumatoid Arthritis," *Clinical Rheumatology*, Vol. 30, No. 1, 2011, pp. 41-47. doi:10.1007/s10067-010-1639-4

[16] H. Visser, S. le Cessie, K. Vos, F. C. Breedveld and J. M. Hazes, "How to Diagnose Rheumatoid Arthritis Early: A Prediction Model for Persistent (Erosive) Arthritis," *Arthritis & Rheumatism*, Vol. 46, No. 2, 2002, pp. 357-365. doi:10.1002/art.10117

[17] M. Schoels, C. Bombardier and D. J. Aletaha, "Diagnostic and Prognostic Value of Antibodies and Soluble Biomarkers in Undifferentiated Peripheral Inflammatory Arthritis: A Systematic Review," *The Journal of Rheumatology*, Vol. 87, 2011, pp. 20-25. doi:10.3899/jrheum.101070

[18] J. Anderson, L. Caplan, J. Yazdany, M. L. Robbins, T. Neogi, K. Michaud, K. G. Saag, J. R. O'Dell and S. Kazi, "Rheumatoid Arthritis Disease Activity Measures: American College of Rheumatology Recommendations for Use in Clinical Practice," *Arthritis Care & Research*, Vol. 64, No. 5, 2012, pp. 640-647. doi:10.1002/acr.21649

[19] C. Gaujoux-Viala, G. Mouterde, A. Baillet, P. Claudepierre, B. Fautrel, X. Le Loët and J. F. Maillefert, "Evaluating Disease Activity in Rheumatoid Arthritis: Which

Composite Index Is Best? A Systematic Literature Analysis of Studies Comparing the Psychometric Properties of the DAS, DAS28, SDAI and CDAI," *Joint Bone Spine*, Vol. 79, No. 2, 2012, pp. 149-155. doi:10.1016/j.jbspin.2011.04.008

[20] M. van den Broek, L. Dirven, J. K. de Vries-Bouwstra, A. J. Dehpoor, Y. P. Goekoop-Ruiterman, A. H. Gerards, P. J. Kerstens, T. W. Huizinga, W. Lems and C. F. Allaart, "Rapid Radiological Progression in the First Year of Early Rheumatoid Arthritis Is Predictive of Disability and Joint Damage Progression during 8 Years of Follow-Up," *Annals of the Rheumatic Diseases*, Vol. 71, No. 9, 2012, pp. 1530-1533. doi:10.1136/annrheumdis-2011-201212

[21] N. Vastesaeger, S. Xu, D. Aletaha, *et al.*, "A Pilot Risk Model for the Prediction of Rapid Radiographic Progression in Rheumatoid Arthritis," *Rheumatology*, Vol. 48, No. 9, 2009, pp. 1114-1121. doi:10.1093/rheumatology/kep155

[22] K. Visser, Y. P. Goekoop-Ruiterman, J. K. de Vries-Bouwstra, *et al.*, "A Matrix Risk Model for the Prediction of Rapid Radiographic Progression in Patients with Rheumatoid Arthritis Receiving Different Dynamic Treatment Strategies: Post Hoc Analyses from the BeSt Study," *Annals of the Rheumatic Diseases*, Vol. 69, No. 7, 2010, pp. 1333-1337. doi:10.1136/ard.2009.121160

[23] D. McGonagle, *et al.*, "The Relationship between Synovitis and Bone Changes in Early Untreated Rheumatoid Arthritis: A Controlled Magnetic Resonance Imaging Study," *Arthritis & Rheumatism*, Vol. 42, No. 8, 1999, pp. 1706-1711. doi:10.1002/1529-0131(199908)42:8<1706::AID-ANR20>3.0.CO;2-Z

[24] E. Olech, J. V. Crues III, D. E. Yocum and J. T. Merrill, "Bone Marrow Edema Is the Most Specific Finding for Rheumatoid Arthritis (RA) on Noncontrast Magnetic Resonance Imaging of the Hands and Wrists: A Comparison of Patients with RA and Healthy Controls," *Journal of Rheumatology*, Vol. 37, No. 2, 2010, pp. 265-274. doi:10.3899/jrheum.090062

[25] A. Filer, *et al.*, "Utility of Ultrasound Joint Counts in the Prediction of Rheumatoid Arthritis in Patients with Very Early Synovitis," *Annals of the Rheumatic Diseases*, Vol. 70, No. 3, 2011, pp. 500-507.

[26] S. Y. Kawashiri, T. Suzuki, A. Okada, S. Yamasaki, M. Tamai, H. Nakamura, T. Origuchi, A. Mizokami, M. Uetani, K. Aoyagi, K. Eguchi and A. Kawakami, "Musculoskeletal Ultrasonography Assists the Diagnostic Performance of the 2010 Classification Criteria for Rheumatoid Arthritis," *Modern Rheumatology*, 2012. doi:10.1007/s10165-012-0628-7

[27] G. Labanauskaite and V. Sarauskas, "Correlation of Power Doppler Sonography with Vascularity of the Synovial Tissue," *Medicina*, Vol. 39, No. 5, 2003, pp. 480-483.

[28] R. J. Wakefield, M. J. Green, H. Marzo-Ortega, P. G. Conaghan, W. W. Gibbon, D. McGonagle, S. Proudman and P. Emery, "Should Oligoarthritis Be Reclassified? Ultrasound Reveals a High Prevalence of Subclinical Disease," *Annals of the Rheumatic Diseases*, Vol. 63, No. 4, 2004, pp. 382-385. doi:10.1136/ard.2003.007062

[29] M. Green, H. Marzo-Ortega, D. McGonagle, R. Wakefield, S. Proudman, P. Conaghan, J. Gooi and P. Emery, "Persistence of Mild, Early Inflammatory Arthritis: The Importance of Disease Duration, Rheumatoid Factor, and the Shared Epitope," *Arthritis & Rheumatism*, Vol. 42, No. 10, 1999, pp. 2184-2188. doi:10.1002/1529-0131(199910)42:10<2184::AID-ANR20>3.0.CO;2-2

[30] V. P. Nell, K. P. Machold, T. A. Stamm, M. Uffmann and J. S. Smolen, "Benefit of Very Early Referral and Very Early Therapy with Disease-Modifying Anti-Rheumatic Drugs in Patients with Early Rheumatoid Arthritis," *Rheumatology*, Vol. 43, No. 7, 2004, pp. 906-914. doi:10.1093/rheumatology/keh199

[31] A. Finckh, M. H. Liang, C. M. van Herckenrode and P. de Pablo, "Long-Term Impact of Early Treatment on Radiographic Progression in Rheumatoid Arthritis: A Meta-Analysis," *Arthritis Care & Research*, Vol. 55, No. 6, 2006, pp. 864-872. doi:10.1002/art.22353

17

Regulation of 11β-Hydroxysteroid Dehydrogenase Types 1 and 2 in Rheumatoid Arthritis

Christine Beyeler[1], Bernhard Dick[2], Howard A. Bird[3], Brigitte M. Frey[2*]

[1]Institute of Medical Education, Department of Rheumatology, Clinical Immunology and Allergology, University Hospital of Berne, Berne, Switzerland; [2]Departments of Nephrology and Hypertension and Clinical Research, University Hospital of Berne, Berne, Switzerland; [3]Academic Department of Musculoskeletal Medicine, University of Leeds, Leeds, UK.
Email: *brigitte.frey@dkf.unibe.ch

ABSTRACT

Objective: The sequential activities of the 11β-hydroxysteroid dehydrogenase enzymes type 1 and 2 have not been investigated so far in patients suffering from rheumatoid arthritis before and after starting treatment though the enzymes balancing cortisol and cortisone levels are involved in regulating various inflammatory diseases. **Methods:** In a retrospective study, a panel of 41 urinary steroid metabolites has been analysed in a group of 18 patients with active rheumatoid arthritis (RA) as they were brought under control with disease modifying drugs. **Results:** No major changes were found in a variety of androgen, oestrogen and progesterone metabolites, however the ratio of THF + 5αTHF/THE as an index of 11β-HSD1 oxidative activity demonstrated down-regulation with modification correlating significantly with change in acute phase reactants as the disease came under control. These findings were supported by a tendency of a reduced ratio of F/E, an index of 11β-HSD2 oxidative activity, resulting in a significant correlation of the two ratios ($p < 0.001$). This parallelism of the two enzymes with functions of clinical laboratory parameters during drug-induced improvement of the disease is novel. **Conclusions:** Urinary steroid metabolites, which alter with disease activity, may provide further insight into the mechanisms by which stress can modify arthritis through hormones.

Keywords: Rheumatoid Arthritis; Basic Clinical Scienc; Hormones; Inflammation; Biomarkers

1. Introduction

11β-hydroxysteroid dehydrogenase (11β-HSD) enzymes type 1 and 2 convert cortisol into receptor inactive cortisone and vice versa (type 1 only). The type 2 isoform, mainly localised in the distal tubule of the kidney, inactivates cortisol to cortisone in a unidirectional manner, while 11β-HSD type 1, mainly localised in the liver, acts bi-directionally and can therefore restore cortisone to active cortisol. The balance between serum cortisol and cortisone is altered during the acute phase response in inflammatory disease, with a shift towards active cortisol [1]. Thus there is evidence that 11β-HSD enzymes play an important role in the modulation of systemic availability of cortisol during acute illness [2,3].

This mechanism may also be relevant for non-inflammatory diseases. Hypothalamic regulation of adiposity is partly mediated through 11β-HSD raising the relevance of this pathway to inflammatory conditions that may be hormonally influenced, such as rheumatoid disease [4]. Moreover, the pathway is also sensitive to influences of various drugs. TNF-α enhances intracellular

glucocorticoid availability [5,6] and interleukin-1β activates the cortisone/cortisol shuttle [7].

11β-HSD enzymes play a pivotal role in the cardiovascular system [8] as well as asthma [9] and, in particular, ulcerative colitis, which can be associated with inflammatory arthritis [10]. Cytokines, hormones and drugs such as ACE inhibitors, furosemide and carbenoxolone act on 11β-HSD enzymes in various ways [11,12]. We have earlier studied urinary 6β-hydroxycortisol excretion in rheumatoid arthritis (RA) as part of a larger pharmacogenetic study to determine whether the activity of the cytochrome P450 isoenzyme CYP3A4 was altered by disease activity in RA [13] Urinary 6β-hydroxycortisol excretions however did not correlate with measurements of disease activity such as plasma viscosity (PV) in 21 closely monitored patients with RA. The ratio also appeared to be unaltered by disease modifying drugs being used at this time (sulphasalazine, sodium aurothiomalate and d-penicillamine) [13]. The recent demonstration that RA synovial cells might have a reduced capacity for reactivation of glucocorticoids [14] prompted us to analyze in a retrospective manner (investigation

*Corresponding author.

performed before year 2000) the urine samples stored from the original study to determine the ratio of the tetrahydro-metabolites of cortisol, THF + 5αTHF, and of cortisone, THE, as an index of 11β-HSD1 activity and the ratio of F and E as an index of 11β-HSD2 activity. We hypothesized based on own observations investigating inflammatory cytokines on steroid metabolism, that untreated inflammatory changes in rheumatoid disease down-regulate the enzyme activity while effective treatment might normalize the ratio of these metabolites [5-7].

2. Patients and Methods

Patients and disease assessments. Patients with RA (ARA criteria) [15] and disease activity sufficient to justify the use of DMARDs were recruited (PV > 1.72 mPa or Ritchie articular index (AI) > 16 or early morning stiffness [16] > 1 h) [17]. Patients with a history of or with laboratory evidence of hepatitis (excessive alcohol intake, infectious, autoimmune or storage diseases) were excluded.

Blinded to the results of steroid metabolites patients were allocated either to sulphasalazine (SASP), sodium aurothiomalate (gold) or d-penicillamine (DPA) according to clinical criteria by the investigating physician. Standard dosage regimens were used [18]. Dosage adjustments, due to toxicity, and concomitant drug therapy, particularly drugs potentially interfering with 11β-HSD activities, were meticulously recorded. Whenever possible the concomitant drug therapy remained constant throughout the study. No patient received systemic steroid therapy or intra articular steroid injections during the three months before the investigation.

At 0, 12 and 24 weeks disease activity of RA and safety of the DMARD treatments were assessed as reported earlier [13,18]. With each clinic visit a 24 h urine collection was obtained. Urinary aliquots were stored at –20°C.

Ethical committee approval was obtained from the Ethics Committee of the Leeds Western Health Authority. All patients gave informed consent.

Laboratory tests. Analysis of urinary steroid metabolites was performed by gas chromatography-mass spectrometry as previously described [19]. Briefly, urine samples were pre-extracted, enzymatic hydrolysed, extracted from the hydrolysis mixture, derivatised and gel filtrated. Medroxyprogesterone was added as a recovery standard. The samples extracted on Sep-Pak C18 columns (Waters Corporation, Milford, Massachusetts USA) were hydrolysed with sulfatase (Sigma-Chemical, St. Louis, Missouri USA) and β-glucuronidase/arylsulfatase (Roche Diagnostics, Rotkreuz, Switzerland). The resulting free steroids were extracted once more on a Sep-Pak C18 cartridge and a mixture of 5α-androstane-3α, 17α-

diol, stigmasterol, cholesteryl butyrate, and 3β5β-tetrahydroaldosterone added as internal standards. Samples were derivatised to form methyloxime-trimethylsilyl ethers. After adding 100 μl of methoxyamine HCl in pyridine (Pierce Biotechnology, Rockford, Illinois USA) the extracts were heated at 60°C for one hour. Then pyridine was evaporated and 100 μl of trimethylsilylimidazole (TMSI) (Pierce) added to form trimethylsilyl ethers. The derivatisation was carried out at 100°C for 16 hours. The derivatives were purified by gel filtration on Lipidex-5000 columns (Perkin Elmer, Boston, Massachusetts USA). Samples were analysed on a gas chromatograph 6890N equipped with an autoinjector 7683a and mass selective detector 5973 (Agilent Technologies, La Jolla, CA USA) by selective ion monitoring (SIM). One characteristic ion was chosen for each compound being measured. Derivatised steroids were analyzed using a temperature-programmed run (210°C - 265°C) over 35-min on a HP-1 MS column (15 m, 0.25 mm I.D., 0.25 μm film thickness) (Agilent). Calibration was performed on a regular basis. Each "ion-peak" abundance was quantified using the corresponding ion-peak of the internal standard stigmasterol. 3α5β-tetrahydroaldosterone was quantified using 3β5β-tetrahydroaldosterone.

Statistical analysis. Statistical analyses included median, interquartile range (IQR) and Wilcoxon matched pair test for differences between paired observations. Linear correlation coefficients (r) were calculated where appropriate. The significance level was set at p = 0.05 with two-sided testing. PV was considered as the primary reference parameter of disease activity. The power to detect difference between week 0 and week 24 was calculated to be 1.000 (albumin), 0.9306 (platelets), 0.8286 (PV), 0.5949 [8] 0.5444, (THF + 5αTHF/THE), 0.3062 (CRP), 0.2602 [16] and 0.0606 (γGT), respectively) [20].

3. Results

Eighteen patients, 1 male and 17 females, suffering from RA of at least 6 months duration (median 11 yr; IQR 7 - 20) were studied. Eight patients were positive for rheumatoid factor, 5 for antinuclear factor and 12 presented extra-articular manifestations, in particular rheumatoid nodules and keratoconjunctivitis. The median age was 58 yrs (IQR 53 - 68) and median weight 59 kg (IQR 53 - 72). Median blood pressure was 140/80 mmHg (IQR 120/70 to 150/85 mmHg). The median creatinine clearance was 60 ml/min/1.73 m^2 at week 0 with no significant change over the 24 weeks period. Five patients were smoking 5 - 30 cigarettes/day (median 20 cigarettes), while 13 patients were non-smokers. Three patients were drinking alcohol > 70 g/week, five patients ≤ 70 g/week and 10 patients denied alcohol consumption. In the past eleven out of the 18 patients (61%) had been treated with a drug regimen conventional at this time, namely DMARD (DPA (n = 3), gold (n = 2), SASP (n = 2), hydroxy-chloroquine (HCQ) (n = 2), auranofin (n = 1) and meth-otrexate (MTX) (n = 1). All 11 patients started a different DMARD allowing a treatment interval of at least three months for gold, one month for MTX and one week for the remainder.

At the beginning of the study all 18 patients were al-located to a new regimen of DMARD treatment. Eight patients were started on gold, 5 on SASP and 5 on DPA. No patient was given furosemide, a known inhibitor of 11β-HSD2 [11]. One patient was taking hydrochlorothi-azide 25 mg/day from week 0 to 24, a questionable in-hibitor of 11β-HSD2 [21]. All other drugs used, such as non-steroidal anti-inflammatory drugs, analgesics, other diuretics, β-blockers, were not reported to influence 11β-HSD2. One patient was taking quinalbarbitone 100 mg/day from week 0 to 24, a well-established inducer of cytochrome P450. Eight patients were given substrates of the CYP3A4 isoenzyme that might influence the 6β-OHC output, such as nifedipine (one patient taking 80 mg/day from week 0 to 24), codeine (one patient taking 24 mg/day at week 12 and one 48 mg/day and 32 mg/day at week 12 and 24 respectively) and dihydrocodeine (two

patients taking between 20 and 40 mg/day from week 0 to 24, one patient with 30 mg/day at week 12, one patient with 120 mg/day at week 0 and, finally, one with 120 mg/day and 60 mg/day at week 12 and 24 respectively). All other drugs used were judged unlikely to influence the CYP3A4 isoenzyme.

Over the 24 weeks period disease activity of RA de-creased significantly (median PV week 0 = 1.85 mPa (IQR 1.76 - 1.90), week 12 = 1.77 (IQR 1.71 - 1.89), week 24 = 1.77 (1.66 - 1.84), $p < 0.01$; median AI week 0 = 24 (IQR 17 - 29), week 12 = 15 (10 - 23), week 24 = 11 (IQR 6 - 23), $p < 0.02$, respectively). Concurrently, significant changes from baseline were found for plate-lets (decrease), haemoglobin (increase), albumin (in-crease), globulins (decrease), IgG, IgA, IgM (decrease), but not for CRP, γGT, leucocytes, lymphocyte count, C3, C4 and EMS (data not shown). No significant changes of urinary steroid metabolite excretion (median values) were detected over the observed time periods (**Tables 1** and **2**) and all urinary steroid levels were in the normal range. Over the same time period the ratio of the tetrahy-dro-metabolites THF + 5αTHF/THE, an index of 11β-HSD1 activity, decreased significantly (median week 0 =

Table 1. Sequential data of urinary sex steroid metabolites (µg/24h). Median and Interquartile range (IQR) of RA patients (n = 18) before (urine 1), 12 (urine 2) and 24 (urine 3) weeks after treatment are given.

METABOLITES	URINE 1 µg/24h			URINE 2 µg/24h			URINE 3 µg/24h		
	IGR			IGR			IGR		
	MEDIAN	LOW	HIGH	MEDIAN	LOW	HIGH	MEDIAN	LOW	HIGH
ANDROGEN									
ANDROSTERONE (AN)	451.2	276.8	784.6	409.3	339.9	658.5	450.4	298.7	602.2
ETIOCHOLANOLONE (ET)	618.6	388.8	912.2	558.6	357.4	978.2	592.0	387.4	1139.7
ANDROSTENEDIOL	92.5	68.3	111.9	67.3	56.3	112.6	67.9	54.6	89.6
11-OXO-ETIOCHOLANOLONE	239.3	106.4	315.0	146.6	99.5	212.0	176.6	130.6	235.8
11β-HYDROXY ANDROSTERONE	594.7	221.5	708.8	468.2	341.9	605.1	468.6	300.8	727.2
11β-HYDROXY ETIOCHOLANOLONE	361.4	122.3	401.2	178.9	107.2	291.7	161.8	103.2	277.6
DEHYDROEPIANDROSTERONE	147.8	56.5	442.1	65.0	29.2	220.4	100.9	33.2	197.4
5-ANDROSTENE-$3\beta,17\beta$-DIOL	144.8	60.2	187.2	86.5	63.8	97.4	70.5	53.0	135.8
16α-HYDROXY-DHEA	201.4	102.2	289.5	107.3	64.1	193.5	145.6	51.7	340.5
5-ANDROSTENE-$3\beta,16\alpha,17\beta$ TRIOL	184.2	136.0	280.7	187.1	104.8	315.7	207.0	108.7	354.7
5-PREGNENE-$3\beta, 16\alpha,17\beta$ TRIOL	117.4	55.2	143.4	87.6	50.0	133.8	108.1	49.5	192.7
TESTOSTERONE	8.0	5.1	18.9	8.8	6.4	14.1	8.7	4.7	12.5
5α-DIHYDROTESTOSTERONE	6.9	2.8	8.9	7.1	3.6	8.7	5.4	3.4	6.1
ESTROGEN									
ESTRIOL	1.6	1.3	2.8	1.9	1.4	2.3	1.9	0.8	4.6
17β-ESTRADIOL	0.8	0.4	3.1	1.4	0.4	2.1	1.7	0.3	4.2
PROGESTERONE									
17-HYDROXYPREGNANOLONE (17HP)	38.1	21.8	45.5	34.7	15.1	52.8	31.7	22.4	48.7
PREGNANEDIOL	134.7	91.2	231.7	80.2	63.2	146.8	128.6	62.1	307.7
PREGNANETRIOL [34]	254.8	166.2	452.6	233.1	145.9	330.4	291.4	147.6	582.6
11-OXO-PREGNANETRIOL (PTONE)	10.1	6.6	14.7	8.1	5.0	13.0	8.7	5.0	18.7

Table 2. Sequential data of urinary glucocorticosteroid and mineralocorticosteroid metabolites (μg/24h). Median and Interquartile range (IQR) of RA patients (n = 18) before (urine 1), 12 (urine 2) and 24 (urine 3) weeks after treatment are given.

METABOLITES	Urine 1 μg/24h IGR			Urine 2 μg/24h IGR			Urine 3 μg/24h IGR		
	Median	Low	High	Median	Low	High	Median	Low	High
CORTISOL									
Cortisone (E)	76.3	42.8	141.8	83.2	68.6	92.8	91.2	52.8	108.5
Tetrahydrocortisone [28]	2662.9	2234.1	3065.2	2478.9	1855.9	3503.3	3325.7	1732.6	4183.5
α-Cortolone	782.9	528.3	1041.1	786.1	611.8	992.5	800.3	484.7	1337.9
β-Cortolone	253.7	194.6	314.2	239.3	164.6	369.5	196.8	152.3	440.4
20α-Dihydrocortisone	7.8	5.3	14.0	8.1	6.0	10.1	8.3	4.7	10.9
20β-Dihydrocortisone	34.5	22.5	47.6	37.1	28.3	50.4	38.9	22.9	52.9
Tetrahydrocortisol (THF)	2087.9	1374.0	2210.5	1626.7	1324.2	2274.1	1813.6	996.4	2833.3
5α-Tetrahydrocortisol (5α-THF)	731.9	404.6	886.3	619.3	462.3	931.9	624.3	462.7	1059.3
α-Cortol	292.1	223.0	420.3	290.4	220.6	441.7	250.7	170.7	469.1
β-Cortol	321.4	201.9	429.6	264.8	207.4	469.2	272.4	192.9	532.3
20α-Dihydrocortisol	27.0	18.0	74.3	35.8	25.2	55.6	32.5	18.6	43.9
20β-Dihydrocortisol	160.9	120.8	188.5	114.2	110.1	147.2	98.1	86.4	115.3
6β-Hydroxycortisol	27.0	12.0	50.3	36.6	17.4	42.4	44.2	13.8	51.2
18-Hydroxycortisol	128.8	81.2	256.9	76.4	54.8	123.9	135.7	107.4	163.6
Totalt F metabolites	4775.4	3609.0	6647.3	5853.2	4046.0	8768.7	6389.1	4919.3	8727.0
CORTICOSTERONE									
TetrahydroDOC (THDOC)	4.8	3.4	11.3	4.0	2.7	8.2	5.6	3.5	10.5
Tetrahydro-11-dehydrocorticosterone (THA)	95.3	73.8	127.2	85.2	55.7	96.5	80.8	54.2	122.1
Tetrahydrocorticosterone (THB)	177.4	114.6	250.2	158.3	99.3	179.2	137.5	82.8	223.2
5α-Tetrahydrocorticosterone, (5α-THB)	184.6	102.1	277.6	181.7	138.7	240.4	181.7	122.4	256.7
18-Hydroxytetrahydro-compound A (18-OH-THA)	65.3	25.1	175.0	46.8	30.9	90.7	46.6	19.4	66.8
11-DEOXYCORTISOL									
Tetrahydrosubstance S (THS)	58.5	34.5	70.2	52.0	31.7	83.9	63.0	43.8	82.6
ALDOSTERONE									
Tetrahydroaldosterone	19.2	12.7	30.6	12.9	10.6	18.3	14.0	10.8	26.6

1.05 (IQR 0.91-1.25), median week 12 = 0.91 (IQR 0.83 - 1.05), median week 24 = 0.85 (IQR 0.77 - 1.17) (**Table 3** and **Figure 1**, $p < 0.05$). Similarly, the ratios of cortoles/cortolones and 11OH-andro + 11OH-etio/11oxo-etio indicated a slightly impaired oxidative activity of 11β-HSD1 (**Figure 1**, $p < 0.05$). Likewise, a tendency, but not significant changes of the 11β-HSD2 and 5α/5β reductase activities were observed (**Figure 1**). Overall a significant correlation of the oxidative activities of the two 11β-HSD enzymes was obtained (**Figure 2**, $p < 0.001$).

Importantly correlations between the ratios of cortisol to cortisone metabolites, (THF + 5aTHF/THE) and F/E as index markers of the activities of 11β-HSD1 and 2, re-

spectively, [22,23], and various clinical and laboratory parameters of disease activity were found (**Figures 3** and **4**). These correlations present evidence, that the enzyme activities are regulated by the disease activity (**Figures 3** and **4**). The ratios are correlating significantly with the PV ($r = 0.482$ and 0.452, $p < 0.001$ for both), platelets ($r = 0.426$ and 0.513, $p < 0.01$ and $p < 0.001$) and albumin ($r = 0.348$ and 0.504, $p < 0.05$ and $p < 0.001$) (**Figures 3** and **4**), CRP ($r = 0.560$ and 0.606, $p < 0.001$ for both), γGT ($r = 0.496$ and 0.564 $p < 0.001$ for both) (data not given). Correlations however with clinical parameters such as AI ($r = 0.010$ and 0.040, ns for both) (**Figures 3** and **4**) and EMS ($r = 0.386$ and 0.254, $p < 0.01$ and ns) (data not given) were less prominent. In addition, a weak

Table 3. Enzyme activities. Median and Interquartile range (IQR) of RA patients (n = 18) before (urine 1), 12 (urine 2) and 24 (urine 3) weeks after treatment are given.

Enzyme Activity	Urine 1			Urine 2			Urine 3		
	IGR			IGR			IGR		
	Median	Low	High	Median	Low	High	Median	Low	High
21-HYDROXYLASE									
17HP/(THE + THF + 5αTHF)	0.008	0.005	0.009	0.005	0.004	0.008	0.005	0.004	0.009
PT/(THE + THF + 5αTHF)	0.051	0.033	0.080	0.053	0.033	0.076	0.054	0.038	0.095
100 × PT'ONE/(THE + THF + 5αTHF)	0.189	0.100	0.263	0.189	0.136	0.199	0.178	0.111	0.330
17-HYDROXYLASE									
(THA + THB + 5αTHB)/(THE + THF + 5αTHF)	0.086	0.073	0.108	0.079	0.065	0.093	0.077	0.064	0.095
(THA + THB + 5αTHB)/(AN + ET)	0.378	0.259	0.617	0.414	0.257	0.550	0.345	0.255	0.550
100 × THDOC/(THE + THF + 5αTHF)	0.111	0.069	0.208	0.105	0.071	0.296	0.094	0.074	0.374
11-HYDROXYLASE									
100 × THS/(THE + THF + 5αTHF)	1.020	0.877	1.636	0.992	0.855	1.527	0.929	0.823	1.360
100 × THDOC/(THE + THF + 5αTHF)	0.111	0.069	0.208	0.105	0.071	0.296	0.104	0.075	0.413
11β-HSD									
F/E	1.009	0.809	1.436	1.017	0.782	1.253	0.895	0.786	1.108
(THF + 5αTHF)/THE	1.049	0.907	1.251	0.906	0.828	1.047	0.854	0.766	1.167
(F + E)/(THE + THF + 5αTHF)	0.033	0.023	0.037	0.030	0.024	0.041	0.026	0.023	0.034

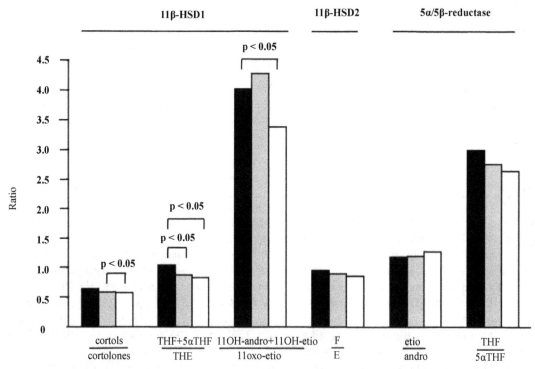

Figure 1. Urinary steroid metabolite ratios from patients with RA before and after treatment for 12 and 24 weeks. Median values of ratios representing oxidative 11β-HSD1 activity decreased significantly ($p < 0.05$) as a function of treatment time, indicating higher amounts of metabolites of the receptor inactive cortisone formed. A similar tendency was observed for 11β-HSD2 and 5α/5β-reductase activities. The median was calculated from 18 patients at week 0 (black column), week 12 (grey column) and week 24 (white column).

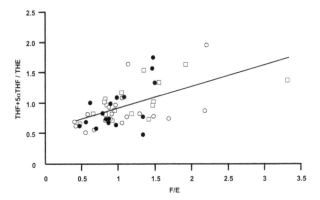

Figure 2. The oxidative activity of 11β-HSD2 correlates with the oxidative activity of 11β-HSD1. The ratios of F/E determined in urine from RA patients after 0 week (closed circle), 12 weeks (open circles) and 24 weeks (open quadrangles) treatment correlated significantly with the ratios of the tetrahydro-metabolites (p < 0.001).

correlation with creatinine clearance was observed, however not reaching significance.

There was no significant correlation with any other laboratory or demographic features studied (haemoglobin, leucocytes, lymphocytes, globulins, IgG, IgA, IgM, C3, C4, age, weight and disease duration, respectively). Notably, the ratio THF + 5αTHF/THE and F/E of the only male studied was within the range of the 17 females.

4. Discussion

To our knowledge this is the first study measuring a large panel of urinary steroid metabolites prospectively in a group of patients with active RA brought under control using a regimen of disease-modifying drugs. Although there was little serial change in the majority of hormones and their metabolites, the correlation of the ratio of cortisol to cortisone tetrahydro-metabolites as an indicator of 11β-HSD1 activity rather than F/E as an indicator of 11β-HSD2 activity was significant for those acute phase reactants proposed to be the most reliable indicators of inflammation in rheumatoid disease (**Figures 1, 3** and **4**). The two ratios correlated significantly in a positive manner plotting the 3 time points of 0, 12 and 24 weeks of treatment (**Figure 2**) indicating a parallel oxidative activity of the two enzymes. In this respect we propose that RA could be added to the list of conditions where altered 11β-HSD regulation might be of pathogenetic importance.

That hormonal changes are important in the progression of rheumatoid arthritis has long been recognised. Evidence for this comes from changes occurring in rheumatoid arthritis during pregnancy [24] and circadian variation [25], presumably because of the intricate association between the hypothalamus, the endocrine system and circulating hormones [26,27]. This probably accounts

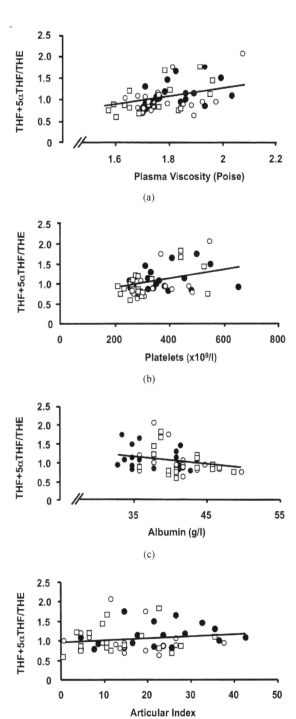

(a)

(b)

(c)

(d)

Figure 3. Correlations of the oxidative 11β-HSD1 activity expressed as the ratio THF + 5αTHF/THE and selected parameters of disease activity. Oxidative 11β-HSD1 activity was correlated to plasma viscosity ((a), p < 0.001)), platelet counts ((b), p < 0.01), plasma albumin levels ((c), p < 0.05) and articular index (d) (ns) in all patients at week 0 (closed circles), week 12 (open circles) and week 24 (open quadrangles). The normal range for plasma viscosity is <1.72 poise, for platelets $1.50 - 4.00 \times 10^{11}$/l, for albumin 37 - 49 g/l and for articular index 0.

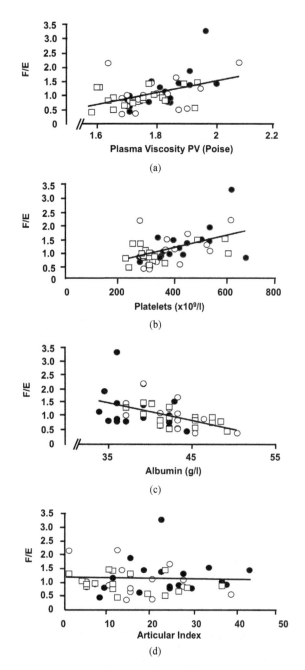

(a)

(b)

(c)

(d)

Figure 4. Correlations of the oxidative 11β-HSD2 activity expressed as the ratio F/E and selected parameters of disease activity. Oxidative 11β-HSD2 activity was correlated to plasma viscosity (a) (p < 0.001)), platelet counts; (b) (p < 0.001), plasma albumin levels; (c) (p < 0.001) and articular index; (d) (ns) in all patients at week 0 (closed circles), week 12 (open circles) and week 24 (open quadrangles). The normal range for plasma viscosity is given on Figure 3.

for diurnal variation in symptoms, particularly grip strength and tiredness, as well as disability [28]. This does not just affect rheumatoid arthritis. In polymyositis, there is a circadian variation in serum myoglobin levels [29] confirming end-organ sensitivity to hormonal change.

The last decade has seen heightened interest in diurnal

variation not just in hormones but also in cytokines. Of necessity, our results derive from an era before cytokines were manipulated as part of conventional therapy for rheumatoid arthritis. Debatably, amongst cytokines, interleukin-6 is one of those displaying most diurnal change, particularly in polymyalgia rheumatica, a rheumatic disease in which diurnal variation is arguably even more pronounced [30]. It would be of interest to repeat this study in a group of rheumatoid patients brought under control not only with TNF-α blockers but also with particular attention to any sub-group requiring the use of interleukin-6 blockade to relieve symptoms.

Surprisingly, and somehow at variance with the literature, amongst the large panel of steroids studied, androgen [14,31,32], oestrogen [16,33] and progesterone [32] metabolites did not display a change in their level as a function of treatment. In part this may be because the group was selected for need of immediate disease control, not because coming from age or gender groups in which hormones might have displayed greater influence. Neither does hormonal influence necessarily need to be mediated through metabolic pathways of disease activity. There is increasing recognition from studies of inherited abnormalities of collagen that progestogens particularly can make previously asymptomatic hyperlax joints symptomatic. If it is accepted that joint laxity exhibits a Gaussian distribution in a normal population without disease, the soil on which the seed of rheumatoid arthritis is sown may also deserve consideration.

There is also no doubting the close relationship between psychological factors and rheumatoid arthritis. Whether rheumatoid arthritis can be precipitated by a psychological event is not certain but the undoubted tiredness, intriguingly often relieved by TNF-α blockade, the undoubted variation in symptoms in some patients in relation to the menstrual cycle and the influence of stress both psychological and physical on the condition [34,35] all represent areas deserving of attention for which variation in all steroid metabolites, measured by means of a urinary test, may provide the sensitive marker we are needing.

It remains a possibility that urinary hormonal metabolite levels might act as a surrogate for monitoring disease progression. Traditionally this had been done with acute phase reactants and quantitative serology. Cytokine levels might provide more refinement but are expensive and not always available. Serial arthroscopy with synovial histology felt to represent the gold standard is invasive and expensive, even though it offers the possibility of histochemical staining demonstrating differential cytokine expression [36,37]. Complementing these existing methods of disease assessment with urinary steroid metabolite analysis might add interesting insight into the mechanisms and periodicity of this disease.

5. Acknowledgements

We thank Miss Susan Dimmock and Mr Robert Addyman for technical assistance, and Dr. Rainer Hofer for statistical advice.

6. Grant Support

This work was supported by grants from the Arthritis Research Campaign (B0132), United Kingdom; the Swiss National Foundation for Scientific Research (3100A0 102153/2 and 320000-122135/1 to B. Frey); Dr Christine Beyeler was in receipt of a Swiss National Foundation Fellowship.

REFERENCES

[1]   M. Vogeser, R. Zachoval, T. W. Felbinger and K. Jacob, "Increased Ratio of Serum Cortisol to Cortisone in Acute-Phase Response," *Hormone Research*, Vol. 58, No. 4, 2002, pp. 172-175. doi:10.1159/000065486

[2]   K. E. Chapman, A. Coutinho, M. Gray, J. S. Gilmour, J. S. Savill and J. R. Seckl, "Local Amplification of Glucocorticoids by 11beta-Hydroxysteroid Dehydrogenase Type 1 and Its Role in the Inflammatory Response," *Annals of the New York Academy of Sciences*, Vol. 1088, 2006, pp. 265-273. doi:10.1196/annals.1366.030

[3]   K. Raza, R. Hardy and M. S. Cooper, "The 11beta-Hydroxysteroid Dehydrogenase Enzymes—Arbiters of the Effects of Glucocorticoids in Synovium and Bone," *Rheumatology*, Vol. 49, No. 11, 2010, pp. 2016-2023. doi:10.1093/rheumatology/keq212

[4]   Z. Hochberg, M. Friedberg, L. Yaniv, T. Bader and D. Tiosano, "Hypothalamic Regulation of Adiposity: The Role of 11beta-Hydroxysteroid Dehydrogenase Type 1," *Hormone and Metabolic Research*, Vol. 36, No. 6, 2004, pp. 365-369. doi:10.1055/s-2004-814570

[5]   C. D. Heiniger, M. K. Rochat, F. J. Frey and B. M. Frey, "TNF-Alpha Enhances Intracellular Glucocorticoid Availability," *Federation of European Biochemical Societies Letters*, Vol. 507, No. 3, 2001, pp. 351-356. doi:10.1016/S0014-5793(01)03004-6

[6]   R. M. Kostadinova, A. R. Nawrocki, F. J. Frey and B. M. Frey, "Tumor Necrosis Factor Alpha and Phorbol 12-Myristate-13-Acetate Down-Regulate Human 11beta-hydroxysteroid Dehydrogenase Type 2 through p50/p50 NF-KappaB Homodimers and Egr-1," *Federation of American Societies for Experimental Biology Journal*, Vol. 19, No. 6, 2005, pp. 650-652.

[7]   G. Escher, I. Galli, B. S. Vishwanath, B. M. Frey and F. J. Frey, "Tumor Necrosis Factor Alpha and Interleukin 1beta Enhance the Cortisone/Cortisol Shuttle," *Journal of Experimental Medicine*, Vol. 186, No. 2, 1997, pp. 189-198. doi:10.1084/jem.186.2.189

[8]   Z. Krozowski and Z. Chai, "The Role of 11beta-Hydroxysteroid Dehydrogenases in the Cardiovascular System," *Endocrinology Journal*, Vol. 50, No. 5, 2003, pp. 485-489.

[9]   B. E. Orsida, Z. S. Krozowski and E. H. Walters, "Clinical Relevance of Airway 11beta-Hydroxysteroid Dehydrogenase Type II Enzyme in Asthma," *American Journal of Respiratory Critical Care Medicine*, Vol. 165, No. 7, 2002, pp. 1010-1014.

[10] K. I. Takahashi, K. Fukushima and H. Sasano, "Type II 11beta-Hydroxysteroid Dehydrogenase Expression in Human Colonic Epithelial Cells of Inflammatory Bowel Disease," *Digestive Diseases and Sciences*, Vol. 44, No. 12, 1999, pp. 2516-2522. doi:10.1023/A:1026699324927

[11] D. Fuster, G. Escher, B. Vogt and F. J. Frey, "Furosemide Inhibits 11beta-Hydroxysteroid Dehydrogenase Type 2," *Endocrinology*, Vol. 139, No. 9, 1998, pp. 3849-3854. doi:10.1210/en.139.9.3849

[12] J. W. Tomlinson and P. M. Stewart, "Cortisol Metabolism and the Role of 11beta-Hydroxysteroid Dehydrogenase," *Best Practice & Research Clinical Endocrinology & Metabolism*, Vol. 15, No. 1, 2001, pp. 61-78. doi:10.1053/beem.2000.0119

[13] C. Beyeler, B. M. Frey and H. A. Bird, "Urinary 6 Beta-Hydroxycortisol Excretion in Rheumatoid Arthritis," *British Journal of Rheumatology*, Vol. 36, No. 1, 1997, pp. 540-558. doi:10.1093/rheumatology/36.1.54

[14] M. Schmidt, C. Weidler, H. Naumann, S. Anders, J. Scholmerich and R. H. Straub, "Reduced Capacity for the Reactivation of Glucocorticoids in Rheumatoid Arthritis Synovial Cells: Possible Role of the Sympathetic Nervous System?" *Arthritis Rheumatism*, Vol. 52, No. 6, 2005, pp. 1711-1720. doi:10.1002/art.21091

[15] F. C. Arnett, S. M. Edworthy and D. A. Bloch, "The American Rheumatism Association 1987 Revised Criteria for the Classification of Rheumatoid Arthritis," *Arthritis Rheumatism*, Vol. 31, No. 3, 1988, pp. 315-324. doi:10.1002/art.1780310302

[16] U. Islander, C. Jochems, M. K. Lagerquist, H. Forsblad-d'Elia and H. Carlsten, "Estrogens in Rheumatoid Arthritis; The Immune System and Bone," *Molecular Cellular Endocrinology*, Vol. 335, No. 1, 2011, pp. 14-29. doi:10.1016/j.mce.2010.05.018

[17] D. M. Ritchie, J. A. Boyle and J. M. McInnes, "Clinical Studies with an Articular Index for the Assessment of Joint Tenderness in Patients with Rheumatoid Arthritis," *Quaterly Journal of Medicine*, Vol. 37, No. 147, 1968, pp. 393-406.

[18] C. Beyeler, A. K. Daly, M. Armstrong, C. Astbury, H. A. Bird and J. R. Idle, "Phenotype/Genotype Relationships for the Cytochrome P450 Enzyme CYP2D6 in Rheumatoid Arthritis: Influence of Drug Therapy and Disease Activity," *Journal of Rheumatoly*, Vol. 21, No. 6, 1994, pp. 1034-1039.

[19] C. Quattropani, B. Vogt, A. Odermatt, B. Dick, B. M. Frey and F. J. Frey, "Reduced Activity of 11 Beta-Hydroxysteroid Dehydrogenase in Patients with Cholestasis," *Journal Clinical Investigation*, Vol. 108, No. 9, 2001, pp. 1299-1305.

[20] B. Kirkwood, "Essentials of Medical Statistics," Wiley-Blackwell, New York, 2003.

[21] M. L. Licketts and P. M. Stewart, "Regulation of 11Beta-Hydroxysteroid Dehydrogenase Type 2 by Diuretics and

the Renin-Angiotensin-Aldosterone Axis," *Clinical Science*, Vol. 96, No. 6, 1999, pp. 669-675.

[22] M. Quinkler, D. Zehnder and J. Lepenies, "Expression of Renal 11beta-Hydroxysteroid Dehydrogenase Type 2 Is Decreased in Patients with Impaired Renal Function," *European Journal of Endocrinology*, Vol. 153, No. 2, 2005, pp. 291-299. doi:10.1530/eje.1.01954

[23] E. A. Walker, A. Ahmed and G. G. Lavery, "11Beta-Hydroxysteroid Dehydrogenase Type 1 Regulation by Intracellular Glucose 6-Phosphate Provides Evidence for a Novel Link between Glucose Metabolism and Hypothalamo-Pituitary-Adrenal Axis Function," *Journal of Biological Chemistry*, Vol. 282, No. 37, 2007, pp. 27030-27036. doi:10.1074/jbc.M704144200

[24] B. H. Scott, "Auto-Immunity and Connective Tissue Disorders," *Oxford Medical Publications*, Oxford University Press, Oxford, 1990.

[25] M. Cutolo, B. Seriolo, C. Craviotto, C. Pizzorni and A. Sulli, "Circadian Rhythms in RA," *Annals of the Rheumatic Diseases*, Vol. 62, No. 7, 2003, pp. 593-596. doi:10.1136/ard.62.7.593

[26] A. K. Bhall, "Hormones and the Immune Response," *Annals of the Rheumatic Diseases*, Vol. 48, No. 1, 1989, pp. 1-6. doi:10.1136/ard.48.1.1

[27] B. W. Kirkham and G. S. Panayi, "Diurnal Periodicity of Cortisol Secretion, Immune Reactivity and Disease Activity in Rheumatoid Arthritis: Implications for Steroid Treatment," *British Journal of Rheumatology*, Vol. 28, No. 2, 1989, pp. 154-157. doi:10.1093/rheumatology/28.2.154

[28] N. Bellamy, R. B. Sothern, J. Campbell and W. W. Buchanan, "Circadian Rhythm in Pain, Stiffness, and Manual Dexterity in Rheumatoid Arthritis: Relation between Discomfort and Disability," *Annals of the Rheumatic Diseases*, Vol. 50, No. 4, 1991, pp. 243-248. doi:10.1136/ard.50.4.243

[29] S. Bombardieri, A. Clerico, L. Riente, M. G. Del Chicca and C. Vitali, "Circadian Variations of Serum Myoglobin Levels in Normal Subjects and Patients with Polymyositis," *Arthritis Rheumatism*, Vol. 25, No. 12, 1982, pp. 1419-1424. doi:10.1002/art.1780251205

[30] M. G. Perry, J. R. Kirwan, D. S. Jessop and L. P. Hunt, "Overnight Variations in Cortisol, Interleukin 6, Tumour Necrosis Factor Alpha and Other Cytokines in People with Rheumatoid Arthritis," *Annals of the Rheumatic Diseases*, Vol. 68, No. 1, 2009, pp. 63-68. doi:10.1136/ard.2007.086561

[31] M. Cutolo, "Androgens in Rheumatoid Arthritis: When Are They Effectors?" *Arthritis Research & Therapy*, Vol. 11, No. 5, 2009, p. 126. doi:10.1186/ar2804

[32] A. Martocchia, M. Stefanelli, S. Cola and P. Falaschi, "Sex Steroids in Autoimmune Diseases," *Current Topics in Medicinal Chemistry*, Vol. 11, No. 13, 2011, pp. 1668-1683. doi:10.2174/156802611796117595

[33] M. Cutolo, B. Villaggio, C. Craviotto, C. Pizzorni, B. Seriolo and A. Sulli, "Sex Hormones and Rheumatoid Arthritis," *Autoimmunity Reviews*, Vol. 1, No. 5, 2002, pp. 284-289. doi:10.1016/S1568-9972(02)00064-2

[34] A. Gupta and A. J. Silman, "Psychological Stress and Fibromyalgia: A Review of the Evidence Suggesting a Neuroendocrine Link," *Arthritis Research & Therapy*, Vol. 6, No. 3, 2004, pp. 98-106. doi:10.1186/ar1176

[35] R. H. Straub, F. S. Dhabhar, J. W. Bijlsma and M. Cutolo, "How Psychological Stress via Hormones and Nerve Fibers May Exacerbate Rheumatoid Arthritis," *Arthritis Rheumatism*, Vol. 52, No. 1, 2005, pp. 16-26. doi:10.1002/art.20747

[36] F. Buttgereit, H. Zhou and M. J. Seibel, "Arthritis and Endogenous Glucocorticoids: The Emerging Role of the 11Beta-HSD Enzymes," *Annals of the Rheumatic Diseases*, Vol. 67, No. 9, 2008, pp. 1201-1203. doi:10.1136/ard.2008.092502

[37] R. Hardy, E. H. Rabbitt and A. Filer, "Local and Systemic Glucocorticoid Metabolism in Inflammatory Arthritis," *Annals of the Rheumatic Diseases*, Vol. 67, No. 9, 2008, pp. 1204-1210. doi:10.1136/ard.2008.090662

18

Pain and fatigue in adult patients with rheumatoid arthritis: Association with body awareness, demographic, disease-related, emotional and psychosocial factors*

Helena Lööf[1,2#], Unn-Britt Johansson[1,2], Elisabet Welin Henriksson[3], Staffan Lindblad[4], Fredrik Saboonchi[2,5,6,7]

[1]Sophiahemmet University, Stockholm, Sweden
[2]Karolinska Institutet, Department of Clinical Sciences, Danderyd Hospital, Division of Medicine, Stockholm, Sweden
[3]Karolinska Institutet, Division of Nursing, Department of Neurobiology and Rheumatology Unit, Karolinska Hospital, Stockholm, Sweden
[4]Karolinska Institutet, Department of Learning Informatics, Management and Ethics, Stockholm, Sweden
[5]Karolinska Institutet, Department of Neuroscience, Division of Insurance Medicine, Stockholm, Sweden
[6]University of Stockholm, Stress Research Institute, Stockholm, Sweden
[7]Red Cross University College, Stockholm, Sweden
Email: [#]helena.loof@sophiahemmethogskola.se

ABSTRACT

Background: Patients and clinicians report pain and fatigue as key outcome measures in rheumatoid arthritis. Fatigue and pain are a major concern to patients. Aim: The objective of this study was to examine fatigue and pain in adult patients with rheumatoid arthritis (RA) and to investigate the association between pain and fatigue with body awareness, demographic, disease-related, emotional and psychosocial factors. Method: Data were collected from a sample of patients with RA ($n = 120$) recruited from a Rheumatology clinic in a large university hospital in Stockholm, Sweden. Eligible for inclusion were patients between 20 - 80 years of age and with a confirmed diagnosis of RA. Fatigue was measured using the Multidimensional Assessment of Fatigue (MAF) scale, while the Visual Analogue Scale (VAS) was used to assess components of pain. A multiple stepwise regression analysis was performed to evaluate factors related to fatigue and pain. In the first step a univariate analysis of variance (ANOVA) was used for all relevant independent factors. In the next step backwards stepwise regression was applied. Result: Fatigue was significantly associated with the Disease Activity Score 28-joints (DAS 28) ($p = 0.049$), the Body Awareness Questionnaire (BAQ) ($p = 0.006$), the Positive Affect (PA) scale ($p = 0.008$) and no smoking ($p = 0.021$). Pain was significantly associated with the EuroQol EQ-5D ($p = 0.008$) and the DAS 28 ($p = 0.001$). The adjusted R-square was 28.6% for fatigue and 50.0% for pain. Conclusion: This study clearly demonstrates that fatigue and pain in patients with RA appear to be associated with disease-related factors. Furthermore, fatigue was related to body awareness and emotional factors, and pain was related to health related quality of life.

Keywords: Pain; Fatigue; Emotional; Psychosocial; Rheumatoid Arthritis

1. INTRODUCTION

Clinically significant fatigue is common in patients with rheumatoid arthritis (RA) [1]. Patients with RA continue to report moderate to severe pain [2], both fatigue and pain are a major concern to patients [3,4]. Patients and clinicians report pain and fatigue as key outcome measures in RA [5,6]. Furthermore, fatigue is recommended [7] as a patient-centered outcome measure in RA. Fatigue predicts quality of life (QoL) [8] and pain impacts QoL [9]. The psychological well-being of the individual living with RA is significantly affected by the fundamental life changes and the complexity of the disease process [10,11].

*This study was supported by research grants from Sophiahemmet University and the Sophiahemmet Foundation, the MSD (Merck Sharp & Dohme, AB Sweden) and the FRS, Association of Rheumatology Nurses in Sweden.
[#]Corresponding author.

Fatigue in RA is associated with the severity of pain, disease activity, functional status [12], comorbidity, disability, multiple social roles and low social support [13-15]. Scientific support is available indicating that sex, disease duration, pain and functional status all influence fatigue in RA [15,16]. In a study [17], the authors report that pain severity, role functioning, depressive mood, self-efficacy on fatigue, helplessness, worrying and non-restorative sleep are factors most strongly associated with fatigue level. Variables described in a review [18] related to fatigue are illness related aspects, physical functioning, cognitive/emotional functioning and social environmental aspects. Some possible consequences of fatigue are psychological distress, reduced QoL and work ability.

The tendency to focus attention on bodily sensations and internal stimuli, *i.e.* body awareness [19] has been associated with an increase in both somatic and emotional distress [20]. A biopsychosocial approach has been suggested to be applicable in the study of chronic diseases in general [21] and RA in particular [22]. In such an approach psychological factors are considered not merely affected by the course of the disease but also important for the patients health and well-being [23]. RA impacts on daily life, especially when performing physical activities. In addition, it has a pronounced effect on mood and social life [24]. Negative emotionality and stress are among major psychological factors that have been associated with RA [25]. The impact of negative emotion in the context can be observed as negative influences on health behavior [26]. Furthermore, emotions have a crucial role in how people adjust to having RA, and in the context of chronic pain in general [27,28]. Negatively toned self-focused bodily attention has been linked to less effective decision-making strategies and worse adherence in patients with other chronic diseases [29].

Because many symptoms of RA (*i.e.* pain and fatigue) are generally evocative of negative emotional responses, elevated body awareness may be associated with worse perceived health. Both emotional and attention related processes in the individual occur in a social context. The objective of this study was to examine fatigue and pain in adult patients with RA and to investigate the association between pain and fatigue with body awareness, demographic, disease-related, emotional and psychosocial factors.

2. METHOD

2.1. Design

This was a cross-sectional questionnaire survey with a descriptive design.

2.2. Population

The study population consisted of a sample of 120 patients with RA attending a physician consultation at the Rheumatology clinic, Karolinska University Hospital, Sweden. Eligible for inclusion were patients aged 20 - 80 years with a confirmed diagnosis of RA according to the American College of Rheumatology (ACR) criteria for RA [30]. The patients should have been diagnosed with RA for at least a period of six months, speak and understand the Swedish language as well as read and comprehend the study instructions. Exclusion criteria were another serious disease (for example, Parkinson or Multiple sclerosis) that could significantly affect the outcome of the study.

2.3. Instrument

The Multidimensional Assessment of Fatigue (MAF) measures four dimensions of fatigue: severity, distress, degree of interference in activities of daily living, and timing. Respondents were asked to reflect on any patterns of fatigue that have occurred over the past week [16]. The Swedish version of MAF has been tested in patients with rheumatic disease (systemic sclerosis) [31].

The VAS was used to assess components of pain occurring over the past week. The patients were asked one question about pain: "*How much pain did you have during the past week because of your rheumatic disease?*" [32].

Demographic data was collected and included sex (female/male), age (year), smoking (yes or no), educational status (compulsory school, upper secondary school, higher education and other education) and marital status (single or common-law). Physical activity per week was categorized into yes = ≥7 days of physical activity per week and no = <7 days of physical activity per week. Working status was categorized into yes = working and no = not working and retired and sick leave.

Disease activity was evaluated using the Disease Activity Score 28-joints (DAS 28). A score, below 3.2 indicates low disease activity and a score above 5.1 indicates high disease activity. DAS 28 is based on erythrocyte sedimentation rate (ESR, mm/h), number of swollen ($n = 28$) and tender ($n = 28$) joints and on the patients perceived general health (VAS, 0 - 100 mm) [33].

The EuroQol, EQ-5D was used to assess components of health related QoL (HRQoL). EQ-5D includes measures related to mobility, hygiene, daily activities, pain/discomfort and anxiety/depression. The questionnaire measures preference-based HRQoL on a 0 to 1 scale, where 0 indicates the worst possible health and 1 full health [34]. It has been suggested to be a valid measure for HRQoL in RA patients [35]

The Body Awareness Questionnaire (BAQ) was used to assess components of body awareness. Higher scores indicate a higher degree of body awareness. The value of Cronbach's alpha has been reported in previous studies to be between 0.80 and 0.88 [19,36]. The Swedish validated version of the BAQ scale was used. In the Swedish version of BAQ Cronbach's alpha was 0.86 [37].

The Emotion Regulation Questionnaire (ERQ) was developed to measure the dispositional use of two specific strategies related to emotion control: reappraisal and suppression. In a previous study on these two emotion regulation processes the value of Cronbach's alpha was 0.79 for reappraisal and 0.73 for suppression [38].

The Perceived Stress Scale 4 (PSS4) was employed to assess components of perceived stress. The scale ranges from 0 - 16, with higher scores indicate of a higher degree of perceived stress. Cronbach's alpha for the Perceived Stress Scale was 0.72 [39]. In our study a Swedish version of PSS4 were included and the Cronbach's alpha was 0.82 [40].

The Positive and Negative Affect Scale (PANAS) was applied to assess components of mood. PANAS includes items relating to a positive affect (PA) domain, and to a negative affect domain (NA) domain. A higher score on the PA domain indicates greater PA, or the extent to which the individual feels enthusiastic, active and alert. A higher score on the NA domain represents a greater negative affect or the extent to which the individual feels aversive mood states and general distress. This measure has been validated in a previous study Cronbach's alpha was 0.86 to 0.90 for the PA domain and 0.84 to 0.87 for the NA domain [41]. In a Swedish study the Cronbach's alpha was 0.86 for PA and 0.85 for NA [42].

The Interview Schedule for Social Interaction (ISSI) was used to assess components of social interaction and support. The ISSI consisting of two scales: one describing the availability of deep emotional relationships and attachments, and the other describing the availability of more peripheral contacts of social networks and integration. In previous work Cronbach's alpha was 0.77 for AVSI scale and 0.80 for AVAT scale [43].

2.4. Data Collection Procedure

A rheumatologist gave verbal and written information about the study to the patients. The information about the study, and question about participation, were given to the patients after consultation with their physician. After the consultation, the patients were informed that they would receive a letter within a week containing written information about the study (together with several questionnaires and a prepaid envelope). The patients were also informed that the completed questionnaires should be returned within two weeks from date of receipt. No reminder was sent to the patients.

2.5. Statistics

Descriptive statistics presented as mean, standard deviation (SD) median, range and percentage were used toassess demographic characteristics of the patients.

To evaluate factors related to fatigue and pain multiple stepwise linear regression analyses were performed. The analyses were performed in two separate models, both performed in two steps. In the first step a univariate ANOVA was conducted on all relevant independent factors. Based on the univariate analyses of variance (ANOVA) all factors with a p-value < 0.2 were entered into the second step. In the second step a backwards stepwise regression was performed with the model selection based on the Akaike information criterion.

When the final model was obtained, the model assumptions were evaluated based on the residual diagnosis. The internal consistency (Cronbach's alpha) for the different measures in our study: 0.86 (BAQ), 0.76 (ERQ-Reappraisal), 0.68 (ERQ-Suppression), 0.90 (PA), 0.89 (NA), 0.76 (AVSI), 0.40 (AVAT) and 0.74 (PSS).

The statistical analyses have been performed in R version 2.14.1 (R Foundation for Statistical Computing, Vienna, Austria) and IBM SPSS Statistics 20 for Windows (IBM SPSS, NY, USA).

2.6. Ethical Consideration

Ethical approval was obtained from the ethics committee of the Regional Ethical Review Board (Dnr. 2010/734-32 and 2009/1795-31/3). All participants gave written informed consent. The anonymity and confidentiality of the participants were guaranteed.

3. RESULTS

3.1. Background Characteristics

In all, 120 (response rate 78%) patients with RA participated in the study; 27 (22.5%) aged <45 years, 51 (42.5%) aged 46 - 65 years and 42 (35%) aged >65 years. The majority of the patients were female (86%). Demographic data are shown in (**Table 1**).

The mean GFI score (MAF total score) was 24.48 ± 10.18 and PAIN 31.58 ± 24.16 for pain. Descriptive statistics of variables included in the univariate analysis are presented in (**Table 2**).

3.2. Univariate Analysis

The univariate analysis identified 7 of 17 independent factors with a p-value of <0.2 (no smoking, no physical activity, DAS 28, BAQ, PA, NA and PSS4) in relation to fatigue. For pain 3 of 17 were identified as significant (EQ-5D, DAS 28, PSS4). The p-values from the univariate analysis for fatigue and pain are listed in (**Table 3**).

3.3. Multiple Regression Analysis

The results from the stepwise multiple regression analy-

Table 1. Demographic characteristics.

			Total
			(*n* = 120)
Sex		*n* (%)	
	Male		17 (14.17)
	Female		103 (85.83)
Age		*n* (%)	
	<45 years		27 (22.50)
	46 - 65 years		51 (42.50)
	>65 years		42 (35.00)
Smoking		*n* (%)	
	Yes		15 (12.61)
	No		104 (87.39)
Marital status		*n* (%)	
	Single		27 (22.50)
	Common-law		93 (77.50)
Working status		*n* (%)	
	Yes		54 (45.76)
	No		39 (33.05)
	Sick leave		25 (21.19)
Educational status		*n* (%)	
	Compulsory school		32 (27)
	Upper secondary school		31 (26)
	Higher education		44 (37)
	Other education		12 (10)
Physical activity		*n* (%)	
	Yes		31 (25.83)

Table 2. Descriptive statistics of variables.

	Mean ± SD	Median	Range	Possible scores
MAF (*n* = 119)	24.48 ± 10.18	25.61	1 to 45	1 - 50
PAIN (*n* = 110)	31.58 ± 24.16	30	0 to 95	0 - 100
BAQ (*n* = 116)	70.00 ± 19.46	71.5	18 to 111	18 - 126
EQ 5D (*n* = 96)	0.78 ± 0.21	0.81	−0.1 to 1	0 - 1
DAS 28 (*n* = 117)	3.17 ± 1.25	2.96	0.68 to 6.99	0 - 10
ERQ-Reappraisal (*n* = 115)	25.77 ± 6.45	26	6 to 41	6 - 42
ERQ-Expressive Suppression (*n* = 116)	11.84 ± 4.88	12	4 to 24	4 - 28
PA (*n* = 112)	31.11 ± 7.29	31	10 to 49	10 - 50
NA (*n* = 112)	14.37 ± 6.13	12	10 to 50	10 - 50
AVSI (*n* = 120)	3.17 ± 1.96	3	0 to 6	0 - 6
AVAT (*n* = 120)	4.68 ± 1.36	5	0 to 6	0 - 6
PSS (*n* = 120)	9.25 ± 2.81	9	4 to 16	0 - 16

Table 3. *p*-values in the univariate analysis of fatigue and pain.

	Fatigue	Pain
Independent variables	*p*-value	*p*-value
Sex	0.376	0.695
Age	0.791	0.308
Smoking	0.104	0.948
Marital status	0.280	0.712
Educational status	0.747	0.051
Physical activity	0.146	0.843
EQ 5D	0.002	<0.001
DAS 28	0.002	<0.001
BAQ	0.056	0.493
ERQ-Reappraisal	0.164	0.522
ERQ-Expressive Suppression	0.807	0.972
PA	0.001	0.248
NA	0.071	0.009
AVSI	0.061	0.868
AVAT	0.033	0.721
PSS	<0.001	0.001
PAIN	0.015	-
MAF	-	0.015

Table 4. Stepwise regression to identify predictors of fatigue.

	Estimate*	95% CI	*p*-value
(Intercept)	21.07	(3.86 - 38.28)	0.017
Smoking (No)	−7.19	(−13.25 - 1.12)	0.021
Physical activity (No)	3.95	(−0.51 - 8.42)	0.082
DAS 28	1.65	(0.01 - 3.29)	0.049
BAQ	0.16	(0.05 - 0.27)	0.006
PA	−0.43	(−0.75 - 0.12)	0.008
NA	−0.27	(−0.60 - 0.07)	0.120
PSS	0.78	(−0.03 - 1.58)	0.058

Adjusted R-square = 28.6%; *Estimated = regression coefficient.

Table 5. Stepwise regression to identify predictors of pain.

	Estimate*	95 % CI	*p*-value
(Intercept)	20.36	(−14.71 - 55.43)	0.252
EQ 5D	−34.98	(−60.51 - 9.46)	0.008
DAS 28	9.32	(5.40 - 13.25)	<0.001
PSS	1.11	(−0.34 - 2.56)	0.131

Adjusted R-square = 50.0%; *Estimated = regression coefficient.

sis for fatigue shows that fatigue was significantly associated with no smoking (*p* = 0.021), DAS 28 (*p* = 0.049), BAQ (*p* = 0.006) and for PA (*p* = 0.008) (**Table 4**).

The results from the stepwise multiple regression analysis for pain shows that pain was significantly associated with the EQ-5D (*p* = 0.008) and DAS 28 (*p* = 0.001). The final models for fatigue and pain were considered acceptable (**Tables 4** and **5**).

Adjusted R-square was 28.6% for fatigue and 50.0% for pain.

4. DISCUSSION

Our study clearly demonstrates that fatigue in RA is associated with increased disease activity, increased body awareness, and decreased PA. Previous studies have confirmed that disease activity and functional status influence RA [15,16]. Psychological factors may play a crucial role in fatigue. For instance, [17] found that severity and depressive mood are factors strongly associated with fatigue level.

The tendency to focus attention on bodily sensations and internal stimuli (*i.e.* body awareness) [19] has been associated with increased somatic and emotional distress [20]. In the present study fatigue was found associated with increased body awareness. Negatively toned self-focused bodily attention has been linked to less effective decision making strategies and worse adherence [29].

The concept of body awareness, as well as its association to fatigue is therefore deserving of further research. Previous study [37] describes that body awareness may

be useful in the management of chronic disease and can be addressed in nursing.

The PA scale is a generic instrument to measure the emotional state of an individual. In the present study decreased PA in patients with RA was associated with fatigue. Previous studies have shown that PA facilitates approach behavior [44] and continued action [45] *i.e.* individuals engage more with their environment and are more willing to take part in different activities. A person with PA feels more enthusiastic, active and alert. Low PA is manifested in decreased arousal, energy and activity, as well as the absence of positive feelings (e.g., sadness, lethargy and boredom) [38]. Negative emotionality and stress are among some of the major psychological factors that have been adversely linked to RA [25]. The impact of negative emotion in this context may be viewed as either through negative influence on health behavior or through a neuroendocrine influence on immune function and health [26]. Moreover, emotions are thought to play a crucial role in the adjustment of people with RA, and in the context of chronic pain in general [21,27].

Pain is a central outcome measure in rheumatoid arthritis [2] and patients themselves have suggested that assessment and management of pain should be prioritized [11]. A study [9] showed that patients with RA, who consider their disease to be "somewhat to completely controlled", continue to report moderate to severe pain. It is therefore important to investigate all potential factors that contribute to pain. In our study pain was associated with decreased HRQoL and increased disease activity. The EQ-5D captures five health dimensions of which the area pain/discomfort is one of these dimensions. Pain/discomfort is also included in the DAS 28. The adjusted R-square value for pain (50% of the model) was fairly high in our study, suggesting that the model is of moderately to high predictive value.

In our study group 54.5% were not working or were on sick leave at the time of the study. A study [46] has shown that RA can affect QoL as well as the ability to do paid or unpaid work.

Furthermore, [47] described the importance of recording socioeconomic status in clinical trials because patients with lower socioeconomic status are more likely to experience higher disease activity, lower physical function, and poorer emotional aspects of mental health, lower QoL, and greater pain. Low level of pain, high levels of physical activity, and good lower extremity function at baseline predicted good general health perception [48]. Our study noted that low levels of pain in RA patients still had some influence on perceived health.

A biopsychosocial approach has been considered appropriate to study chronic diseases in general [21] and RA in particular [22]. According to such an approach, psychological factors are not merely affected by the course of the disease, but are also important for the patients general health and well-being [23]. To emphasize a health-oriented and salutogenic theoretical perspective the individuals health-relevant pattern of goals and expectations, social needs and resources, as well as emotions, attention, and activities needs to be addressed. In a study [18] the findings underlined the importance of targeting psychological factors to enhance HRQoL issues in the clinical management of RA patients.

The findings in our study confirm that there is an association between negative PA and fatigue, and that pain was associated with decreased HRQoL and increased disease activity. To apply the biopsychosocial approach to clinical practice, it is of importance that the clinician elict the patients history in the context of life circumstances. The clinician should also determine which aspect of biological, psychological, and social domains that is most important to understanding and promoting the patients health and well-being [49,50].

4.1. Method Discussion and Limitations

The present study has limitations. One limitation is that we did not include biological markers of RA. A second limitations concerns using a generic instrument to measure fatigue, which means we could have missed dimensions important to patients with RA. Furthermore, we have no information about the non-respondents (22%) though the response rate of 78% can be considered fairly high for this kind of study.

There are a number of problems, in inferring changes and trends over time, using a cross-sectional study [51]. This study found several factors significantly associated with fatigue, the adjusted R-square value (28.6 of the model) was moderate, suggesting that the model is of limited predictive value. In further research it is of importance to include other predictors as quality of sleep and several psychological factors [17,18] which could increase the predictive value.

The authors [18] describe that it is a need of prospective longitudinal studies to find out more about the multicausal pathways of fatigue in RA. In addition, it would also be interesting to use other methods to get a deeper understanding of pain, fatigue and body awareness in adult patients with rheumatoid arthritis. In our experience this is the first study investigating the association between fatigue, pain and body awareness.

In the present study a sample from one geographical region was used. However, the sample was demographically comparable to the sample in a population study carried out in southern Sweden [52]. Still, these results need to be interpreted with caution because of the fairly small sample size ($n = 120$).

4.2. Conclusion

In conclusion, this study shows that fatigue and pain in patients with RA appear to be associated with disease-related factors. Fatigue was also related to body awareness and emotional factors, and pain was related to health related quality of life. This relation requires further research.

4.3. Practice Implications

The tendency to focus attention on bodily sensations and internal stimuli (*i.e.* body awareness) has been associated with increased somatic and emotional distress. In the present study fatigue was found associated with increased body awareness. Negatively toned self-focused bodily attention has been linked to less effective decision-making strategies and worse adherence. In future research it is of importance to highlight and address the concept of body awareness.

5. ACKNOWLEDGEMENTS

The authors wish to thank Inga Lodin, Birgitta Nordmark, Anders Harju, and Sofia Ernestam at Karolinska University Hospital, Solna and Huddinge, Sweden, for help with the administration of this study. The authors are also grateful to Marcus Thuresson Statisticon AB for assistance with the statistical analysis.

REFERENCES

[1]   Wolfe, F., Hawley, D.J. and Wilson, K. (1996) The

prevalence and meaning of fatigue in rheumatic disease. *Journal of Rheumatology*, **23**, 1407-1417.

[2] Taylor, P., Manger, B., Alvaro-Gracia, J., Johnstone, R., Gomez-Reino, J., Eberhardt, E., Wolfe, F., Schwartzman, S., Furfaro, N. and Kavanaugh, A. (2010) A patient perceptions concerning pain management in the treatment of rheumatoid arthritis. *The Journal of International Medical Research*, **8**, 1213-1224.
doi:10.1177/147323001003800402

[3] Carr, A., Hewlett, S. and Huges, R. (2003) Rheumatology outcomes: The patient's perspective. *Journal of Rheumatology*, **30**, 880-883.

[4] Heiberg, T., Finset, A., Uhlig, T. and Kvien, T.K. (2005) Seven year changes in health status and priorities for improvement of health in patients with rheumatoid arthritis. *Annuals Rheumatic Diseases*, **64**, 191-195.
doi:10.1136/ard.2004.022699

[5] Felson, D.T., Andersson, J.J. and Boers, M. (1993) The American College of Rheumatology preliminary core set of disease activity measures for rheumatoid arthritis clinical trials. *Arthritis & Rheumatism*, **36**, 729-740.
doi:10.1002/art.1780360601

[6] Minnock, P., FitzGerald, O. and Bresnihan, B. (2003) Women with established rheumatoid arthritis perceive pain as the predominant impairment of health status. *Rheumatology*, **41**, 995-1000.
doi:10.1093/rheumatology/keg281

[7] Kirwan, J.R., Minnock, P., Adebajo, A., *et al.* (2006) Patient's perspective: Fatigue as a recommended patient centered outcome measure in rheumatoid arthritis. *Journal of Rheumatology*, **34**, 1174-1777.

[8] Rupp, I., Boshuizen, H.C., Jacobi, C.E., *et al.* (2004) Impact of fatigue on health-related quality of life in rheumatoid arthritis. *Arthritis & Rheumatism*, **51**, 578-585.
doi:10.1002/art.20539

[9] Read, E., Mc Eachern, C. and Mitchell, T. (2001) Psychological wellbeing of patients with rheumatoid arthritis. *British Journal of Nursing*, **10**, 1385-1391.

[10] Davis, R.M., Wagner, E.G. and Groves, T. (2000) Advances in managing chronic illness. *British Medical Journal*, **320**, 525-526. doi:10.1136/bmj.320.7234.525

[11] Husted, J., Gladman, D., Farewell, V. and Cook, R. (2001) Health related quality of life of patients with psoriatic arthritis: A comparison with patients with rheumatoid and arthritis. *Arthritis Care Research*, **45**, 151-158.
doi:10.1002/1529-0131(200104)45:2<151::AID-ANR168>3.0.CO;2-T

[12] Garip, Y., Eser, F., Aktenkin, L. and Bodur, H. (2011) Fatigue in rheumatoid arthritis: Association with severity of pain. Disease activity and functional status. *Acta Reumatologica Portuguesa*, **36**, 364-369.

[13] Croby, L.J. (1991) Factors which contribute to fatigue associated with rheumatoid arthritis. *Journal of Advanced Nursing*, **16**, 974-981.
doi:10.1111/j.1365-2648.1991.tb01803.x

[14] Fifield, J., Tennen, H., Reisine, S. and McQuillan, J. (1998) Depression and the long-term risk of pain, fatigue, and disability in patients with rheumatoid arthritis. *Ar-*

thritis & Rheumatism, **41**, 1851-1857.
doi:10.1002/1529-0131(199810)41:10<1851::AID-ART18>3.0.CO;2-I

[15] Huyser, B.A., Parker, J.C., Thoreson, R., Smarr, K.L., Johnson, J.C. and Hoffman, R. (1998) Predictors of subjective fatigue among individuals with rheumatoid arthritis. *Arthritis & Rheumatism*, **41**, 2230-2237.
doi:10.1002/1529-0131(199812)41:12<2230::AID-ART19>3.0.CO;2-D

[16] Belza, B.L., Henke, C.J., Yelin, E.H., Epstein, W.V. and Gilliss, C.L. (1993) Correlates of fatigue in older adults with rheumatoid arthritis. *Nursing research*, **42**, 93-99.
doi:10.1097/00006199-199303000-00006

[17] Van Hoogmoed, D., Fransen, J.J., Bleiienberg, G., *et al.* (2010) Physical and psychosocial correlates of severe fatigue in rheumatoid arthritis. *Rheumatology*, **49**, 1294-1302. doi:10.1093/rheumatology/keq043

[18] Nikolaus, S., Bode, C., Taal, E. and van de Laar, M. (2012) Which factors are related to fatigue in rheumatoid arthritis? *Annals of the Rheumatic Diseases. The EULAR Journal*, **71**, 740-741.

[19] Shields, S.A., Mallroy, M.E. and Simon, A. (1989) The body awareness questionnaire: Reliability and validity. *Journal of Personality Assessment*, **53**, 802-815.
doi:10.1207/s15327752jpa5304_16

[20] Ingram, R.E. (1990) Self-focused attention in clinical disorders: Review and conceptual model. *Psychological Bullentin*, **107**, 156-176. doi:10.1037/0033-2909.107.2.156

[21] Hamilton, N.A. and Malcarne, V.L. (2004) Cognition, emotion, and chronic illness. *Cognitive Therapy and Research*, **28**, 555-557. doi:10.1023/B:COTR.0000045564.11322.53

[22] Zautra, A.J. (2003) Comment on "Stress-vulnerabiliy factors as long-term predictors of disease activity in early rheumatoid arthritis". *Journal of Psychosomatics Research*, **55**, 303-304.
doi:10.1016/S0022-3999(03)00035-7

[23] Keefe, F.J., Smith, S.J., Buffington, A.L., Gibson, J., Studts, J.L. and Caldwell, D.S. (2002) Recent advances and future directions in the biopsychosocial assessment and treatment of arthritis. *Journal of Consulting and Clinical Psychology*, **70**, 640-655.
doi:10.1037/0022-006X.70.3.640

[24] Nyman, S.C. and Lutzen, K. (1999) Caring needs of patients with rheumatoid arthritis. *Nursing Science Quarterly*, **12**, 164-169.

[25] Dickenset, C., Jackson, J., Tomenson, B., Hay, E. and Creed, F. (2004) Association of depression and rheumatoid arthritis. *Psychosomatics*, **44**, 209-215.
doi:10.1176/appi.psy.44.3.209

[26] Kiecolt-Glaser, J.K., McGuire, L., Robles, T.F. and Glaser, R. (2002) Psychoneuroimmunology: Psychological influences on immune function and health. *Journal of Consulting and Clinical Psychology*, **70**, 537-547.
doi:10.1037/0022-006X.70.3.537

[27] Hamilton, N., Zautra, A., Alex, J. and Reich, J.W. (2005) Affect and pain in rheumatoid arthritis: Do individual differences in affective regulation and affective intensity predict emotional recovery from pain? *Annals of behavior*

Medicine, **29**, 216-224.
doi:10.1207/s15324796abm2903_8

[28] Hamilton, N.A., Karoly, P. and Kitzman, H. (2004) Self-regulation and chronic pain: The role of emotion. *Cognitive Therapy and Research*, **28**, 559-576.
doi:10.1023/B:COTR.0000045565.88145.76

[29] Christensen, A.J., Wiebe, J.S., Edwards, D.L., Micheles, J.D. and Lawton, W.J. (1996) Body consciousness, illness-related impairment, and patient adherence in hemodialysis. *Journal of Consulting Clinical Psychology*, **64**, 147-152. doi:10.1037/0022-006X.64.1.147

[30] Arnett, F.C., Edworthy, S.M. and Bloch, D.A. (American Rheumatism Association) (1987) A revised criteria for classification of rheumatoid arthritis, from 1998. *Arthritis & Rheumatism*, **31**, 315-324. doi:10.1002/art.1780310302

[31] Sandqvist, G., Archenholtz, B., Scheja, A. and Hesselstrand, R. (2011) The Swedish version of the Multidimensional Assessment of Fatigue (MAF) in systemic sclerosis: Reproducibility and correlations to other fatigue instruments. *Scandinavian Journal of Rheumatology*, **40**, 493-494. doi:10.3109/03009742.2011.605395

[32] Dixon, J.S. and Bird, H.A. (1981) Reproducibility along a 10 cm vertical visual analogue scale. *Annals of the Rheumatic Diseases*, **40**, 87-89. doi:10.1136/ard.40.1.87

[33] Prevoo, M.L., van't Hof, M.A., Kuper, H.H., van Leeuwen, M.A., van dePutte, L.B. and van Riel, P.L. (1995) Modified disease activity scores that include twenty-eight-joint counts. Development and validation in a prospective longitudinal study of patients with rheumatoid arthritis. *Arthritis & Rheumatism*, **38**, 44-48.
doi:10.1002/art.1780380107

[34] EuroQol Group (1990) EuroQol: A new facility for the measurement of health-related quality of life. *Health Policy*, **16**, 199-208. doi:10.1016/0168-8510(90)90421-9

[35] Hurst, N.P., Kind, P., Ruta, D., Hunter, M., and Stubbings, A. (1997) Measuring health-related quality of life in rheumatoid arthritis: Validity, responsiveness and reliability of EuroQol (EQ-5D). *British Journal of Rheumatology*, **36**, 551-559. doi:10.1093/rheumatology/36.5.551

[36] Baas, L.S., Berry, T.A., Allen, G., Wizer, M. and Wagoner, L.E. (2004) An exploratory study of body awareness in persons with heart failure treated medically or with transplantation. *Journal of Cardiovascular Nursing*, **19**, 32-40.

[37] Lööf, H., Johansson, U.-B., Welin Henriksson, E., Lindblad, S. and Saboonchi, F. (2012) Development and psychometric testing of the Swedish version of the body awareness questionnaire. *Journal of Advanced Nursing*.
doi:10.1111/jan.12020

[38] Gross, J.J. and John, O.P. (2003) Individual differences in two emotion regulation processes: Implications for affect, relationships, and well-being. *Journal of Personality and Social Psychology*, **85**, 348-362.
doi:10.1037/0022-3514.85.2.348

[39] Cohen, S., Kamarck, T. and Mermelstein, R. (1983) A global measure of perceived stress. *Journal of Health Social Behavior*, **24**, 385-396. doi:10.2307/2136404

[40] Eskin, M. and Parr, D. (1996) Introducing a Swedish version of an instrument measuring mental stress. Reports from the Department of Psychology, Stockholm University, Stockholm.

[41] Watson, D., Clark, L.A. and Tellegen, A. (1988) Development and validation of brief measures of positive and negative affect: The PANAS scales. *Journal of Personality and Social Psychology*, **54**, 1063-1070.
doi:10.1037/0022-3514.54.6.1063

[42] Nahlén, C. and Saboonchi, F. (2010) Coping, sense of coherence and the dimensions of affect in patients with chronic heart failure. *European Journal of Cardiovascular Nursing*. **9**, 118-125.
doi:10.1016/j.ejcnurse.2009.11.006

[43] Undén, A.L. and Orth-Gomer, K. (1989) Development of a social support instrument for use in population surveys. *Social Science and Medicine*, **29**, 1387-1392.
doi:10.1016/0277-9536(89)90240-2

[44] Davidson, R.J. (1993) The neuropsychology of emotion and affective style. In: M. Lewis and J. M. Haviland, Eds., Handbook of Emotion, Guilford Press, New York, 143-154.

[45] Carver, C.S. and Scheier, M.F. (1990) Principles of self-regulation: Action and emotion. In: E. T. Higgins and R. M. Sorrentino, Eds., *Handbook of Motivation and Cognition: Foundations of Social Behavior*, The Guilford Press, New York, 3-52.

[46] Strand, V. and Khanna, D. (2010) The impact of rheumatoid arthritis and treatment on patients' lives. *Clinical and Experimental Rheumatology*, **28**, 32-40.

[47] Harrison, M.J., Tricker, K.J., Davies, L., Hassell, A., Dawes, P., Scott, D.L., Knight, S., Davis, M., Mulherin, D. and Symmons, D.P.M. (2005) The relationship between social deprivation, disease outcome measures, and response to treatment in patients with stable, long-standing rheumatoid arthritis. *Journal of Rheumatology*, **32**, 2330-2336.

[48] Eurenius, E., Brodin, N., Lindblad, S., Opava, C., and PARA Study Group (2007) Predicting physical activity and general health perception among patients with rheumatoid arthritis. *Journal of Rheumatology*, **34**, 10-15.

[49] Engel, G.L. (1980) The clinical application of the biopsychosocial model. *American Journal of Psychiatry*, **137**, 535-544.

[50] Frankel, R.M., Quill, T.E. and McDaniel, S.H. (2003) The biopsychosocial approach: Past, present, and future. University of Rochester Press, Rochester.

[51] Polit, D.F. and Beck, C.T. (2012) Nursing research: Generating and assessing evidence for nursing practice. 9th Edition, Wolters Kluwe Health/Lippincott Williams & Wilkins, Philadelphia.

[52] Englund, M., Joud, A., Geborek, P., Felson, D.T., Jacobsson, L.T. and Petersson, I.F. (2010) Prevalence and incidence of rheumatoid arthritis in southern Sweden 2008 and their relation to prescribed biologics. *Rheumatology*, **49**, 1563-1569. doi:10.1093/rheumatology/keq127

19

Unmet Needs in the Treatment of Rheumatoid Arthritis[*]

Janet Pope[1,2], Bernard Combe[3]

[1]Schulich School of Medicine & Dentistry, University of Western Ontario, London, Canada; [2]St. Joseph's Health Care, London, Canada; [3]Department of Rheumatology, Lapeyronie Hospital, CHU Montpellier, Montpellier 1 University, Montpellier, France.
Email: janet.pope@sjhc.london.on.ca

ABSTRACT

Biologics have greatly improved the management of rheumatoid arthritis (RA), demonstrating efficacy and safety in alleviating symptoms, inhibiting bone erosion, and preventing loss of function. Unmet therapeutic needs in RA remain; however, further advances require an understanding of issues left unaddressed under the current treatment paradigm. Most biologic-naïve and biologic-pretreated patients who initiate a biologic therapy, for example, do not reach American College of Rheumatology 50% (ACR50) response, and few achieve remission. Responses are often not durable, prompting frequent treatment switching. Predictive markers are unavailable to guide therapy selection, and clinical trial data are lacking on whether a tumor necrosis factor inhibitor (TNFi) is the best first-line biologic and on the optimal sequence of use for the different biologics. Risk of serious infection is the major safety concern. Translating preclinical and clinical findings into new therapeutics may help address unmet needs. An increasing body of evidence indicates that the cytokine interleukin (IL)-17A represents an important therapeutic target; ongoing trials with IL-17A inhibitors will determine whether these agents can address some of the unmet needs associated with current biologics.

Keywords: Rheumatoid Arthritis; Biologics; Tumor Necrosis Factor Inhibitors; Unmet Need; Interleukin-17A; IL-17 Inhibitors; Treatment Challenges

1. Introduction

Rheumatoid arthritis (RA) is a chronic inflammatory disease associated with progressive joint damage, disability, and systemic complications [1]. RA has considerable interpatient variability in clinical course and severity, which may be due to genetics or environmental factors. The goal of RA treatment is clinical remission, defined by the absence of signs and symptoms of inflammation. When remission is not possible, the target should be low disease activity, particularly in patients with established disease [2]. To achieve these goals, European League Against Rheumatism (EULAR) guidelines recommend starting therapy with synthetic disease-modifying antirheumatic drugs (DMARDs) as soon as possible after diagnosis [3]. In patients with an inadequate response to synthetic DMARDs, a biologic should be added when poor prognostic features are present (*i.e.*, presence of

rheumatoid factor [RF] or anti-cyclic citrullinated peptide [anti-CCP] antibodies, high disease activity despite synthetic DMARD treatment, or early erosions), and in others after failure of more than one DMARD. The Canadian Rheumatology Association (CRA) and the American College of Rheumatology (ACR) have recently published similar treatment recommendations [4,5]. It is common practice to initiate a tumor necrosis factor inhibitor (TNFi) as the first biologic and, if this is ineffective, to switch to another TNFi or to an alternative biologic with a different mechanism of action. The reason for starting biologic therapy with a TNFi may be historical, in that TNFi agents were the first biologic class approved for RA and clinicians now have more than a decade of experience with these agents. Although the advent of biologic therapy has greatly improved RA management, there are still unmet needs. This paper reviews unmet needs with the currently available biologics and then describes an investigational approach targeting interleukin (IL)-17A, which may have the potential to address some of the challenges in the current treatment of RA.

[*]Declaration of Interest: Dr. Pope has no conflicts of interest to declare. Dr. Combe has received compensation for speaking, consultancy, and/or advisory board participation from BMS, Celgene, Merck, Novartis, Pfizer, Roche, and UCB and received grant support from Pfizer, Roche and UCB.

2. Literature Search

Areas of potential unmet needs with respect to efficacy, safety, and treatment persistence were identified based on the authors' clinical experience, and literature searches were then conducted on Medline to identify relevant articles published in English from January 2000 to June 2012. Search terms included "RA" in combination with biologic by class ("TNF blocker" or "TNF inhibitor") and by individual drug ("adalimumab", "certolizumab pegol", "etanercept", "golimumab", "infliximab", "abatacept", "rituximab", "tocilizumab") and biologic by class or individual drug in combination with "safety", "infection", "malignancy", "autoimmune", "cardiovascular", "adherence", and "persistence". The term "IL-17" was also searched, with particular attention paid to articles relevant to arthritis. Reference lists in selected articles and recent meeting abstracts were also reviewed. Preference in selecting articles was given to randomized controlled trials, meta-analyses, and large observational registries.

3. Adequacy of Responses to Current Biologics

3.1. Response Rates and Durability of Response

Biologics may be more effective than synthetic DMARDs, but a substantial proportion of patients achieve only partial responses and not remission. In randomized clinical trials, the addition of a TNFi to methotrexate (MTX) produced higher response rates than MTX alone in MTX-inadequate responders [6-9]. The TNFi-MTX combination also significantly improved other efficacy measures: disease activity as assessed by the 28-item Disease Activity Score (DAS28), tender joint counts, swollen joint counts, and C-reactive protein (CRP); function as measured by the Health Assessment Questionnaire-Disability Index (HAQ-DI); and radiographical joint damage as evaluated on serial X-rays. However, most patients treated with a TNFi plus MTX failed to achieve ACR50 or ACR70 responses or remission (**Table 1**). Radiographical analyses showed the combination slowed or arrested progressive joint damage; however, erosions usually did not heal during the observation period [10-12]. Moreover, good responses were often subsequently lost, with an estimated 20% to 25% of patients per year discontinuing treatment [13-15].

Observational registries suggest that response rates achieved in daily clinical practice may be lower than those reported in randomized clinical trials [16,17]. Several reasons may contribute to this disparity, including differences in patient selection (specific enrollment criteria versus all-comers), use of a washout period in randomized clinical trials (which may increase disease activity at baseline), differences in disease activity (real-world patients often start treatment with lower disease activity and therefore may not achieve high ACR responses), and differences in drug doses and adherence rates [18]. However, for some measures, such as HAQ-DI, the minimally important difference observed in clinical practice is smaller than that observed in randomized clinical trials, indicating that real-world patients indeed experience relevant

Table 1. Proportion of patients with inadequate response to MTX who did not meet major ACR response criteria in key phase III clinical trials of a TNFi plus MTX.

Study	Treatments	N	Assessment Time (weeks)	Percentage of Patients Who Did Not Achieve Response	
				ACR50	ACR70
ATTRACT [6]	Infliximab 3 mg/kg q8w[a] + MTX	83		73[b]	92[c]
	Infliximab 3 mg/kg q4w[a] + MTX	85		71[b]	89[c]
	Infliximab 10 mg/kg q8w[a] + MTX	85	30	69[b]	82[c]
	Infliximab 10 mg/kg q4w[a] + MTX	80		74[b]	89[c]
	Placebo + MTX	84		95	100
ARMADA [7]	Adalimumab 20 mg q2w + MTX	69		68[c]	90
	Adalimumab 40 mg q2w + MTX	67	24	45[b]	73[b]
	Adalimumab 80 mg q2w + MTX	73		58[b]	81[d]
	Placebo + MTX	62		92	95
GO-FORWARD [8]	Golimumab 50 mg q4w + MTX	89		63[b]	80[b]
	Golimumab 100 mg q4w + MTX	89	24	67[b]	85[d]
	Golimumab 100 mg q4w + Placebo	133		80	89
	Placebo + MTX	133		86	95
RAPID 2 [9]	Certolizumab pegol 200 mg q2w[e] + MTX	246		68[b]	84[c]
	Certolizumab pegol 400 mg q2w + MTX	246	24	67[b]	89[c]
	Placebo + MTX	127		97	99

ACR, American College of Rheumatology; ARMADA, Anti-TNF Research Study Program of the Monoclonal Antibody D2E7 in Patients with Rheumatoid Arthritis; ATTRACT, Anti-Tumor Necrosis Factor Trial in Rheumatoid Arthritis with Concomitant Therapy; GO-FORWARD, GOlimumab FOR Subjects With Active RA Despite MTX; MTX, methotrexate; RAPID 2, Rheumatoid Arthritis PreventIon Damage 2; TNFi, tumor necrosis factor inhibitor. [a]Patients received infliximab at the indicated dose at weeks 0, 2, and 6, and then every 4 or 8 weeks as indicated. [b]$p < 0.001$ versus placebo + MTX group. [c]$p < 0.01$. [d]$p < 0.05$. [e]Patients in this group received certolizumab pegol 400 mg at weeks 0, 2, and 4 and then 200 mg every 2 weeks.

improvement with available biologic agents [19]. When registry patients meeting clinical trial enrollment criteria are considered separately, response rates approach those achieved in the clinical trials [16,17]. Nevertheless, only a small proportion of patients in clinical practice achieve remission as defined by the new ACR/EULAR Boolean criteria [20].

Several other biologics and small molecules have emerged for RA treatment, including abatacept (a CTLA4-Fc fusion protein that modulates T-cell costimulation), rituximab (an anti-CD20 monoclonal antibody that depletes B cells), tocilizumab (an anti-IL-6 receptor monoclonal antibody), Janus kinase (JAK) inhibitors such as tofacitinib and baricitinib, and the spleen tyrosine kinase (Syk) inhibitor fostamatinib [21]. However, these agents also exhibit a ceiling for response rates, with only a minority of patients reaching ACR50 or ACR70 responses.

3.2. Switching Biologic Therapy

Patients who do not respond to a TNFi or who lose their initial response may still benefit from another TNFi, or they may respond to other biologics with different mechanisms of action. In general, ACR50 and ACR70 response rates are decreased with the next biologic after use of a TNFi. Additionally, the reason for discontinuing the initial TNFi can predict the results of the next treatment. In a meta-analysis of 19 studies, switching to a second TNFi was associated with a slightly higher ACR50 rate if the switch had been prompted by adverse events (43%) rather than by lack of efficacy (31%), although the EULAR responses were similar in both subgroups [22].

Within the TNFi class, differences in molecular structure provide a rationale for switching to a second or even a third TNFi [23]. Choices include the TNF receptor fusion protein etanercept, the chimeric anti-TNFα monoclonal antibody infliximab, the fully human anti-TNFα monoclonal antibodies adalimumab and golimumab, and the pegylated humanized anti-TNFα Fab' fragment certolizumab pegol. The benefit of switching to a second TNFi is illustrated by the golimumab in patients with active rheumatoid arthritis after treatment with TNFα inhibitors (GO-AFTER) trial, in which 461 patients with active RA who discontinued their previous TNFi were randomized to receive golimumab 50 or 100 mg subcutaneously (SC) or placebo every 4 weeks, with or without background DMARDs. Compared with placebo, golimumab significantly increased ACR50 responses at week 14 (18% versus 6%; $p < 0.001$) [24]. Fifty-one percent of the patients continued treatment for 3 years. In this subgroup, ACR50 and ACR70 response rates were 40% and 19%, respectively, at the end of the 3-year period, but it is important to recognize that these rates exclude patients who discontinued before 3 years [25].

Rituximab, tocilizumab, and abatacept, other available biologic options with distinct mechanisms of action, are often initiated following TNFi failure. The recombinant IL-1 receptor antagonist anakinra is also approved for use in RA but will not be discussed further here as it is generally less effective than other options and not recommended in EULAR guidelines as a major biologic in RA [3]. Rituximab, tocilizumab, and abatacept significantly increased response rates compared with placebo when added to background MTX in patients who had failed one or more TNFi agents. ACR20, ACR50, and ACR70 response rates at week 24 were 51% versus 18%, 27% versus 5%, and 12% versus 1%, respectively, with rituximab versus placebo (all $p < 0.001$) in the Randomized Evaluation of Long-Term Efficacy of rituximab in RA (REFLEX) trial [26]; 50% versus 10%, 29% versus 4%, and 12% versus 1%, respectively, with tocilizumab 8 mg/kg versus placebo (all $p < 0.001$) in the Research on Actemra Determining efficacy after Anti-TNF failures (RADIATE) trial [27]; and 50% versus 20%, 20% versus 4%, and 10% versus 2%, respectively, with abatacept versus placebo (all $p \leq 0.003$) in the Abatacept Trial in Treatment of Anti-TNF Inadequate Responders (ATTAIN) trial [28]. Significant improvements in other efficacy measures, including HAQ-DI, DAS28 remission, and health-related quality of life measured by SF-36 were also reported in one or more of these trials. Rituximab also showed a trend for slowing progression of radiographical damage [26].

In a recent meta-analysis, the probability of achieving an ACR50 response did not differ among golimumab, rituximab, tocilizumab, and abatacept in patients with inadequate responses to a prior TNFi (TNF-IR) [29]. As initial biologic therapy in MTX-inadequate responders, TNFi agents were significantly more likely to produce an ACR50 response than abatacept but not rituximab or tocilizumab [29]. However, the results of several recently reported trials call the latter conclusion into question, in that no differences in response rates were seen with abatacept SC compared with adalimumab in MTX-inadequate responders in the Abatacept Versus Adalimumab Comparison in Biologic-Naive rheumatoid arthritis Subjects With Background Methotrexate (AMPLE) trial [30] or between abatacept 10 mg/kg every 4 weeks and infliximab 3 mg/kg every 8 weeks in the Abatacept or infliximab versus placebo, a Trial for Tolerability, Efficacy and Safety in Treating RA (ATTEST) trial [31]. Moreover, monotherapy with tocilizumab (8 mg/kg IV every 4 weeks) was superior to monotherapy with adalimumab in patients who were intolerant of MTX or for whom continued MTX was inappropriate in the ADalimumab ACTemrA (ADACTA) study [32].

In summary, available clinical data indicate the utility of switching therapy in patients who have an inadequate response to their current agent but provide little guidance on selection of the next therapy.

4. Predictive Clinical Characteristics and Biomarkers

Predictive clinical characteristics and biomarkers are needed to help identify which agents should be used in individual patients as initial biologic therapy or following failure of TNFi therapy. Clinical and observational studies indicate that concurrent use of a synthetic DMARD (especially MTX) and nonsmoking status are predictive of better response to TNFi therapy [33-35]. Beyond that, other baseline factors associated with good response depend on the efficacy measure being evaluated. High disease activity at baseline was associated with better ACR50 and ACR70 responses, which is not unexpected given that higher baseline activity offers a greater window for showing a treatment effect [36]. In contrast, low baseline disease activity was associated with DAS28 remission rate, which is also logical given that it is much easier to produce remission when disease is less active. Numerous genetic markers, including TNFα gene polymorphisms, and protein markers, including RF and anti-CCP antibodies, have been evaluated, but to date, none has shown robust and consistent predictive value for TNFi response [36] The presence of RF and/or anti-CCP antibodies appears predictive of better responses with rituximab [37]. Other studies suggest that the reason prompting biologic switching and the number of previous biologics may influence treatment response. In the observational Swiss Clinical Quality Management RA cohort, switching to rituximab was more effective than switching to a second or third TNFi when the change in therapy was prompted by inadequate response to the initial TNFi, but switching to rituximab or to another TNFi had comparable efficacy when the switch was prompted by other reasons [38,39]. However, it is important to remember that observational studies are limited by potential patient selection and prescribing biases. Whereas rituximab may be most effective when used after zero to one TNFi, the efficacy of tocilizumab was independent of the number of previous TNFi agents in the RADIATE trial [27]. In a large Canadian observational cohort, abatacept produced similar changes in HAQ-DI as initial biologic therapy and after previous TNFi therapy; however, the durability of response to abatacept was greater when it was used as the first biologic [40].

5. Safety Profiles of Current Agents

5.1. Serious Infection

Serious infection is the most important safety concern with biologic therapy. In a meta-analysis of 160 randomized clinical trials and 46 extension studies, biologics as a group in the standard-dose model were significantly

associated with increased risk of serious infection compared with control treatment (odds ratio 1.37, 95% confidence interval [CI] 1.04 - 1.82) [41]. The risk of serious infection with the individual biologics is shown in **Figure 1**; most showed odds ratios above 1 but had 95% CIs overlapping with unity. However, recent data from several observational registries suggest that TNFi therapy (etanercept, infliximab, and adalimumab) is associated with a small but significantly increased risk of serious infection in daily clinical practice. In an analysis of the Consortium of Rheumatology Researchers in North America (CORRONA) registry involving 7971 RA patients, TNFi use tended to increase the risk of opportunistic infections (incidence rate ratio 1.67, 95% CI 0.95 - 2.94) [42]. Similarly, in the British Society for Rheumatology Biologics Register (BSRBR), involving 15,396 RA patients, TNFi therapy was associated with risk of serious infection compared with nonbiologic DMARDs (hazard ratio [HR] = 1.2, 95% CI 1.1 - 1.5); this association was most pronounced during the first 6 months of treatment (HR = 1.8, 95% CI 1.3 - 2.6) but then declined over time [43]. Finally, in the French RATIO (Recherche Axée sur la Tolérance des Biothérapies) registry, risk of nontuberculosis opportunistic infections was substantially higher with the anti-TNF monoclonal antibodies infliximab and adalimumab than with the TNF receptor fusion protein etanercept [44].

5.2. Tuberculosis Reactivation

TNFi therapy is associated with increased risk of tuberculosis due to reactivation of latent disease [45], with the anti-TNF monoclonal antibodies carrying a higher risk than etanercept [46,47]. As a result, screening for latent tuberculosis before initiation of any TNFi has become standard practice and has resulted in substantial reduction in tuberculosis risk [48]. With this practice in place,

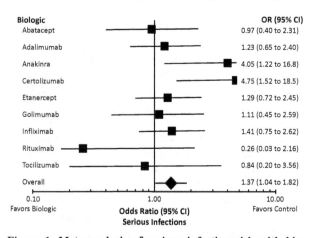

Figure 1. Meta-analysis of serious infection risk with biologics [41]. Reproduced with permission. Copyright © 2010 The Cochrane Collaboration. Published by John Wiley & Sons, Ltd.

tuberculosis risk with newer agents appears low [49,50]. Recommendations are in place for country-specific tuberculosis screening for TNFi agents, tocilizumab, and abatacept, but screening is not necessary for rituximab. TNFi agents are also associated with increased risk of nontuberculosis mycobacterial infections. These infections, which are most commonly caused by *Mycobacterium avium*, are difficult to diagnose and no screening tests for them are as yet available [51].

5.3. Malignancy

RA patients are at higher risk of certain malignancies, notably, lymphomas and lung cancer [52]. Given that the molecular targets of biologic therapy may be important in tumor surveillance and control, there is concern about increased cancer risk. Evidence supporting this concern is limited. A meta-analysis of clinical trials with infliximab and adalimumab found a higher malignancy risk, particularly with higher doses of these agents [53]. In addition, several studies suggest that TNFi therapy is associated with risk of melanoma and nonmelanoma skin cancers [54,55]. However, large meta-analyses and observational registries suggest that TNFi agents are not associated with increased risk of malignancy overall [41,55-57]. Similarly, pooled analyses of clinical trials suggest that rituximab, tocilizumab, and abatacept are not associated with increased malignancy risk in RA, although additional long-term follow-up data are needed [58-60].

Limited information is available on malignancy risk in patients with a history of cancer, because these patients were typically excluded from randomized clinical trials. The incidence of new cancers was not increased by TNFi agents compared with synthetic DMARDs in a cohort of 293 patients with prior malignancy in the BSRBR, but these findings may have been biased by the fact that patients are more likely to be selected for biologic therapy if a prior malignancy is considered to have a good prognosis [61].

5.4. Immune Reactions

TNFi agents are associated with the production of antinuclear antibodies (ANA) and, less frequently, with anti-double stranded DNA (anti-dsDNA) antibodies [62,63]. Although such antibodies have been associated with the development of systemic lupus erythematosus and other immune conditions, these events are uncommon in patients treated with TNFi agents or abatacept [64,65]. For example, 22 of 156 infliximab-treated patients (14%) developed anti-dsDNA, but only one of them had symptoms suggestive of a drug-induced lupus syndrome [62].

5.5. Cardiovascular Risk

Cardiovascular disease is common in patients with RA.

TNFα is involved in all stages of atherosclerosis, from plaque generation through plaque rupture, and may stimulate several cardiovascular risk factors, including dyslipidemia and insulin resistance [66]. Consistent with this profile, multiple observational registries and meta-analyses have shown that TNFi therapy is associated with significant reductions in risk of major cardiovascular events [67-69]. Of note, some evidence suggests that the cardiovascular benefit may be restricted to RA patients who respond to TNFi [70].

The risk of congestive heart failure (CHF) with TNFi therapy remains controversial. TNFα levels are known to be elevated in CHF patients [71], which prompted clinical trials of TNFi agents in this population. Two clinical trials of etanercept in CHF patients were stopped early, with a pooled analysis showing a small, nonsignificant trend toward increased hospitalization and mortality at higher doses [72]. Similarly, infliximab was ineffective in CHF patients, with the higher dose (10 mg/kg) associated with a significant increase in risk of mortality or CHF hospitalization [73]. However, observational studies have not convincingly shown that TNFi agents increase CHF risk in RA patients, particularly in the absence of pre-existing cardiovascular disease [69,74,75]. Nevertheless, caution appears warranted when these agents are used in RA patients with CHF.

Information about the cardiovascular risk profile of the other available biologics is limited. Evidence from long-term extension studies suggests that they do not have a beneficial or a detrimental effect on cardiovascular outcomes [66]. Differences among biologics in associated cardiovascular risk could reflect differences in underlying risk factors. For example, TNFi agents may increase total cholesterol and high-density lipoprotein (HDL) cholesterol [76], and tocilizumab raises total cholesterol and low-density lipoprotein (LDL) lipid parameters with or without increases in HDL [77,78].

6. Persistence and Adherence with Current Therapies

Despite the effectiveness of biologics, patients may discontinue treatment for a variety of reasons, including lack of efficacy, loss of treatment response, adverse events, personal preference, and achievement of remission. Treatment persistence is defined by treatment continuation for a given time period without significant gaps in treatment and/or without switching between biologics. In a recent systematic review, median drug survival across all biologics was typically between 32 and 39 months [79]. For example, median drug survival was 37 months in a cohort of 2364 patients treated initially with infliximab, etanercept, or adalimumab [80]. Median drug survival decreased with each subsequent TNFi to 21 months for the second agent and 13 months for the third agent

[80]. In the BSRBR registry, discontinuation of a TNFi due to lack of efficacy was associated with an increased rate of discontinuation of a second TNFi due to lack of efficacy [81]. Similarly, discontinuation due to toxicity from the first agent was associated with an increased rate of discontinuation of the second drug for toxicity. Persistence with abatacept averaged 26.8 months in a Canadian observational cohort and was significantly longer among biologic-naive patients than among those treated previously with TNFi therapy [40].

Whereas persistence measures drug continuation, treatment adherence reflects whether the patient takes a medication according to the prescription. Measures of adherence vary across studies, as do adherence rates. When measured as the proportion of patients with a medication possession ratio ≥ 0.8, adherence rates with TNFi agents ranged from 41% to 81% in four studies, and the mean medication possession ratio for treatment with a biologic plus MTX was 0.64 to 0.72 [79]. In general, higher rates of adherence with biologics in RA are associated with a belief in the medication's necessity for health and with lower out-of-pocket costs, whereas lower adherence is associated with concern about toxicity [82,83]. Patients who are adherent to the prescribed dosing of a TNFi seem to have a more durable response, consistent with observations relating adherence to treatment benefits in other therapeutic areas.

7. IL-17A Inhibitors: Novel Investigational Agents with Potential to Address Unmet Needs

The TNFi agents were developed at a time when RA was thought to be a Th1-mediated disease leading to the production of monocyte-/macrophage-derived cytokines, such as TNFα, IL-1β, and IL-6. In 2005, a new subset of T-helper cells, known as Th17 cells, was discovered, whose effector functions are mediated predominantly by IL-17A [84,85]. IL-17A plays a key role in host defense against extracellular bacteria and fungi; this role is distinct from the role of the Th1 pathway and its monocyte-derived cytokines in host defense against intracellular pathogens and certain fungi [86].

IL-17A is thought to play an important role in RA according to both preclinical and clinical data and therefore may be a viable therapeutic target. As shown in **Figure 2**, IL-17A is produced by multiple cell types and causes a range of biological effects culminating in joint inflammation, cartilage degradation, and bone erosion.

These effects are reproduced in experimental models associated with IL-17A overexpression [94], whereas they are blocked in IL-17A-deficient animals [95] and by the use of IL-17A inhibitors [96,97]. In RA patients, IL-17A levels are elevated in serum and synovial fluid and appear to be associated with greater disease activity

[98-101]. Moreover, IL-17A has been associated with impaired microvascular function and arterial compliance in RA and therefore may contribute to comorbid cardiovascular risk [101].

IL-17A inhibitors have been developed and evaluated in early clinical trials. Secukinumab (previously known as AIN457), a fully human IgG1α anti-IL-17A monoclonal antibody, was initially assessed in a randomized, placebo-controlled, proof-of-concept trial involving 52 RA patients on stable background MTX [102]. Administered at 10 mg/kg IV at weeks 0 and 3, secukinumab significantly improved the area under the treatment response-time curve for ACR20 ($p = 0.011$), the adjusted DAS28 score ($p = 0.027$), and the baseline-adjusted CRP level ($p = 0.002$), with effects evident by 1 week and maintained throughout the 16-week trial. Secukinumab was subsequently evaluated in a randomized, double-blind, placebo-controlled phase II trial, in which 237 RA patients with active disease despite stable MTX were allocated to monthly treatment at a dose of 25, 75, 150, or 300 mg SC [103]. Doses of 75 to 300 mg produced higher ACR20 response rates than placebo at the week 16 primary endpoint (47% - 54% versus 36%), although statistical significance was not demonstrated. Patients with ACR20 responses received the same dose of secukinumab through week 52, whereas in patients who did not show a response by week 16, the dose was escalated at week 20. For responders who remained on the 150 mg dose for the entire study, ACR20 response rates improved to 75% at week 24 and to 90% at week 52, with corresponding improvements in ACR70 response rates to 20% and 40%, respectively. Responders who remained on the 150 mg dose also had sustained improvements in DAS28-CRP and HAQ-DI. In contrast, week 16 nonresponders derived little benefit from dose escalation. Adverse events were mostly mild to moderate in severity and led to discontinuation in 6.9% of patients.

Ixekizumab (previously known as LY2439821), a humanized IgG4 anti-IL-17A monoclonal antibody, was evaluated in proof-of-concept and phase II trials. In the former, patients on one or more synthetic DMARDs received ixekizumab 0.2, 0.6, or 2 mg/kg IV at weeks 0, 2, 4, 6, and 8 [104]. Ixekizumab (all doses combined) significantly reduced DAS28 compared with placebo at week 10 (−2.3 versus −1.7; $p \leq 0.05$) and showed activity by 1 week that was maintained at the final week 16 assessment. In a subsequent phase II trial, patients on background DMARD therapy received placebo or ixekizumab at doses of 3 to 180 mg SC if naïve to biologic therapy and 80 or 180 mg SC if previously treated with a TNFi [105]. Treatment was given at weeks 0, 1, and 2 and then every other week through week 10. Ixekizumab produced an ACR70 response rate of 14% at the dose levels of 10, 30, and 180 mg in the biologic-naïve cohort

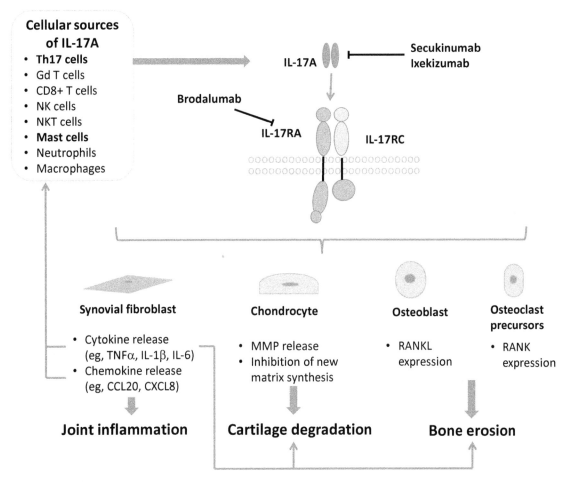

Figure 2. Role of interleukin (IL)-17A in rheumatoid arthritis (RA) pathogenesis. IL-17A is produced by Th17 cells and binds to a receptor complex consisting of IL-17RA and IL-17RC subunits on target cells [86,87]. IL-17A is also produced by cells of the innate immune system, of which mast cells may be the most important in the rheumatoid synovium [86,88-91]. IL-17A acts on synovial fibroblasts to increase chemokine and cytokine production, leading to joint inflammation, on chondrocytes to stimulate release of cartilage-degrading matrix metalloproteinases (MMPs) and block new matrix synthesis, and on osteoblasts and osteoclast precursors to stimulate expression of RANKL and RANK, respectively, leading to bone erosion. The products released promote further effects in the joint (e.g., CCL20 may promote recruitment of Th17 and dendritic cells; tumor necrosis factor (TNF)-α acts on chondrocytes and osteoclast precursors to promote joint damage) [86,92,93]. Secukinumab and ixekizumab are monoclonal antibodies directed against IL-17A, whereas brodalumab is a monoclonal antibody directed against the IL-17RA subunit.

(all $p < 0.05$ versus placebo) and 10% at a dose of 180 mg in TNFi-pretreated patients ($p = 0.11$ versus placebo). Although infection rates were slightly higher with ixekizumab than with placebo, no mycobacterial or systemic fungal infections were observed.

Brodalumab (previously AMG-827) differs mechanistically from secukinumab and ixekizumab; it is a fully human monoclonal antibody directed against IL-17RA [106], which is a subunit of the receptor through which IL-17A produces its biological effects [87,107]. IL-17RA also mediates the effects of IL-17F, another Th17 cytokine, with similar but less potent effects than IL-17A, and IL-17RA is also a subunit of the receptor for IL-17E (also known as IL-25), which may be involved in Th2-mediated eosinophil recruitment. A phase II study of

brodalumab in biologic-naïve RA patients on background MTX yielded negative results [108]. A total of 252 participants who had previously experienced an inadequate response to MTX were randomized to additional treatment with brodalumab (70, 140, or 210 mg) or placebo subcutaneously at day 1 and weeks 1, 2, 4, 6, 8, and 10. The percentage of patients who achieved ACR50 response at week 12, the primary endpoint, did not significantly differ between any brodalumab-treated group and placebo: 70 mg (16%), 140 mg (16%), 210 mg (10%), placebo (13%). Differences in ACR20 and ACR70 response were nonsignificant for any brodalumab group versus placebo. Incidences of adverse events, including serious adverse events, were similar across treatment groups.

Blocking IL-17A potentially raises the risk of infection and immune-mediated disorders, given the role of IL-17A in host defense. Several different genetic disorders have been identified that result in a deficiency of IL-17RA or IL-17F or lead to autoantibody production against IL-17A and other Th17 cytokines [109-111]. Affected patients develop chronic mucocutaneous candidiasis characterized by recurrent or persistent skin, nail, and mucosal infections caused by *Candida albicans*. Therefore, mucocutaneous candidiasis is a theoretical risk with IL-17A inhibitors, but its occurrence should require complete blockade of IL-17A function rather than the partial inhibition likely to be achieved with therapeutic doses.

8. Conclusions

Despite the treatment advances achieved with biologics, most patients do not reach ACR50 or ACR70 responses, and few actually achieve remission. Moreover, responses are often not durable, prompting frequent treatment switching. These issues are evident in both biologic-naïve and TNF-IR patients and underscore the need for new agents that allow a greater proportion of patients to reach treatment goals than currently available biologics (*i.e.*, higher rates of ACR70 response, DAS28 remission, and ACR/EULAR remission) and that produce longer-lasting responses. The new agents should ideally also improve other features of RA, such as fatigue, function, pain, joint damage, and disability.

On the basis of available data, it is difficult to know which biologic to choose, and in which order, after failure of MTX as well as after failure of a TNFi. Common practice dictates starting biologic therapy with a TNFi, but other drug classes may be perfectly acceptable alternatives, as illustrated by meta-analyses and recent clinical trial findings [29,30]. With multiple biologic options, there is a need for strong predictive biomarkers to determine which drug is most likely to be effective (and which will likely be ineffective), safe, and durable in a given individual. The fact that available biologics are not effective in all patients attests to the heterogeneity of RA and implies that the underlying pathophysiology likely varies across patients and disease stages. Seropositivity appears to predict better responses to rituximab [37], but overall, robust predictive markers for use in clinical practice remain elusive.

From a safety perspective, the risks of serious infection and malignancy are significant concerns with available biologics. Most safety data focus on the TNFi class, and specifically on the first three members that were available—etanercept, infliximab, and adalimumab. In general, the safety data from meta-analyses and observational registries suggest that TNFi agents increase the risk of serious infection and skin cancer but not that of malignancy overall. Importantly, the adoption of appropriate clinical practices, such as tuberculosis screening prior to initiating biologic therapy, has helped to reduce serious infection risk. With the newer biologics, pooled analyses of clinical trial databases provide an initial step in assessing their safety, but additional long-term data are needed to adequately define their overall safety profiles. On the basis of available safety information, there is still a need for new agents with a lower risk of serious infection, particularly for patients with certain comorbidities (e.g., diabetes, bronchiectasis, prednisone use), and a lower risk of potential immune-mediated adverse events. Given the potential cardioprotective effects of TNFi agents, it would be preferable for new agents to retain this feature, particularly because cardiovascular disease is increased in RA. However, it is unknown whether effective RA treatment is sufficient for lowering cardiovascular risk and whether intrinsic factors associated with TNFi contribute to risk reduction.

To address these unmet needs, innovation is needed to translate preclinical and clinical evidence into viable therapeutics. Along these lines, significant progress has been made in identifying IL-17A as a therapeutic target and in developing IL-17 inhibitors for RA. Early clinical trial results are as yet mixed, and further evaluation is ongoing in phase II and III studies. It is still too soon to determine whether the IL-17 inhibitors will address some of the unmet needs associated with current agents.

9. Acknowledgements

This article was supported by a grant from Novartis Pharma AG. BioScience Communications, New York, USA, provided writing and editorial assistance in the development of this manuscript, supported by Novartis Pharma AG.

REFERENCES

[1] I. B. McInnes and G. Schett, "The Pathogenesis of Rheumatoid Arthritis," *New England Journal of Medicine*, Vol. 365, No. 23, 2011, pp. 2205-2219. doi:10.1056/NEJMra1004965

[2] J. S. Smolen, D. Aletaha, J. W. Bijlsma, F. C. Breedveld, D. Boumpas, G. Burmester, *et al.*, "Treating Rheumatoid Arthritis to Target: Recommendations of an International Task Force," *Annals of the Rheumatic Diseases*, Vol. 69, No. 4, 2010, pp. 631-637. doi:10.1136/ard.2009.123919

[3] J. S. Smolen, R. Landewé, F. C. Breedveld, M. Dougados, P. Emery, C. Gaujoux-Viala, *et al.*, "EULAR Recommendations for the Management of Rheumatoid Arthritis with Synthetic and Biological Disease-Modifying Antirheumatic Drugs," *Annals of the Rheumatic Diseases*, Vol. 69, No. 6, 2010, pp. 964-975. doi:10.1136/ard.2009.126532

[4] V. P. Bykerk, P. Akhavan, G. S. Hazlewood, O. Schier, A. Dooley, B. Haraoui, *et al.*, "Canadian Rheumatology Association Recommendations for Pharmacological Man-

agement of Rheumatoid Arthritis with Traditional and Biologic Disease-Modifying Antirheumatic Drugs," *Journal of Rheumatology*, Vol. 39, No. 8, 2012, pp. 1559-1582. doi:10.3899/jrheum.110207

[5] J. A. Singh, D. E. Furst, A. Bharat, J. R. Curtis, A. F. Kavanaugh, J. M. Kremer, *et al.*, "2012 Update of the 2008 American College of Rheumatology Recommendations for the Use of Disease-Modifying Antirheumatic Drugs and Biologic Agents in the Treatment of Rheumatoid Arthritis," *Arthritis Care & Research*, Vol. 64, No. 5, 2012, pp. 625-639. doi:10.1002/acr.21641

[6] R. Maini, E. W. St. Clair, F. Breedeveld, D. Furst, J. Kalden, M. Weisman, *et al.*, "Infliximab (Chimeric Anti-Tumour Necrosis Factor Alpha Monoclonal Antibody) versus Placebo in Rheumatoid Arthritis Patients Receiving Concomitant Methotrexate: A Randomized Phase III Trial," *Lancet*, Vol. 354, No. 9194, 1999, pp. 1932-1939. doi:10.1016/S0140-6736(99)05246-0

[7] M. E. Weinblatt, E. C. Keystone, D. E. Furst, L. W. Moreland, M. H. Weisman, C. A. Birbara, *et al.*, "Adalimumab, a Fully Human Anti-Tumor Necrosis Factor α Monoclonal Antibody, for the Treatment of Rheumatoid Arthritis in Patients Taking Concomitant Methotrexate: The ARMADA Trial," *Arthritis and Rheumatism*, Vol. 48, No. 1, 2003, pp. 35-45. doi:10.1002/art.10697

[8] E. C. Keystone, M. C. Genovese, L. Klareskog, E. C. Hsia, S. T. Hall, P. C. Miranda, *et al.*, "Golimumab, a Human Antibody to Tumour Necrosis Factor α Given by Monthly Subcutaneous Injections, in Active Rheumatoid Arthritis Despite Methotrexate Therapy: The GO-FORWARD Study," Annals of the Rheumatic Diseases, Vol. 68, No. 6, 2009, pp. 789-796. doi:10.1136/ard.2008.099010

[9] J. Smolen, R. B. Landewé, P. Mease, J. Brzezicki, D. Mason, K. Luijtens, *et al.*, "Efficacy and Safety of Certolizumab Pegol plus Methotrexate in Active Rheumatoid Arthritis: The RAPID 2 Study. A Randomised Controlled Trial," *Annals of the Rheumatic Diseases*, Vol. 68, No. 6, 2009, pp. 797-804. doi:10.1136/ard.2008.101659

[10] R. N. Maini, F. C. Breedveld, J. R. Kalden, J. S. Smolen, D. Furst, M. H. Weisman, *et al.*, "Sustained Improvement over Two Years in Physical Function, Structural Damage, and Signs and Symptoms among Patients with Rheumatoid Arthritis Treated with Infliximab and Methotrexate," *Arthritis and Rheumatism*, Vol. 50, No. 4, 2004, pp. 1051-1065. doi:10.1002/art.20159

[11] E. C. Keystone, A. F. Kavanaugh, J. T. Sharp, H. Tannenbaum, Y. Hua, L. S. Teoh, *et al.*, "Radiographic, Clinical and Functional Outcomes of Treatment with Adalimumab (a Human Anti-Tumor Necrosis Factor Monoclonal Antibody) in Patients with Active Rheumatoid Arthritis Receiving Concomitant Methotrexate Therapy: A Randomized, Placebo-Controlled, 52-Week Trial," Arthritis and Rheumatism, Vol. 50, No. 5, 2004, pp. 1400-1411. doi:10.1002/art.20217

[12] E. Keystone, D. van der Heijde, D. Mason Jr., R. Landewé, R. V. Vollenhoven, B. Combe, *et al.*, "Certolizumab Pegol plus Methotrexate Is Significantly More Effective than Placebo plus Methotrexate in Active Rheumatoid Arthritis: Findings of a Fifty-Two-Week, Phase III, Multicenter, Randomized, Double-Blind, Placebo-Controlled, Parallel-Group Study," *Arthritis and Rheumatism*, Vol. 58, No. 11, 2008, pp. 3319-3329. doi:10.1002/art.23964

[13] A. Finckh, J. F. Simard, C. Gabay, P. A. Guerne and SCQM Physicians, "Evidence for Differential Acquired Drug Resistance to Anti-Tumour Necrosis Factor Agents in Rheumatoid Arthritis," *Annals of the Rheumatic Diseases*, Vol. 65, No. 6, 2006, pp. 746-752. doi:10.1136/ard.2005.045062

[14] L. Barra, J. E. Pope and M. Payne, "Real-World Anti-Tumor Necrosis Factor Treatment in Rheumatoid Arthritis, Psoriatic Arthritis, and Ankylosing Spondylitis: Cost-Effectiveness Based on Number Needed to Treat to Improve Health Assessment Questionnaire," *Journal of Rheumatology*, Vol. 36, No. 7, 2009, pp. 1421-1428. doi:10.3899/jrheum.081122

[15] J. D. Greenberg, G. Reed, D. Decktor, L. Harrold, D. Furst, A. Gibofsky, *et al.*, "A Comparative Effectiveness Study of Adalimumab, Etanercept and Infliximab in Biologically Naive and Switched Rheumatoid Arthritis Patients: Results from the US CORRONA Registry," *Annals of the Rheumatic Diseases*, Vol. 71, No. 7, 2012, pp. 1134-1142. doi:10.1136/annrheumdis-2011-150573

[16] A. Zink, A. Strangfeld, M. Schneider, P. Herzer, F. Hierse, M. Stoyanova-Scholz, *et al.*, "Effectiveness of Tumor Necrosis Factor Inhibitors in Rheumatoid Arthritis in an Observational Cohort Study: Comparison of Patients according to Their Eligibility for Major Randomized Clinical Trials," *Arthritis and Rheumatism*, Vol. 54, No. 11, 2006, pp. 3399-3407. doi:10.1002/art.22193

[17] W. Kievit, J. Fransen, A. J. Oerlemans, H. H. Kuper, M. A. van der Laar, D. J. de Rooij, *et al.*, "The Efficacy of Anti-TNF in Rheumatoid Arthritis, a Comparison between Randomised Controlled Trials and Clinical Practice," *Annals of the Rheumatic Diseases*, Vol. 66, No. 11, 2007, pp. 1473-1478. doi:10.1136/ard.2007.072447

[18] R. Caporali, F. B. Pallavicini, M. Filippini, R. Gorla, A. Marchesoni, E. G. Favalli, *et al.*, "Treatment of Rheumatoid Arthritis with Anti-TNF-Alpha Agents: A Reappraisal," *Autoimmunity Reviews*, Vol. 8, No. 3, 2009, pp. 274-280. doi:10.1016/j.autrev.2008.11.003

[19] J. E. Pope, D. Khanna, D. Norrie and J. M. Ouimet, "The Minimally Important Difference for the Health Assessment Questionnaire in Rheumatoid Arthritis Clinical Practice Is Smaller than in Randomized Controlled Trials," *Journal of Rheumatology*, Vol. 36, No. 2, 2009, pp. 254-259. doi:10.3899/jrheum.080479

[20] S. H. Shahouri, K. Michaud, T. R. Mikuls, L. Caplan, T. S. Shaver, J. D. Anderson, *et al.*, "Remission of Rheumatoid Arthritis in Clinical Practice: Application of the American College of Rheumatology/European League Against Rheumatism 2011 Remission Criteria," *Arthritis and Rheumatism*, Vol. 63, No. 11, 2011, pp. 3204-3215. doi:10.1002/art.30524

[21] M. H. Buch and P. Emery, "New Therapies in the Management of Rheumatoid Arthritis," *Current Opinion in Rheumatology*, Vol. 23, No. 3, 2011, pp. 245-251. doi:10.1097/BOR.0b013e3283454124

[22] A. Rémy, J. Avouac, L. Gossec and B. Combe, "Clinical Relevance of Switching to a Second Tumour Necrosis Factor-Alpha Inhibitor after Discontinuation of a First tumour Necrosis Factor-Alpha Inhibitor in Rheumatoid Arthritis: A Systematic Literature Review and Meta-Analysis," *Clinical and Experimental Rheumatology*, Vol. 29, No. 1, 2011, pp. 96-103.

[23] M. H. Buch, "Sequential Use of Biologic Therapy in Rheumatoid Arthritis," *Current Opinion in Rheumatology*, Vol. 22, No. 3, 2010, pp. 321-329. doi:10.1097/BOR.0b013e328337bd01

[24] J. S. Smolen, J. Kay, M. K. Doyle, R. Landewé, E. L. Matteson, J. Wollenhaupt, *et al.*, "Golimumab in Patients with Active Rheumatoid Arthritis after Treatment with Tumour Necrosis Factor Alpha Inhibitors (GO-AFTER study): A Multicentre, Randomised, Double-Blind, Placebo-Controlled, Phase III Trial," *Lancet*, Vol. 374, No. 9685, 2009, pp. 210-221. doi:10.1016/S0140-6736(09)60506-7

[25] J. S. Smolen, J. Kay, R. Landewé, N. Gaylis, J. Wollenhaupt, F. T. Murphy, *et al.*, "Golimumab in Patients with Active Rheumatoid Arthritis Who Have Previous Experience with Tumour Necrosis Factor Inhibitors: Results of a Long-Term Extension of the Randomised, Double-Blind, Placebo-Controlled GO-AFTER Study through Week 160," *Annals of the Rheumatic Diseases*, Vol. 71, No. 10, 2012, pp. 1671-1679. doi:10.1136/annrheumdis-2011-200956

[26] S. B. Cohen, P. Emery, M. W. Greenwald, M. Dougados, R. A. Furie, M. C. Genovese, *et al.*, "Rituximab for Rheumatoid Arthritis Refractory to Anti-Tumor Necrosis Factor Therapy: Results of a Multicenter, Randomized, Double-Blind, Placebo-Controlled, Phase III Trial Evaluating Primary Efficacy and Safety at Twenty-Four Weeks," *Arthritis and Rheumatism*, Vol. 54, No. 9, 2006, pp. 2793-2806. doi:10.1002/art.22025

[27] P. Emery, E. Keystone, H. P. Tony, A. Cantagrel, R. van Vollenhoven, A. Sanchez, *et al.*, "IL-6 Receptor Inhibition with Tocilizumab Improves Treatment Outcomes in Patients with Rheumatoid Arthritis Refractory to Anti-Tumour Necrosis Factor Biologicals: Results from a 24-Week Multicentre Randomised Placebo-Controlled Trial," *Annals of the Rheumatic Diseases*, Vol. 67, No. 11, 2008, pp. 1516-1523. doi:10.1136/ard.2008.092932

[28] M. C. Genovese, J. C. Becker, M. Schiff, M. Luggen, Y. Sherrer, J. Kremer, *et al.*, "Abatacept for Rheumatoid arthritis Refractory to Tumor Necrosis Factor α Inhibition," *New England Journal of Medicine*, Vol. 353, No. 11, 2005, pp. 1114-1123. doi:10.1056/NEJMoa050524

[29] C. Salliot, A. Finckh, W. Katchamart, Y. Lu, Y. Sun, C. Bombardier, *et al.*, "Indirect Comparisons of the Efficacy of Biological Antirheumatic Agents in Rheumatoid Arthritis in Patients with an Inadequate Response to Conventional Disease-Modifying Antirheumatic Drugs or to an Anti-Tumour Necrosis Factor Agent: A Meta-Analysis," *Annals of the Rheumatic Diseases*, Vol. 70, No. 2, 2011, pp. 266-271. doi:10.1136/ard.2010.132134

[30] M. Schiff, R. Fleischmann, M. Weinblatt, R. Valente, D. van der Heijde, G. Citera, *et al.*, "Abatacept sc versus Adalimumab on Background Methotrexate in RA: One Year Results from the AMPLE Study," *Annals of the Rheumatic Diseases*, Vol. 71, Suppl. 3, 2012, p. 60.

[31] M. Schiff, M. Keiserman, C. Codding, S. Songcharoen, A. Berman, S. Nayiager, *et al.*, "Efficacy and Safety of Abatacept or Infliximab vs Placebo in ATTEST: A Phase III, Multi-Centre, Randomised, Double-Blind, Placebo-Controlled Study in Patients with Rheumatoid Arthritis and an Inadequate Response to Methotrexate," *Annals of the Rheumatic Diseases*, Vol. 67, No. 8, 2008, pp. 1096-1103. doi:10.1136/ard.2007.080002

[32] C. Gabay, P. Emery, R. van Vollenhoven, A. Dikranian, R. Alten, M. Klearman, *et al.*, "Tocilizumab (TCZ) Monotherapy Is Superior to Adalimumab (ADA) Monotherapy in Reducing Disease Activity in Patients with Rheumatoid Arthritis (RA): 24-Week Data from the Phase 4 ADACTA Trial," *Annals of the Rheumatic Diseases*, Vol. 71, Suppl. 3, 2012, p. 152.

[33] K. L. Hyrich, K. D. Watson, A. J. Silman, D. P. Symmons and British Society for Rheumatology Biologics Register, "Predictors of Response to Anti-TNF-α Therapy among Patients with Rheumatoid Arthritis: Results from the British Society for Rheumatology Biologics Register," *Rheumatology*, Vol. 45, No. 12, 2006, pp. 1558-1565. doi:10.1093/rheumatology/kel149

[34] L. Mancarella, F. Bobbio-Pallavicini, F. Ceccarelli, P. C. Falappone, A. Ferrante, D. Malesci, *et al.*, "Good Clinical Response, Remission, and Predictors of Remission in Rheumatoid Arthritis Patients Treated with Tumor Necrosis Factor-Alpha Blockers: The GISEA Study," *Journal of Rheumatology*, Vol. 34, No. 8, 2007, pp. 1670-1673.

[35] L. E. Kristensen, M. C. Kapetanovic, A. Gülfe, M. Söderlin, T. Saxne and P. Geborek, "Predictors of Response to Anti-TNF Therapy according to ACR and EULAR Criteria in Patients with Established RA: Results from the South Swedish Arthritis Treatment Group Register," *Rheumatology*, Vol. 47, No. 4, 2008, pp. 495-499. doi:10.1093/rheumatology/ken002

[36] P. Emery and T. Dörner, "Optimising Treatment of Rheumatoid Arthritis: A Review of Potential Biological Markers of Response," *Annals of the Rheumatic Diseases*, Vol. 70, No. 12, 2011, pp. 2063-2070. doi:10.1136/ard.2010.148015

[37] K. Chatzidionysiou, E. Lie, E. Nasonov, G. Lukina, M. L. Hetland, U. Tarp, *et al.*, "Highest Clinical Effectiveness of Rituximab in Autoantibody-Positive Patients with Rheumatoid Arthritis and in Those for Whom No more than One Previous TNF Antagonist Has Failed: Pooled Data from 10 European Registries," *Annals of the Rheumatic Diseases*, Vol. 70, No. 9, 2011, pp. 1575-1580. doi:10.1136/ard.2010.148759

[38] A. Finckh, A. Ciurea, L. Brulhart, D. Kyburz, B. Möller, S. Dehler, *et al.*, "B Cell Depletion May Be more Effective than Switching to an Alternative Anti-Tumor Necrosis Factor Agent in Rheumatoid Arthritis Patients with Inadequate Response to Anti-Tumor Necrosis Factor Agents," *Arthritis and Rheumatism*, Vol. 56, No. 5, 2007, pp. 1417-1423. doi:10.1002/art.22520

[39] A. Finckh, A. Ciurea, L. Brulhart, B. Möller, U. A. Walker, D. Courvoiser, *et al.*, "Which Subgroup of Pa-

tients with Rheumatoid Arthritis Benefits from Switching to Rituximab versus Alternative Anti-Tumour Necrosis Factor (TNF) Agents after Previous Failure of an Anti-TNF Agent?" *Annals of the Rheumatic Diseases*, Vol. 69, No. 2, 2010, pp. 387-393. doi:10.1136/ard.2008.105064

[40] J. Pope, E. Rampakakis, J. Sampalis and O. Desjardins, "The Effectiveness of Abatacept in a Large RA Real World Practice: Changes in the HAQ over Time and Durability of Response [Abstract and Poster]," *Arthritis and Rheumatism*, Vol. 63, No. S10, 2011, pp. S476-S477.

[41] J. A. Singh, G. A. Wells, R. Christensen, E. Tajong-Ghogomu, L. Maxwell, J. K. Macdonald, *et al.*, "Adverse Effects of Biologics: A Network Meta-Analysis and Cochrane Overview," *Cochrane Database of Systematic Reviews*, Vol. 16, No. 2, 2011, Article ID: CD008794.

[42] J. D. Greenberg, G. Reed, J. M. Kremer, E. Tindall, A. Kavanaugh, C. Zheng, *et al.*, "Association of Methotrexate and Tumour Necrosis Factor Antagonists with Risk of Infectious Outcomes including Opportunistic Infections in the CORRONA Registry," *Annals of the Rheumatic Diseases*, Vol. 69, No. 2, 2010, pp. 380-386. doi:10.1136/ard.2008.089276

[43] J. B. Galloway, K. L. Hyrich, L. K. Mercer, W. G. Dixon, B. Fu, A. P. Ustianowski, *et al.*, "Anti-TNF Therapy Is Associated with an Increased Risk of Serious Infections in Patients with Rheumatoid Arthritis especially in the First 6 Months of Treatment: Updated Results from the British Society for Rheumatology Biologics Register with Special Emphasis on Risks in the Elderly," *Rheumatology (Oxford)*, Vol. 50, No. 1, 2011, pp. 124-131. doi:10.1093/rheumatology/keq242

[44] D. Salmon-Ceron, F. Tubach, O. Lortholary, O. Chosidow, S. Bretagne, N. Nicolas, *et al.*, "Drug-Specific Risk of Non-Tuberculosis Opportunistic Infections in Patients Receiving Anti-TNF Therapy Reported to the 3-Year Prospective French RATIO Registry," *Annals of the Rheumatic Diseases*, Vol. 70, No. 4, 2011, pp. 616-623. doi:10.1136/ard.2010.137422

[45] J. J. Gómez-Reino, L. Carmona, V. R. Valverde, E. M. Mola and M. D. Montero(BIOBADASER Group), "Treatment of Rheumatoid Arthritis with Tumor Necrosis Factor Inhibitors may Predispose to Significant Increase in Tuberculosis Risk: A Multicenter Active-Surveillance Report," *Arthritis and Rheumatism*, Vol. 48, No. 8, 2003, pp. 2122-2127. doi:10.1002/art.11137

[46] F. Tubach, D. Salmon, P. Ravaud, Y. Allanore, P. Goupille, M. Bréban, *et al.*, "Risk of Tuberculosis Is Higher with Anti-Tumor Necrosis Factor Monoclonal Antibody Therapy than with Soluble Tumor Necrosis Factor Receptor Therapy: The Three-Year Prospective French Research Axed on Tolerance of Biotherapies Registry," *Arthritis and Rheumatism*, Vol. 60, No. 7, 2009, pp. 1884-1894. doi:10.1002/art.24632

[47] W. G, Dixon, K. L. Hyrich, K. D. Watson, M. Lunt, J. Galloway, A. Ustianowski, *et al.*, "Drug-Specific Risk of Tuberculosis in Patients with Rheumatoid Arthritis Treated with Anti-TNF Therapy: Results from the British Society for Rheumatology Biologics Register (BSRBR)," *Annals of the Rheumatic Diseases*, Vol. 69, No. 3, 2010,

pp. 522-528. doi:10.1136/ard.2009.118935

[48] L. Carmona, J. J. Gómez-Reino, V. Rodriguez-Valverde, D. Montero, E. Pascual-Gómez, E. M. Mola, *et al.*, "Effectiveness of Recommendations to Prevent Reactivation of Latent Tuberculosis Infection in Patients Treated with Tumor Necrosis Factor Antagonists," *Arthritis and Rheumatism*, Vol. 52, No. 6, 2005, pp. 1766-1772. doi:10.1002/art.21043

[49] C, Salliot, M. Dougados and L. Gossec, "Risk of Serious Infections during Rituximab, Abatacept and Anakinra Treatments for Rheumatoid Arthritis: Meta-Analyses of Randomised Placebo-Controlled Trials," *Annals of the Rheumatic Diseases*, Vol. 68, No. 1, 2009, pp. 25-32. doi:10.1136/ard.2007.083188

[50] L. Campbell, C. Chen, S. S. Bhagat, R. A. Parker and A. J. Östör, "Risk of Adverse Events including Serious Infections in Rheumatoid Arthritis Patients Treated with Tocilizumab: A Systematic Literature Review and Meta-Analysis of Randomized Controlled Trials," *Rheumatology (Oxford)*, Vol. 50, No. 3, 2011, pp. 552-562. doi:10.1093/rheumatology/keq343

[51] K. L. Winthrop, E. Chang, S. Yamashita, M. F. Iademarco and P. A. LoBue, "Nontuberculous Mycobacteria Infections and Anti-Tumor Necrosis Factor-α Therapy," *Emerging Infectious Diseases*, Vol. 15, No. 15, 2009, pp. 1556-1561. doi:10.3201/eid1510.090310

[52] A. L. Smitten, T. A. Simon, M. C. Hochberg and S. Suissa, "A Meta-Analysis of the Incidence of Malignancy in Adult Patients with Rheumatoid Arthritis," *Arthritis Research & Therapy*, Vol. 10, No. 2, 2008, p. R45. doi:10.1186/ar2404

[53] T. Bongartz, A. J. Sutton, M. J. Sweeting, I. Buchan, E. L. Matteson and V. Montori," Anti-TNF Antibody Therapy in Rheumatoid Arthritis and the Risk of Serious Infections and Malignancies: Systematic Review and Meta-Analysis of Rare Harmful Effects in Randomized Controlled Trials," *Journal of the American Medical Association*, Vol. 295, No. 19, 2006, pp. 2275-2285. doi:10.1001/jama.295.19.2275

[54] F. Wolfe and K. Michaud, "Biologic Treatment of Rheumatoid Arthritis and the Risk of Malignancy: Analyses from a Large US Observational Study," *Arthritis and Rheumatism*, Vol. 56, No. 9, 2007, pp. 2886-2895. doi:10.1002/art.22864

[55] X. Mariette, M. Matucci-Cerinic, K. Pavelka, P. Taylor, R. van Vollenhoven, R. Heatley, *et al.*, "Malignancies Associated with Tumor Necrosis Factor Inhibitors in Registries and Prospective Observational Studies: A Systematic Review and Meta-Analysis," *Annals of the Rheumatic Diseases*, Vol. 70, No. 11, 2011, pp. 1895-1904. doi:10.1136/ard.2010.149419

[56] J. Askling, E. Baecklund, F. Granath, P. Geborek, M. Fored, C. Backlin, *et al.*, "Anti-Tumour Necrosis Factor Therapy in Rheumatoid Arthritis and Risk of Malignant Lymphomas: Relative Risks and Time Trends in the Swedish Biologics Register," *Annals of the Rheumatic Diseases*, Vol. 68, No. 5, 2009, pp. 648-653. doi:10.1136/ard.2007.085852

[57] A. E. Thompson, S. W. Rieder and J. E. Pope, "Tumor

Necrosis Factor Therapy and the Risk of Serious Infection and Malignancy in Patients with Early Rheumatoid Arthritis: A Meta-Analysis of Randomized Controlled Trials," *Arthritis and Rheumatism*, Vol. 63, No. 6, 2011, pp. 1479-1485. doi:10.1002/art.30310

[58] R. F. van Vollenhoven, P. Emery, C. O. Bingham III, E. C. Keystone, R. Fleischmann, D. E. Furst, *et al*., "Long-Term Safety of Patients Receiving Rituximab in Rheumatoid Arthritis Clinical Trials," *Journal of Rheumatology*, Vol. 37, No. 3, 2010, pp. 558-567. doi:10.3899/jrheum.090856

[59] M. H. Schiff, J. M. Kremer, A. Jahreis, E. Vernon, J. D. Isaacs and R. F. van Vollenhoven, "Integrated Safety in Tocilizumab Clinical Trials," *Arthritis Research & Therapy*, Vol. 13, No. 5, 2011, p. R141. doi:10.1186/ar3455

[60] T. A. Simon, A. L. Smitten, J. Franklin, J. Askling, D. Lacaille, F. Wolfe, *et al*., "Malignancies in the Rheumatoid Arthritis Abatacept Clinical Development Programme: An Epidemiological Assessment," *Annals of the Rheumatic Diseases*, Vol. 68, No. 12, 2009, pp. 1819-1826. doi:10.1136/ard.2008.097527

[61] W. G. Dixon, K. D. Watson, M. Lunt, L. K. Mercer, K. L. Hyrich, D. P Symmons, *et al*., "Influence of Anti-Tumor Necrosis Factor Therapy on Cancer Incidence in Patients with Rheumatoid Arthritis Who Have Had a Prior Malignancy: Results from the British Society for Rheumatology Biologics Register," *Arthritis Care & Research*, Vol. 62, No. 6, 2010, pp. 755-763. doi:10.1002/acr.20129

[62] P. J. Charles, R. J. Smeenk, J. De Jong, M. Feldmann and R. N. Maini, "Assessment of Antibodies to Double-Stranded DNA Induced in Rheumatoid Arthritis Patients Following Treatment with Infliximab, a Monoclonal Antibody to Tumor Necrosis Factor α: Findings In Open-Label and Randomized Placebo-Controlled Trials," *Arthritis and Rheumatism*, Vol. 43, No. 11, 2000, pp. 2383-2390. doi:10.1002/1529-0131(200011)43:11<2383::AID-ANR2>3.0.CO;2-D

[63] F. Atzeni, M. Turiel, F. Capsoni, A. Doria, P. Meroni and P. Sarzi-Puttini, "Autoimmunity and Anti-TNF-α Agents," *Annals of the New York Academy of Science*, Vol. 1051, 2005, pp. 559-569. doi:10.1196/annals.1361.100

[64] H. Bacquet-Deschryver, F. Jouen, M. Quillard, J. F. Ménard, V. Goëb, T. Lequerré, *et al*., "Impact of Three Anti-TNFα Biologics on Existing and Emergent Autoimmunity in Rheumatoid Arthritis and Spondylarthropathy Patients," *Journal of Clinical Immunology*, Vol. 28, No. 5, 2008, pp. 445-455. doi:10.1007/s10875-008-9214-3

[65] J. Sibilia and R. Westhovens, "Safety of T-cell Co-Stimulation Modulation with Abatacept in Patients with Rheumatoid Arthritis," *Clinical and Experimental Rheumatology*, Vol. 25, No. S5, 2007, pp. S46-S56.

[66] J. D. Greenberg, V. Furer and M. E. Farkouh, "Cardiovascular Safety of Biologic Therapies for the Treatment of RA," *Nature Reviews. Rheumatology*, Vol. 8, No. 1, 2012, pp. 13-21.

[67] C, Barnabe, B. J. Martin and W. A. Ghali, "Systematic Review and Meta-Analysis: Anti-Tumor Necrosis Factor

α Therapy and Cardiovascular Events in Rheumatoid Arthritis," *Arthritis Care & Research*, Vol. 63, No. 4, 2011, pp. 522-529. doi:10.1002/acr.20371

[68] J. D. Greenberg, J. M. Kremer, J. R. Curtis, M. C. Hochberg, G. Reed, P. Tsao, *et al*., "Tumour Necrosis Factor Antagonist Use and Associated Risk Reduction of Cardiovascular Events among Patients with Rheumatoid Arthritis," *Annals of the Rheumatic Diseases*, Vol. 70, No. 4, 2011, pp. 576-582. doi:10.1136/ard.2010.129916

[69] S. L. Westlake, A. N. Colebatch, J. Baird, N. Curzen, P. Kiely, M. Quinn, *et al*., "Tumour Necrosis Factor Antagonists and the Risk of Cardiovascular Disease in Patients with Rheumatoid Arthritis: A Systemic Literature Review," *Rheumatology (Oxford)*, Vol. 50, No. 3, 2011, pp. 518-531. doi:10.1093/rheumatology/keq316

[70] W. G. Dixon, K. D. Watson, M. Lunt, K. L. Hyrich, A. J. Silman and D. P. Symmons, "Reduction in the Incidence of Myocardial Infarction in Patients with Rheumatoid Arthritis who Respond to Anti-Tumor Necrosis Factor α Therapy: Results from the British Society for Rheumatology Biologics Register," *Arthritis and Rheumatism*, Vol. 56, No. 9, 2007, pp. 2905-2912. doi:10.1002/art.22809

[71] B. Levine, J. Kalman, L. Mayer, H. M. Fillit and M. Packer, "Elevated Circulating Levels of Tumor Necrosis Factor in Severe Chronic Heart Failure," *New England Journal of Medicine*, Vol. 323, No. 4, 1990, pp. 236-241. doi:10.1056/NEJM199007263230405

[72] D. L. Mann, J. J. McMurray, M. Packer, K. Swedberg, J. S. Borer, W. S. Colucci, *et al*., "Targeted Anticytokine Therapy in Patients with Chronic Heart Failure: Results of the Randomized Etanercept Worldwide Evaluation (RENEWAL)," *Circulation*, Vol. 109, No. 13, 2004, pp. 1594-1602. doi:10.1161/01.CIR.0000124490.27666.B2

[73] E. S. Chung, M. Packer, K. H. Lo, A. A. Fasanmade and J. T. Willerson, "Anti-TNF Therapy Against Congestive Heart Failure Investigators. Randomized, Double-Blind, Placebo-Controlled, Pilot Trial of Infliximab, a Chimeric Monoclonal Antibody to Tumor Necrosis Factor-α, in Patients with Moderate-to-Severe Heart Failure: Results of the Anti-TNF Therapy Against Congestive Heart Failure (ATTACH) Trial," *Circulation*, Vol. 107, No. 25, 2003, pp. 3133-3140. doi:10.1161/01.CIR.0000077913.60364.D2

[74] F. Wolfe and K. Michaud, "Heart Failure in Rheumatoid Arthritis: Rates, Predictors, and the Effect of Anti-Tumor Necrosis Factor Therapy," *American Journal of Medicine*, Vol. 116, No. 5, 2004, pp. 305-311. doi:10.1016/j.amjmed.2003.09.039

[75] J. Listing, A. Strangfeld, J. Kekow, M. Schneider, A. Kapelle, S. Wassenberg, *et al*., "Does Tumor Necrosis Factor α Inhibition Promote or Prevent Heart Failure in Patients with Rheumatoid Arthritis?" *Arthritis and Rheumatism*, Vol. 58, No. 3, 2008, pp. 667-677. doi:10.1002/art.23281

[76] C. I. Daïen, Y. Duny, T. Barnetche, J. P. Daurès, B. Combe and J. Morel, "Effect of TNF Inhibitors on Lipid Profile in Rheumatoid Arthritis: A Systematic Review with Meta-Analysis," *Annals of the Rheumatic Diseases*, Vol. 71, No. 6, 2012, pp. 862-868.

doi:10.1136/annrheumdis-2011-201148

[77] R. N. Maini, P. C Taylor, J. Szechinski, K. Pavelka, J. Bröll, G. Balint, *et al.*, "Double-Blind Randomized Controlled Clinical Trial of the Interleukin-6 Receptor Antagonist, Tocilizumab, in European Patients with Rheumatoid Arthritis who Had an Incomplete Response to Methotrexate," *Arthritis and Rheumatism*, Vol. 54, No. 9, 2006, pp. 2817-2829. doi:10.1002/art.22033

[78] M. C. Genovese, J. D. McKay, E. L. Nasonov, E. F. Mysler, N. A. da Silva, E. Alecock, *et al.*, "Interleukin-6 Receptor Inhibition with Tocilizumab Reduces Disease Activity in Rheumatoid Arthritis with Inadequate Response to Disease-Modifying Antirheumatic Drugs: the Tocilizumab in Combination with Traditional Disease-Modifying Antirheumatic Drug Therapy Study," *Arthritis and Rheumatism*, Vol. 58, No. 10, 2008, pp. 2968-2980. doi:10.1002/art.23940

[79] M. A. Blum, D. Koo and J. A. Doshi, "Measurement and Rates of Persistence with and Adherence to Biologics for Rheumatoid Arthritis," *Clinical Therapeutics*, Vol. 33, No. 7, 2011, pp. 901-913. doi:10.1016/j.clinthera.2011.06.001

[80] S. M, Du Pan, S. Dehler, A. Ciurea, H. R. Ziswiler, C. Gabay, A. Finckh, *et al.*, "Comparison of Drug Retention Rates and Causes of Drug Discontinuation between Anti-Tumor Necrosis Factor Agents in Rheumatoid Arthritis," *Arthritis and Rheumatism*, Vol. 61, No. 5, 2009, pp. 560-568. doi:10.1002/art.24463

[81] K. L, Hyrich, M. Lunt, K. D. Watson, D. P. Symmons and A. J. Silman, "British Society for Rheumatology Biologics Register. Outcomes after Switching from One Anti-Tumor Necrosis Factor α Agent to a Second Anti-Tumor Necrosis Factor α Agent in Patients with Rheumatoid Arthritis: Results from a Large UK National Cohort Study," *Arthritis and Rheumatism*, Vol. 56, No. 1, 2007, pp. 13-20. doi:10.1002/art.22331

[82] S. Curkendall, V. Patel, M. Gleeson, R. S. Campbell, M. Zagari and R. Dubois, "Compliance with Biologic Therapies for Rheumatoid Arthritis: Do Patient Out-of-Pocket Payments Matter?" *Arthritis and Rheumatism*, Vol. 59, No. 10, 2008, pp. 1519-1526. doi:10.1002/art.24114

[83] J. L. Barton, "Patient Preferences and Satisfaction in the Treatment of Rheumatoid Arthritis with Biologic Therapy," *Patient Preference and Adherence*, Vol. 3, 2009, pp. 335-344. doi:10.2147/PPA.S5835

[84] L. E. Harrington, R. D. Hatton, P. R. Mangan, H. Turner, T. L. Murphy, K. M. Murphy, *et al.*, "Interleukin 17-Producing CD4+ Effector T Cells Develop a Lineage Distinct from the T Helper Type 1 and 2 Lineages," *Nature Immunology*, Vol. 6, No. 11, 2005, pp. 1123-1132.

[85] C. L. Langrish, Y. Chen, W. M. Blumenschein, J. Mattson, B. Basham, J. D. Sedgwick, *et al.*, "IL-23 Drives a Pathogenic T Cell Population that Induces Auto-Immune Inflammation," *Journal of Experimental Medicine*, Vol. 201, No. 2, 2005, pp. 233-240. doi:10.1084/jem.20041257

[86] P. Miossec, T. Korn and V. K. Kuchroo, "Interleukin-17 and Type 17 Helper T Cells," *New England Journal of Medicine*, Vol. 361, No. 9, 2009, pp. 888-898.

doi:10.1056/NEJMra0707449

[87] S. L. Gaffen, "Structure and Signalling in the IL-17 Receptor Family," *Nature Reviews. Immunology*, Vol. 9, No. 8, 2009, pp. 556-567. doi:10.1038/nri2586

[88] R. M. Onishi and S. L. Gaffen, "Interleukin-17 and Its Target Genes: Mechanisms of Interleukin-17 Function in Disease," *Immunology*, Vol. 129, No. 3, 2010, pp. 311-321. doi:10.1111/j.1365-2567.2009.03240.x

[89] A. J. Hueber, D. L. Asquith, A. M. Miller, J. Reilly, S. Kerr, J. Leipe, *et al.*, "Mast Cells Express IL-17A in Rheumatoid Arthritis Synovium," *Journal of Immunology*, Vol. 184, No. 7, 2010, pp. 3336-3340. doi:10.4049/jimmunol.0903566

[90] A. M. Lin, C. J. Rubin, R. Khandpur, J. Y. Wang, M. Riblett, S. Yalavarthi, *et al.*, "Mast Cells and Neutrophils Release IL-17 through Extracellular Trap Formation in Psoriasis," *Journal of Immunology*, Vol. 187, No. 1, 2011, pp. 490-500. doi:10.4049/jimmunol.1100123

[91] C. T. Weaver, R. D. Hatton, P. R. Mangan and L. E. Harrington, "IL-17 Family Cytokines and the Expanding Diversity of Effector T Cell Lineages," *Annual Review of Immunology*, Vol. 25, 2007, pp. 821-852. doi:10.1146/annurev.immunol.25.022106.141557

[92] E. Lubberts, "Th17 Cytokines and Arthritis," *Seminars in Immunopathology*, Vol. 32, No. 1, 2010, pp. 43-53. doi:10.1007/s00281-009-0189-9

[93] S. Kotake, T. Yago, M. Kawamoto and Y. Nanke, "Role of Osteoclasts and Interleukin-17 in the Pathogenesis of Rheumatoid Arthritis: Crucial 'Human Osteoclastology'," *Journal of Bone and Mineral Metabolism*, Vol. 30, No. 2, 2012, pp. 125-135.

[94] E. Lubberts, L. A. Joosten, B. Oppers, L. van den Bersselaar, C. J. Coenen-de Roo, J. K. Kolls, *et al.*, "IL-1-Independent Role of IL-17 in Synovial Inflammation and Joint Destruction during Collagen-Induced Arthritis," *Journal of Immunology*, Vol. 167, No. 2, 2001, pp. 1004-1013.

[95] S. Nakae, A. Nambu, K. Sudo and Y. Iwakura, "Suppression of Immune Induction of Collagen-Induced Arthritis in IL-17-Deficient Mice," *Journal of Immunology*, Vol. 171, No. 11, 2003, pp. 6173-6177.

[96] E. Lubberts, M. I. Koenders, B. Oppers-Walgreen, L. van den Bersselaar, C. J. Coenen-de Roo, L. A. B. Joosten, *et al.*, "Treatment with a Neutralizing Anti-Murine Interleukin-17 Antibody after the Onset of Collagen-Induced Arthritis Reduces Joint Inflammation, Cartilage Destruction, and Bone Erosion," *Arthritis and Rheumatism*, Vol. 50, No. 2, 2004, pp. 650-659. doi:10.1002/art.20001

[97] M. I. Koenders, E. Lubberts, B. Oppers-Walgreen, L. van den Bersselaar, M. M. Helsen, F. E. Di Padova, *et al.*, "Blocking of Interleukin-17 during Reactivation of Experimental Arthritis Prevents Joint Inflammation and Bone Erosion by Decreasing RANKL and Interleukin-1," *American Journal of Pathology*, Vol. 167, No. 1, 2005, pp. 141-149. doi:10.1016/S0002-9440(10)62961-6

[98] M. Ziolkowska, A. Koc, G. Luszczykiewicz, K. Ksiezopolska-Pietrzak, E. Klimczak, H. Chwalinska-Sadowska, *et al.*, "High Levels of IL-17 in Rheumatoid Arthritis Patients: IL-15 Triggers *in vitro* IL-17 Production

via Cyclosporine A-Sensitive Mechanism," *Journal of Immunology*, Vol. 164, No. 5, 2000, pp. 2832-2838.

[99] S. A. Metawi, D. Abbas, M. M. Kamal and M. K. Ibrahim, "Serum and Synovial Fluid Levels of Interleukin-17 in Correlation with Disease Activity in Patients with RA," *Clinical Rheumatology*, Vol. 30, No. 9, 2011, pp. 1201-1207. doi:10.1007/s10067-011-1737-y

[100] J. Suurmond, A. L. Dorjée, M. R. Boon, E. F. Knol, T. W. Huizinga, R. E. Toes, *et al.*, "Mast Cells Are the Main Interleukin 17-Positive Cells in Anticitrullinated Protein Antibody-Positive and -Negative Rheumatoid Arthritis and Osteoarthritis Synovium," *Arthritis Research & Therapy*, Vol. 13, No. 5, 2011, p. R150. doi:10.1186/ar3466

[101] W. Marder, S. Khalatbari, J. D. Myles, R. Hench, S. Yalavarthi, S. Lustig, *et al.*, "Interleukin 17 as a Novel Predictor of Vascular Function in Rheumatoid Arthritis," *Annals of the Rheumatic Diseases*, Vol. 70, No. 9, 2011, pp. 1550-1555. doi:10.1136/ard.2010.148031

[102] W. Hueber, D. D. Patel, T. Dryja, A. M. Wright, I. Koroleva, G. Bruin, *et al.*, "Effects of AIN457, a Fully Human Antibody to Interleukin-17A, on Psoriasis, Rheumatoid Arthritis, and Uveitis," *Science Translational Medicine*, Vol. 2, No. 52, 2010, p. 52ra72. doi:10.1126/scitranslmed.3001107

[103] M. C. Genovese, P. Durez, H. B. Richards, J. Supronik, E. Dokoupilova, J. A. Aelion, *et al.*, "One Year Efficacy and Safety Results of a Phase II Trial of Secukinumab in Patients with Rheumatoid Arthritis [abstract]," *Arthritis and Rheumatism*, Vol. 63, No. S10, 2011, pp. S149-S150.

[104] M. C. Genovese, F. Van den Bosch, S. A. Roberson, S. Bojin, I. M. Biagini, P. Ryan, *et al.*, "LY2439821, a Humanized Anti-Interleukin-17 Monoclonal Antibody, in the Treatment of Patients with Rheumatoid Arthritis. A Phase I Randomized, Double-Blind, Placebo-Controlled, Proof-of-Concept Study," *Arthritis and Rheumatism*, Vol. 62, No. 4, 2010, pp. 929-939. doi:10.1002/art.27334

[105] M. C. Genovese, M. W. Greenwald, C. S. Cho, A. Berman, L. Jin, G. Cameron, *et al.*, "A Phase 2 Study of Multiple Subcutaneous Doses of LY2439821, an Anti-IL-17

Monoclonal Antibody, in Patients with Rheumatoid Arthritis in Two Populations: Naïve to Biologic Therapy or Inadequate Responders to Tumor Necrosis Factor Alpha Inhibitors [abstract]," *Arthritis and Rheumatism*, Vol. 63, No. S10, 2011, p. S1017.

[106] K. A. Papp, C. Leonardi, A. Menter, J. P. Ortonne, J. G. Krueger, G. Kricorian, *et al.*, "Brodalumab, an Anti-Interleukin-17—Receptor Antibody for Psoriasis," *New England Journal of Medicine*, Vol. 366, No. 13, 2012, pp. 1181-1189. doi:10.1056/NEJMoa1109017

[107] Y. Iwakura, H. Ishigame, S. Saijo and S. Nakae, "Functional Specialization of Interleukin-17 Family Members," *Immunity*, Vol. 34, No. 2, 2011, pp. 149-162. doi:10.1016/j.immuni.2011.02.012

[108] K. Pavelka, Y. Chon, R. Newmark, N. Erondu and S. L. Lin, "A Randomized, Double-Blind, Placebo-Controlled, Multiple-Dose Study to Evaluate the Safety, Tolerability, and Efficacy of Brodalumab (AMG 827) in Subjects with Rheumatoid Arthritis and an Inadequate Response to Methotrexate," *Arthritis and Rheumatism*, Vol. 64, No. S10, 2012, p. S362.

[109] A. Puel, R. Döffinger, A. Natividad, M. Chrabieh, G. Barcenas-Morales, C. Picard, *et al.*, "Autoantibodies against IL-17A, IL-17F, and IL-22 in Patients with Chronic Mucocutaneous Candidiasis and Autoimmune Polyendocrine Syndrome Type I," *Journal of Experimental Medicine*, Vol. 207, No. 2, 2010, pp. 291-297. doi:10.1084/jem.20091983

[110] A. Puel, S. Cypowyj, J. Bustamante, J. F. Wright, L. Liu, H. K. Lim, *et al.*, "Chronic Mucocutaneous Candidiasis in Humans with Inborn Errors of Interleukin-17 Immunity," *Science*, Vol. 332, No. 6025, 2011, pp. 65-68. doi:10.1126/science.1200439

[111] K. Kisand, A. S. Bøe Wolff, K. T. Podkrajsek, L. Tserel, M. Link, K. V. Kisand, *et al.*, "Chronic Mucocutaneous Candidiasis in APECED or Thymoma Patients Correlates with Autoimmunity to Th17-Associated Cytokines," *Journal of Experimental Medicine*, Vol. 207, No. 2, 2010, pp. 299-308. doi:10.1084/jem.20091669

20

Association of a cytosine-adenine repeat polymorphism in the estrogen receptor β gene with occurrence and severity of rheumatoid arthritis

Kanako Watanabe[1*], Hiromi Sato[1*#], Ayano Ito[1], Tomomi Sato[1], Aránzazu González-Canga[2], Hana Sugai[1], Masahiko Suzuki[3], Takao Namiki[4], Koichi Ueno[1]

[1]Department of Geriatric Pharmacology and Therapeutics, Graduate School of Pharmaceutical Sciences, Chiba University, Chiba, Japan
[2]Assessment Area, Medicines for Veterinary Use Department, Agencia Española de Medicamentosy Productos Sanitarios (AEMPS), Madrid, Spain
[3]Research Center for Frontier Medical Engineering, Chiba University, Chiba, Japan
[4]Department of Frontier Japanese-Oriental (Kampo) Medicine, Graduate School of Medicine, Chiba University, Chiba, Japan
Email: hiromi-s@chiba-u.jp

ABSTRACT

We investigated the influence of the cytosine-adenine (CA) dinucleotide repeat polymorphism in intron 6 of estrogen receptor β (ERβ) gene on rheumatoid arthritis (RA) risk. One hundred and ninety-three RA patients and 77 control subjects with osteoarthritis (OA) were recruited. The CA repeat polymorphism was assayed by a dye-terminator cycle sequencing analysis. No statistically significant difference in the mean number of CA repeats between the RA and OA patients was observed (RA: 21.47, OA: 21.23, $P = 0.324$). The alleles were categorized according to the number of repeats: short (S, $\leqq 21$) and long (L, $\geqq 22$), in which the genotypes SS, SL, and LL were observed. No significant differences were observed for the allele and genotype distributions of this polymorphism in both patient groups. The RA patients were classified according to RA severity: mild (least erosive disease) and severe (more erosive and mutilating disease). Again, no significant difference in genotype frequency between these groups was observed, even after stratifying by sex. The present study indicates that additional studies are needed to clarify the roles of this polymorphism, estrogen, and ER in the development of autoimmune diseases.

Keywords: Polymorphism; Rheumatoid Arthritis; Sex; Estrogen Receptor β; CA Repeat

1. INTRODUCTION

Rheumatoid arthritis (RA) is the most common chronic autoimmune disorder, characterized by chronic inflammation and destruction of the synovial joints, leading to progressive joint deterioration and disability [1]. RA is characterized as a complex genetic disease, meaning that several genes and environmental and stochastic (chance) factors act in concert to cause the pathological events [2]. Principal among the list of known risk factors is sex, as the rate of RA in females is 2 to 3 times higher than that in males [3]. The underlying immune response in RA seems to be influenced by sex hormones, which have been shown to modulate the onset and progression of connective tissue diseases, including RA, in clinical and in vivo studies [4]. In addition, some studies have suggested that female sex hormones and pregnancy are factors possibly associated with RA symptoms. For example, amelioration of RA occurs in approximately three quarters of pregnancies. In these cases, most women who improve experience initial relief in the first trimester, but RA almost invariably recurs within 3 or 4 months after delivery [5]. Another investigation concluded that the menopausal state could be responsible for the major part of the differences in outcome of RA between men and women [6].

To understand the functional role of estrogens in RA development, it is important to study not only estrogens but also the estrogen receptor (ER). Two types of ERs have been identified and cloned: ERα and ERβ [7]. ERα and ERβ are both expressed in synovial tissue, but ERβ has been identified as the predominant ER subtype in normal human synovial tissue [8]. The relative ERα/ERβ messenger RNA expression ratio was reported to be significantly lower in RA than in non-inflamed synovial tissue [9].

Several studies have investigated the potential roles of

*Kanako Watanabe and Hiromi Sato contributed equally to this work.
#Corresponding author.

ERβ (14q22 - 24) genetic polymorphisms in disease. For example, a cytosine-adenine (CA) dinucleotide repeat in intron 6 and the single nucleotide polymorphism (SNP) rs1256049 (Rsa polymorphism) have been studied in the context of various human phenotypes, including osteoarthritis [10], bone mineral density [11], and climacteric disorder [12]. In RA, we previously reported that longer CA repeats in the intron 6 of ERβ and the GG genotype at SNP rs1256049 were potential risk factors for RA [13, 14].

In this study, we investigated the association between the CA repeat polymorphism in the intron 6 of the ERβ gene and RA in men and women and compared the results obtained with those found in OA patients. In addition, we investigated the relationship between RA severity and CA repeat polymorphism.

2. SUBJECTS AND METHODS

2.1. Subjects and Study Design

The protocols and procedures for this experiment were approved by the ethics committee of the Graduate School of Pharmaceutical Sciences of Chiba University. All the genetic information used in this study remains confidential.

A total of 270 Japanese patients (222 women and 48 men) from the Chiba University Hospital, Japan, were recruited to participate in this study. These patients belong to 2 groups of subjects: those with rheumatoid arthritis (n = 193; 150 women and 43 men) and those recruited from the same geographical area and who had osteoarthritis (n = 77; 72 women and 5 men), designated as the control subjects. Informed consent was obtained from all subjects who participated in this study.

2.2. Analysis of the CA Repeat Polymorphisms

Genomic DNA was extracted from human peripheral blood leukocytes using the QIAamp DNA Mini Kit (Qiagen, Inc., Hilden, Germany) according to the manufacturer's protocol. Polymerase chain reaction (PCR) was performed in 75 μL of reaction mixture with the following components: 150 ng of human genomic DNA, oligonucleotide primers designed to amplify polymorphic CA repeats in the intron 6 of the human ERβ gene (forward: 5'-CAA TTC CCA ATT CTA AGC CT-3' and reverse: 5'-ATT CTT CTT TAG GCC AGG CA-3') at 0.4 μM, dNTP mixture (TaKaRa Bio, Inc., Otsu, Japan) at 200 μM, 7.5 μL of 10× Reaction Buffer (containing 15 mM MgSO$_4$) (Transgenomic, Inc., Omaha, USA), and 2.5 U of Optimase Polymerase (Transgenomic, Inc.). The reactions were brought to a total volume of 75 μL by adding MilliQ water. The amplification profiles were as follows: 35 cycles of denaturing at 94°C for 30 seconds, annealing at 60°C for 30 seconds, and extension at 72°C for 30

seconds. The PCR products were purified with the QIAquick PCR Purification Kit (Qiagen) and used in the following analysis.

The analysis of the CA repeat polymorphisms was conducted by dye-terminator cycle sequencing using the Dye Terminator Cycle Sequencing Quick Start Kit (Beckman Coulter, Inc. Fullerton, USA) and the CEQ2000 DNA Analysis System (Beckman Coulter, Inc.) according to the manufacturers' protocols.

2.3. Statistical Analysis

The allele and genotype frequencies were compared between the patient groups using the Fisher's exact probability test, except for 2 groups (age and the mean numbers of CA repeats), which were compared using the student's t test. $P < 0.05$ was considered to represent statistically significant differences for all the analyses.

3. RESULTS

The characteristics of the RA and OA patients are shown in **Table 1**. Significant differences were detected between the RA and OA patients with respect to sex, although in both groups of patients, the occurrence of disease in the women was higher than that in men. In addition, in the female and male groups, the RA patients were significantly younger than the OA patients. We used the same

Table 1. Characteristics of the RA and OA patients.

	RA	OA	P value
Characteristic			
All patients (n)	193	77	
Sex (n (%))			
Women	150 (77.7)	72 (93.5)	0.001[a]
Men	43 (22.3)	5 (6.5)	
Age (mean (SD, range))			
Women	61.0 ± 10.8 (24 - 86)	70.0 ± 9.33 (50 - 91)	0.000[b]
Men	61.9 ± 11.00 (38 - 83)	73.4 ± 14.15 (51 - 89)	0.037[b]
Total	61.2 ± 10.83 (24 - 86)	70.2 ± 9.62 (50 - 91)	0.000[b]
Severity (n (%))			
LES	48 (24.9)	-	
MES	135 (69.9)	-	
MUD	10 (5.2)	-	

P values are shown for comparisons between RA and OA by [a]the Fisher's exact probability test and [b]student's t test. Differences were considered significant at $P < 0.05$. LES, least erosive subset; MES, more erosive subset; MUD, mutilating disease.

criteria as those used by Ochi *et al.* [15] to classify our patients into 3 severity types (least erosive disease, LES; more erosive disease, MES; and mutilating disease, MUD). These severity classifications were determined by orthopedic specialists based on long-term observation data. Most of the patients in the study were classified as MES, similar to those in our previous study [14].

Figure 1 shows the frequency distribution of the CA repeats in the RA and OA patients. In the RA patients, the number of CA repeats ranged in length from 15 to 28, with a mean value of 21.47 and a median of 22. In the OA patients, the number of CA repeats ranged in length from 15 repeats to 29 repeats, with a mean value of 21.23 and a median of 22. The mean numbers of CA repeats were not statistically different between the RA and OA patients ($P = 0.324$). In addition, we categorized 2 allelic types according to the median number of CA repeats: $\leqq 21$ repeats (short allele, S), and $\geqq 22$ repeats (long allele, L). The cutoff value was based on that used in previous studies [10,12,13]. Based on these alleles, 3 genotypes (SS, SL and LL) were identified.

The allele and genotype frequency distributions for the ERβ CA repeat polymorphism in the RA and OA patients are shown in **Table 2**. There were no significant differences observed between the RA and OA patients in this respect. The RA patients were also classified and divided according to sex and RA severity: mild (LES) and severe (MES and MUD). No significant differences in genotype frequency between the RA severity classes were observed before or after stratifying these groups by sex (**Table 3**).

Table 2. Comparison of genotype and allele frequencies for the ERβ CA repeat polymorphism in the RA and OA patients.

Genotype	RA	OA	Genotype distribution	Allele S vs allele L	
	n (%)	n (%)	P value	OR (95% CI)	P value
SS	48 (24.9)	22 (28.6)	0.703	0.801	0.446
SL	78 (40.4)	32 (41.5)		(0.45 - 1.42)	
LL	67 (34.7)	23 (29.9)			

Differences were considered significant at $P < 0.05$ using the Fisher's exact test. OR: Odds ratio; 95% CI: 95% confidence interval.

Table 3. Comparison of the genotype and allele frequencies for the ERβ CA repeat polymorphism between mild (LES) RA, severe (MUD + MES) RA, and OA patients.

		RA (LES)	RA (MES + MUD)	OA	Genotype distribution
		n (%)	n (%)	n (%)	P value
Female	SS	7 (19.4)	30 (26.3)	20 (27.8)	0.455
	SL	21 (58.3)	46 (40.4)	31 (43.0)	
	LL	8 (22.2)	38 (33.3)	21 (29.2)	
Male	SS	3 (25.0)	8 (25.8)	2 (40.0)	0.985
	SL	3 (25.0)	8 (25.8)	1 (20.0)	
	LL	6 (50.0)	15 (48.4)	2 (40.0)	

Differences were considered significant at $P < 0.05$ using the Fisher's exact test. LES: Least erosive subset; MES: More erosive subset; MUD: Mutilating disease.

4. DISCUSSION

We investigated the association of the CA repeat polymorphism in the intron 6 of the ERβ gene with RA and OA to follow up on the findings from a previous report [13]; however, our results did not reveal significant differences between RA and OA patients with respect to allele and genotype frequencies identified at this locus.

Based on the patient characteristics (**Table 1**), we evaluated the degree of severity of RA in the patients according to Ochi *et al.* [15]. Because this evaluation is primarily dependent on the stages and progress of joint deterioration (e.g., mild or rapid, and oligo arthritis or multi joint), classifications of disease severity are not influenced by differences in sensitivity to drug treatment. Most of the patients enrolled in this study were classified as MES RA, which was consistent with the findings of the previous study by Sato *et al.* investigating the effects of the ERβ Rsa polymorphism on RA [14]. Furthermore, in this study, we found that the OA patients were older than the RA patients, which is perhaps not surprising given that OA pathologic features is closely associated with aging. These findings were also similar to those reported by Sato *et al.* [14]. In the present study, we ana-

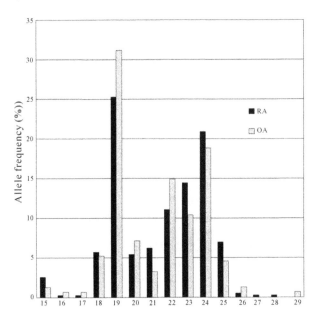

Figure 1. Frequency distribution of alleles at the CA repeat polymorphism in the estrogen receptor β gene for the RA and OA patients.

lyzed the CA repeat polymorphism by direct sequencing, a method typically used for the analysis of microsatellite polymorphisms. The mean CA repeat length observed for the RA patients was the same as that reported in a previous study [13]. Thus, neither the patient background nor the methods used for the analyses in the present study are likely to have resulted in the lack of association observed here. Similar patient cohorts were recently used to identify the association between the Rsa polymorphism in the ERβ gene and RA risk [14]. Considering this, it could be suggested that the Rsa and CA repeat polymorphisms are functionally different, a finding that would not be surprising given that the Rsa polymorphism resides within an exon and the CA repeat polymorphism resides within an intron; however, additional studies are needed to investigate this further.

To date, only a single study has investigated the potential association between the ERβ CA repeat polymorphism and RA [13]. Wang et al. [16] recently reported that shorter alleles (S, <23 repeats) were marginally associated with increased risk of systemic lupus eryhtematosus (SLE) compared with longer alleles (L, $\geqq$ 23 repeats). While it is well known that, like RA, SLE is an autoimmune disease, a link between this polymorphism and RA should not be inferred based solely on the association to SLE [16] given that many differences are known to exist between SLE and RA, such as age at onset and sex differences [17]. Furthermore, Dziedziejko et al. [18] examined the association of SNPs in ERα and ERβ gene with RA but did not observe any significant differences in the distributions of genotypes and alleles between RA patients and controls and no significant association of the genotypes with rheumatoid factor (RF), erosive disease, extra-articular manifestations, or anticyclic citrullinated peptide (anti-CCP) antibodies [18]. In a subsequent study, Dziedziejko et al. [19] also examined potential associations of these SNPs with response to treatment with leflunomide in RA patients but did not reveal a significant association in ERβ SNPs [19]. Engdahl et al. [20] reported that ERα, but not ERβ or GPR-30 signaling, was shown to ameliorate disease and associated development of osteoporosis in a well-established model of postmenopausal RA. These results indicate that the role of ERβ in the pathogenesis of RA should be reconsidered.

Furthermore, the effects of estrogen on the development and severity of RA remain controversial, as pro-inflammatory and anti-inflammatory effects have been reported. For example, some selective ERβ agonists like ERB-041 are reported to have potent anti-inflammatory effects in animal arthritis models [21], but in a clinical trial, ERB-041 failed to demonstrate anti-inflammatory efficacy in RA patients despite the evidence of strong activity in a preclinical study [22]. Randomized controlled trials conducted by the Women's Health Initiative revealed that there was no significant evidence for a dif-

ference in the hazard rate of RA incidence or symptom severity between postmenopausal hormone therapy and placebo groups [23]. Ganesan et al. [24] recently reported protective effects of estrogen and testosterone. This study showed that estrogen had a higher potency in rat arthritic synovial fibroblasts, whereas progesterone was not observed to inhibit TNF-α-induced change [24].

In addition to estrogen, other sex hormones have also been implicated in the etiology of RA. For example, the level of dehydroepiandrosterone (DHEA) and DHEA sulfate (DHEAS), the major androgen in women, were associated with the onset of RA [1]. Karlson et al. [25] investigated potential association between androgen levels; polymorphisms in ERβ, PGR, and CYP19 genes; and risk of RA, but no significant associations were observed [25]. To the best of our knowledge, there have been no reported associations between the ERβ CA repeat polymorphism and sex hormones. Thus, studies assessing potential combinatorial effects of multiple genetic polymorphisms and hormone levels on the risk of RA are warranted.

5. CONCLUSION

In conclusion, the results of the present study did not reveal a significant association between alleles at the CA repeat polymorphism in the intron 6 of the ERβ gene and RA severity. Additional studies are needed to further clarify potential roles of this polymorphism, as well as roles for estrogen and ER in the pathogenesis and severity of autoimmune diseases.

6. ACKNOWLEDGEMENTS

We wish to thank Dr. Yoichi Suzuki of the Medical Faculty of Chiba University for the invaluable help with the genotype analysis. This study was funded by a Grant-in-Aid for Scientific Research (C) from the Japan Society for the Promotion of Sciences and Health Labor Sciences Research Grant.

REFERENCES

[1]   Härle, P., Bongartz, T., Schölmerich, J., Müller-Ladner, U. and Straub, R.H. (2005) Predictive and potentially predictive factors in early arthritis: A multidisciplinary approach. *Rheumatology (Oxford)*, **44**, 426-433. doi:10.1093/rheumatology/keh530

[2]   Klareskog, L., Catrina, A.I. and Paget, S. (2009) Rheumatoid arthritis. *Lancet*, **373**, 659-672. doi:10.1016/S0140-6736(09)60008-8

[3]   Whitacre, C.C. (2001) Sex differences in autoimmune disease. *Nature Immunology*, **2**, 777-780. doi:10.1038/ni0901-777

[4]   Cutolo, M., Straub, R.H. and Bijlsma, J.W. (2007) Neuroendocrine-immune interactions in synovitis. *Nature Clinical Practice. Rheumatology*, **3**, 627-634. doi:10.1038/ncprheum0601

[5] Nelson, J.L. and Ostensen, M. (1997) Pregnancy and rheumatoid arthritis. *Rheumatic Diseases Clinics of North America*, **23**, 195-212. doi:10.1016/S0889-857X(05)70323-9

[6] Kuiper, S., van Gestel, A.M., Swinkels, H.L., de Boo, T.M., da Silva, J.A. and van Riel, P.L. (2001) Influence of sex, age, and menopausal state on the course of early rheumatoid arthritis. *The Journal of Rheumatology*, **28**, 1809-1816.

[7] Mosselman, S., Polman, J. and Dijkema, R. (1996) ERβ: Identification and characterization of a novel human estrogen receptor. *FEBS Letters*, **392**, 49-53. doi:10.1016/0014-5793(96)00782-X

[8] Dietrich, W., Haitel, A., Holzer, G., Huber, J.C., Kolbus, A. and Tschugguel, W. (2006) Estrogen receptor-β is the predominant estrogen receptor subtype in normal human synovia. *Journal of the Society for Gynecologic Investigation*, **13**, 512-517.

[9] Ishizuka, M., Hatori, M., Suzuki, T., Miki, Y., Darnel, A.D., Tazawa, C., Sawai, T., Uzuki, M., Tanaka, Y., Kokubun, S. and Sasano, H. (2004) Sex steroid receptors in rheumatoid arthritis. *Clinical Science*, **106**, 293-300. doi:10.1042/CS20030317

[10] Fytili, P., Giannatou, E., Papanikolaou, V., Stripeli, F., Karachalios, T., Malizos, K. and Tsezou, A. (2005) Association of repeat polymorphisms in the estrogen receptors α, β, and androgen receptor genes with knee osteoarthritis. *Clinical Genetics*, **68**, 268-277. doi:10.1111/j.1399-0004.2005.00495.x

[11] Shearman, A.M., Karasik, D., Gruenthal, K.M., Demissie, S., Cupples, L.A., Housman, D.E. and Kiel, D.P. (2004) Estrogen receptor beta polymorphisms are associated with bone mass in women and men: The Framingham Study. *Journal of Bone and Mineral Research*, **19**, 773-781. doi:10.1359/jbmr.0301258

[12] Negishi, E., Takeo, C., Nakajima, A., Hisamitsu, K., Amano, K., Hirai, A. and Ueno, K. (2006) Analysis of correlation between prescription drugs for climacteric disorders and CA repeat polymorphism of estrogen receptor β gene. *Japanese Journal of Pharmaceutical Health Care and Sciences*, **32**, 21-26. doi:10.5649/jjphcs.32.21

[13] Gonzalez-Canga, A., Ugai, K., Okuzawa, H., Suzuki, M., Okuzawa, H., Negishi, E. and Uneo, K. (2010) Association of cytosin-adenine repeat polymorphism of the estrogen receptor-β gene withrheumatoid arthritis symptoms. *Rheumatology International*, **30**, 1259-1262. doi:10.1007/s00296-010-1423-4

[14] Sato, H., Ito, A., González-Canga, A., Okuzawa, H., Ugai, K., Suzuki, M., Namiki, T. and Ueno, K. (2011) Association of Rsa polymorphism of the estrogen receptor-β gene with rheumatoid arthritis. *Rheumatology International*, **32**, 2143-2148. doi:10.1007/s00296-011-1947-2

[15] Ochi, T., Iwase, R., Yonemasu, K., Matsukawa, M., Yoneda, M., Yukioka, M. and Ono, K. (1988) Natural course of joint destruction and fluctuation of serum C1q levels in patients with rheumatoid arthritis. *Arthritis and Rheumatism*, **31**, 37-43. doi:10.1002/art.1780310106

[16] Wang, J., Nuite, M. and McAlindon, T.E. (2010) Association of estrogen and aromatase gene polymorphisms with systemic lupus erythematosus. *Lupus*, **19**, 734-740. doi:10.1177/0961203309359517

[17] Oliver, J.E. and Silman, A.J. (2009) Why are women predisposed to autoimmune rheumatic diseases? *Arthritis Research & Therapy*, **11**, 252. doi:10.1186/ar2825

[18] Dziedziejko, V., Kurzawski, M., Safranow, K., Drozdzik, M., Chlubek, D. and Pawlik, A. (2011) Oestrogen recaptor polymorphisms in female patients with rheumatoid arthritis. *Scandinavian Journal of Rheumatology*, **40**, 329-333. doi:10.3109/03009742.2011.563752

[19] Dziedziejko, V., Kurzawski, M., Safranow, K., Chlubek, D. and Pawlik, A. (2011) The effect of ESR1 and ESR2 gene polymorphisms on the outcome of rheumatoid arthritis treatment with leflunomide. *Pharmacogenomics*, **12**, 41-47. doi:10.2217/pgs.10.164

[20] Engdahl, C., Jochems, C., Windahl, S.H., Börjesson, A.E., Ohlsson, C., Carlsten, H. and Lagerquist, M.K. (2010) Amelioration of collagen-induced arthritis and immune-associated bone loss through signaling via estrogen receptor, and not estrogen receptor or G protein-coupled receptor 30. *Arthritis and Rheumatism*, **62**, 524-533.

[21] Cvoro, A., Tatomer, D., Tee, M.K., Zogovic, T., Harris, H.A. and Leitman, D.C. (2008) Selective estrogen recaptor-beta agonists repress transcription of proinflammatory genes. *Journal of Immunology*, **180**, 630-636.

[22] Roman-Blas, J.A., Castañeda, S., Cutolo, M. and Herrero-Beaumont, G. (2010) Efficacy and safety of a selective estrogen receptor agonist, ERB-041, in patients with rheumatoid arthritis: A 12-week, randomized, placebo-controlled, phase II Study. *Arthritis Care & Research*, **62**, 1588-1593. doi:10.1002/acr.20275

[23] Walitt, B., Pettinger, M., Weinstein, A., Katz, J., Torner, J., Wasko, M.C., Howard, B.V. and Women's Health Initiative Investigators (2008) Effects of postmenopausal hormone therapy on rheumatoid arthritis: The women's health initiative randomized controlled trials. *Arthritis and Rheumatism*, **59**, 302-310. doi:10.1002/art.23325

[24] Ganesan, K., Balachandran, C., Manohar, B.M. and Puvanakrishnan, R. (2011) Effects of testosterone, estrogen and progesterone on TNF-α mediated cellular damage in rat arthritic synovial fibroblasts. *Rheumatology International*, **32**, 3181-3188. doi:10.1007/s00296-011-2146-x

[25] Karlson, E.W., Chibnik, L.B., McGrath, M., Chang, S.-C., Keenan, B.T., Costenbader, K.H., Fraser, P.A., Tworoger, S., Hankinson, S.E., Lee, I.-M., Buring, J. and De Vivo, I. (2009) A prospective study of androgen levels, hormone-related genes and risk of rheumatoid arthritis. *Arthritis Research & Therapy*, **11**, R97. doi:10.1186/ar2742

21

Leukotriene-A4-Hydrolase and Basic Aminopeptidase Activities Are Related with Collagen-Induced Arthritis in a Compartment-Dependent Manner

Mariana Trivilin Mendes[1,2], Paulo Flavio Silveira[1]

[1]Laboratory of Pharmacology, Unit of Translational Endocrine Physiology and Pharmacology, Instituto Butantan, São Paulo, Brazil;
[2]Department of Physiology, Instituto de Biociências, Universidade de São Paulo, São Paulo, Brazil.
Email: paulo.silveira@butantan.gov.br

ABSTRACT

Objective: Previous study demonstrated the involvement of basic aminopeptidase (APB) activity in the development of collagen-induced arthritis (CIA). Two zinc dependent metalloenzymes (EC 3.4.11.6 and EC 3.3.2.6) are known to exhibit concomitantly APB and leukotriene-A4-hydrolase (LT-A4-H) activities. Influence of the interrelationship between both activities on arthritic processes, however, is presently uncertain. This study aimed to compare these activities in CIA. **Methods:** CIA was induced in rats and arthritis was assessed macroscopically. Ultracentrifugation was used to separate soluble (S) and solubilized membrane-bound (M) fractions from peripheral blood mononuclear cells (PBMCs) and synovial tissue (ST). Enzyme immunoassay was used to measure LT-A4-H activity, and Real Time Polymerase Chain Reaction was used for evaluating EC 3.4.11.6 and EC 3.3.2.6 gene expressions. **Results:** The existence of genes for EC 3.3.2.6 and EC 3.4.11.6 was demonstrated in the ST. Compared with control, LT-A4-H activity increased in synovial fluid (SF) and in S-PBMCs of CIA-arthritic and CIA-resistant and in M-ST of CIA-resistant, while it decreased in M-PBMCs of CIA-arthritic and CIA-resistant. In all these locations APB activity remained unchanged or inversely correlated with LT-A4-H activity. **Conclusions:** LT-A4-H and APB activities in joint-related samples are associated, for the first time, with EC 3.3.2.6 and EC 3.4.11.6 genes, exhibiting a compartment-dependent differential modulation of their specificity, efficiency and/or affinity or an inverse concurrent pattern. Changes in LT-A4-H activity have implications for development or resistance to arthritis in CIA model with a potential to be a diagnostic tool.

Keywords: Aminopeptidase; Ether Hydrolase; Bifunctional Enzyme; Eicosanoids

1. Introduction

Rheumatoid arthritis (RA) is characterized by peripheral polyarthritis with cartilage and bone erosions, resulting in deformity and joint destruction [1]. This process is associated with inflammatory hyperplasia of the synovial membrane, also known as pannus [2]. What happens is the neovascularization, which occurs after the infiltration of inflammatory cells into the synovial membrane [3] and the immune response against cartilage components, among them the type II collagen (CII) has been most commonly associated with this response [1]. The arthritis induced by CII (CIA) [4-9] generates an erosive polyarthritis [5,8,10] that has been intensively studied due to its similarities with the RA [4,6,9-11], mainly regarding

the development of synovitis, progressive pannus formation, marginal erosion of bone and cartilage destruction [4,6,8]. In CIA model the symptoms in rats and mice begin about 21 days after the CII injection at currently used dose [9].

The role of enzymes in the etiology of inflammatory diseases, such as RA and osteoarthritis, has been the focus of many investigations [12-14]. Two zinc dependent metalloenzymes [15-18], leukotriene (LT)-A4 hydrolase (LT-A4-H) (EC 3.3.2.6) and basic aminopeptidase (APB) (EC 3.4.11.6), seem to exhibit concomitant hydrolytic activities on L-arginyl-β-naphthylamide (ArgNA) and on LT-A4 [18-23].

EC 3.4.11.6 preferentially hydrolyzes basic residues (Arg and Lys) of peptides [17,18,24,25], being ArgNA its preferential synthetic substrate [26]. This enzyme is structurally similar to EC 3.3.2.6 (33% identity and 48% similarity) and it has also been reported to exhibit LT-A4-H activity [16,17,27]. Whether there is a reciprocal interference of peptide and eicosanoid substrates in each one of these possible catalytic activities of EC 3.4.11.6 is not known. Mantle *et al.* [22] suggest that changes in LTs generate changes in the APB activity. Although the EC 3.4.11.6 gene expression has not yet been evaluated in joint-related samples, the APB activity [28] and other aminopeptidase activities, such as neutral and dipeptidyl peptidase IV [29], have already been implicated in the etiology and development of arthritis in CIA model. The potential importance of APB activity in RA could be related to their participation in the peptides processing [30]. One hypothesis is its association with the post-translational maturation in the trans-Golgi network, and with the regulatory processes in the plasma membrane, which includes extracellular hydrolysis of several peptide substrates. Moreover, APB can participate in the final stages of processing of hormones precursors [15]. The significance and even the existence of the two catalytic functions of EC 3.4.11.6 remain unknown [15,17,25], but its hydrolytic ability in a wide pH range is suggestive of its adaptability to various cellular sub-compartments, which has been reinforced by some reports about its involvement in a broad spectrum of pathophysiological processes [15,17], including the RA [28].

EC 3.3.2.6 from human and rodent is a soluble and monomeric enzyme [18,31], with at least one report also showing a membrane-bound LT-A4-H activity in hepatocytes [32]. In addition to the epoxide hydrolase activity upon LT-A4, the EC 3.3.2.6 also seems to exhibit activity upon ArgNA [19]. Both catalytic activities of EC 3.3.2.6 were reported to be inhibited by divalent cations, while only aminopeptidase activity was stimulated by monovalent anions such as chloride [18,21]. Although the involvement of EC 3.3.2.6 in RA by means of the LT-B4 (acid 5[S], 12[R]-dihydroxy-6,14-*cis*-8,10-*trans*eicosatetraenoic) formation is an attractive and predictable hypothesis, studies in this direction are rare [33]. In addition, EC 3.3.2.6 gene expression has also not yet been evaluated in joint-related samples. The LT-B4 is a potent pro-inflammatory mediator synthesized by immune cells, such as eosinophils, neutrophils and macrophages, which stimulates the production of several cytokines [16] and it has been recognized as a potent chemotactic factor during early inflammation [34,35]. Moreover, it promotes degranulation, increased release of lysosomal enzymes and superoxide production by neutrophils [36,37].

To know the possible changes in LT-A4-H activity in CIA model, as well as to infer its involvement in the pa-

thophysiology and its potential to be a RA biomarker are important tasks. In addition, the knowledge of the gene expression of EC 3.3.2.6 and EC 3.4.11.6 and the comparative analysis of the catalytic activities upon LT-A4 and ArgNA in CIA model may contribute to the identification of interrelation pattern of these catalytic functions in both proteins. For this purposes this study evaluates the gene expression of EC 3.3.2.6 and EC 3.4.11.6, as well as the levels of LT-A4-H activity (LT-A4 hydrolysis) in comparison with APB activity levels (ArgNA hydrolysis) reported by Mendes *et al.* [28].

2. Materials and Methods

2.1. Animals and Treatments

Adult male Wistar rats, weighing 160 - 180 g and maintained in polyethylene cages with food and tap water *ad libitum* in a container with controlled temperature of 25°C, relative humidity of 65.3% ± 0.9% and 12 h:12 h photoperiod light:dark (lights on at 6:00 am), were subjected to the following procedures approved by the Ethics Committee on Animal Use of Butantan Institute (682/09). Based on Cremer method (1998), modified by Mendes *et al.* [28], the animals were injected with CII from chicken (Sigma, USA) dissolved in 0.01M acetic acid and emulsified in equal volume of Freund's incomplete adjuvant (Sigma) (prepared at 4°C just before use), via single intradermal dose of 0.4 mg/0.2 mL/animal, into the proximal one-third of the tail (induced animals), or with 0.9% saline at the same scheme of administration (sham induction). All animals that received the emulsion or saline were previously anesthetized with a solution of ketamine (3.75%) (Fort Dodge, USA) and xylazine (0.5%) (Vetbrands, Brasil) at a dose of 0.2 mL/100 g body weight, via intraperitoneal (ip). All these procedures mentioned above, as well as the evaluation of edema, erythema and cyanosis, and the collection of samples were carried out in the morning.

2.2. Macroscopic Assessment of Arthritis

Erythema and cyanosis were observed, and dorsal-plantar thickness of the hind paws in the region of the metatarsus was quantified with paquimeter (Mitutoyo, USA). Both paws were measured and mean thickness for each animal was calculated. This measurement was performed immediately before the euthanasia and sample collection.

2.3. Sample Collection

On 41st day after treatments, the animals were anesthetized using the same scheme specified above and thus the following experimental groups were formed: Control (all animals submitted to sham induction); Arthritic (induced animals with hind paw thickness > 5.7 mm that also present erythema and cyanosis); Resistant (induced animals without erythema and cyanosis and with hind paw thickness similar to control). Thus, blood was withdrawal from the left ventricle with heparinized syringes and used to obtain peripheral blood mononuclear cells (PBMCs) or centrifuged (at 200 × g for 10 min at at 4˚C) to obtain plasma. The SF and ST were subsequently removed from both knees of each animal as follows: 200 μL of 0.9% NaCl was injected intraarticularly into each knee with an ultrafine needle (0.45 × 13 mm) and aspirated with a syringe and, after such washing, the ST was excised together with the connective tissue of the joint capsule.

2.4. Gene Expressions of EC 3.4.11.6 and EC 3.3.2.6

2.4.1. RNA Extraction

The RNA of ST suspension for each control healthy animal was extracted using the sound RiboPure™ Kit (Applied Biosystems, USA) as recommended by the manufacturer. Briefly, the ST samples were homogenized on ice with TriReagent® (Applied Biosystems) (1 mL TriReagent® for each 0.05 to 0.1 mg of original tissue) on Polytron® 11,000 rpm and sequentially incubated for 5 min at 25˚C and centrifuged at 12,000 × g for 10 min at 4˚C. Afterward, 200 μL chloroform were added to each 1 mL of sample and mixed by a vortex at a maximum speed for 15 sec and then incubated for 5 min at 25˚C and centrifuged at 12,000 × g for 10 min at 4˚C. Three layers were formed after this centrifugation: a top, or aqueous phase, composed of RNA; an intermediate phase, composed of DNA; and a lower, or phenol phase, composed of protein. 400 μL of aqueous phase were transferred to a new tube, and thus mixed with 200 μL ethanol (99.5%) and homogenized by a vortex mixer for 15 sec and transferred to a Filter Cartridge-Collection Tube. Subsequently, this apparatus was centrifuged at 12,000 × g for 30 sec at 25˚C and the liquid drained into the collector tube was discarded, while the filter containing the RNA was placed in the same collector tube and washed with 500 μL of wash solution. This washing was repeated twice more. Subsequently, the filter was centrifuged at 12,000 × g for 30 sec at 25˚C to remove residual wash solution and then the filter was transferred to a new collector tube where 100 μL of elution buffer were added. After incubation for 2 min at 25˚C, this Filter Cartridge coupled with this new Collection Tube were centrifuged at 12,000 × g for 30 sec at 25˚C and the final eluate containing the RNA was obtained and stored at −20˚C until used.

2.4.2. Quantitative Real Time Polymerase Chain Reaction (qPCR)

The total RNA isolated was quantified and its purity was evaluated by Synergy™ H1 using the software Gen5™. The adequate quality of total RNA was checked by the existence of bands corresponding to 25S and 18S ribosomal RNA, obtained in 1% agarose (Amersham Bioscience, Sao Paulo, SP, Brazil) gel electrophoresis (wt/v), prepared in Tris/sodium acetate/EDTA 1x buffer, pH 8.0, under constant voltage (80 V), and stained with ethidium bromide solution (0.5 μg/mL) under ultraviolet light. As recommended by manufacturer, until 2 μg of total RNA in a maximum volume of 9 μL were used for reverse transcription procedure using the High Capacity RNA-to-cDNA kit (Applied Biosystems). Briefly, 10 μL of reaction buffer, 1 μL of enzyme mix and the sample at final volume of 20 μL in 0.01% diethylpyrocarbonate (DEPC) (Sigma) in sterile deionized water were placed in the thermal cycler for 60 min at 37˚C and for 5 min at 95˚C. Them, the samples were stored at −80˚C. The expression of APB and LT-A4-H mRNAs was measured with Taqman system®. In addition to the primers, a probe that selectively hybridizes with cDNA was used. The thermal cycler conditions for the PCR reaction were: 1 cycle of 2 min at 50˚C, 1 cycle of 10 min at 95˚C, followed by 40 cycles: 15 sec at 95˚C and 1 min at 60˚C. APB (Rn 00579477_m1, GenBank: NM_020216) and LT-A4-H (Rn01503878_m1, acess number to GenBank: NM_001030031) primers and probes and GAPDH (GenBank: NM_017008) (positive control) used were purchased from Life Technologies (Brazil). Relative gene expression was determined using the $\Delta\Delta C_T$ method ($\Delta C_{T(sample)}$ - $\Delta C_{T(reference)}$, threshold cycle). The comparative C_T method is a mathematical model that consists of normalizing the number of target gene copies to an endogenous reference gene (GAPDH) and compare it to control sample (that with highest cycle threshold and, consequently, lowest gene expression) designed as the calibrator.

2.5. Obtaining PBMCs

According to the method of Grage-Griebenow et al. [38], heparinized blood was carefully layered on Percoll (density = 1.077 g/mL) (GE—Healthcare, USA) in PBS (56%) at a proportion of 5:3 (v/v) and subsequently centrifuged (1000 × g for 40 min at 25˚C). The layer containing the PBMCs was then removed from the tube and transferred to microtubes to be immediately used.

2.6. PBMCs Counting and Viability

20-μL aliquots of PBMCs suspension were diluted with Turk's fluid (1:20, v/v). The cell viability was assessed using 40 μL aliquots of this suspension diluted in equal volume of Trypan. Cell counting was performed in a Neubauer chamber under optical microscopy.

2.7. Fractionation of ST and PBMCs

As previously described by Mendes *et al.* [28], the ST from both knees of each animal was homogenized in 10 mM Tris-HCl buffer, pH 7.4 (0.1 g tissue/3.0 mL) for 3 min at 15,000 rpm (homogenizer Polytron-Aggregate, Kinematica, Switzerland). PBMCs homogenates were sonicated in 10 mM Tris-HCl, pH 7.4 (3.0×10^6 cells/mL), for 10 sec at amplitude level of 40 μm at a constant frequency of 20 kHz. These samples were then ultracentrifuged at $100,000 \times$ g for 35 min (ultracentrifuge Hitachi CP60E). The resulting supernatants correspond to soluble (S) fraction. The resulting pellets were washed twice with the same buffer and ultracentrifuged at $100,000 \times$ g for 35 min, to assure the complet removal of S. The pellet was homogenized for 3 min at 800 rpm (homogenizer Tecnal TE 099) with the same volume of the same buffer plus Triton X-100 (Sigma) (0.1%) and ultracentrifuged again ($100,000 \times$ g for 35 min). The resulting supernatants correspond to solubilized membrane-bound (M) fraction. All procedures were carried out at 4°C. The efficiency of this fractionation in both materials was previously demonstrated using lactate dehydrogenase activity as a marker [28,29].

2.8. LT-A4-H Activity

2.8.1. Incubation of Samples with or without LT-A4

Based on the methodology of Mendes *et al.* [20], 1 μL of LT-A4 solution (Sigma) (100 μg/mL) was diluted in 1499 μL of 50 mM HEPES buffer (Sigma), pH 7.5, containing 0.0625% glycerol (USB Co., USA) and 1% dimethyl sulfoxide (DMSO) (Sigma). Alternatively, 1 μL of LT-A4 solution was substituted by 1 μL 0.9% NaCl in this mixture. 50 μL of plasma, SF, and S and M from ST and PBMCs and 250 μL of buffer solution mentioned above containing or not LT-A4 (LT-A4 final concentration = 166.66 nM) were pipetted into each microplate well (96 wells) (Corning) and then incubated (25°C) under orbital shaking (250 rpm) for 10 min. Thus, 10 μL of each incubated were transferred to a microtube containing 190 μL of ice-cold assay buffer (EIA buffer) from EIA kit for LT-B4 (Leukotriene B4 EIA kit using monoclonal antibody produced in mice against LT-B4 rabbit, Cayman Chemical, USA).

2.8.2. Enzyme Immunoassay (EIA)

The absorbance at $\lambda = 412$ nm of each samples obtained as described above was read against two HEPES buffer solutions, with or without LT-A4, both considered the "blank" of each kind of incubation, and also against the "blank" supplied with the kit.

2.8.3. Catalytic Activity

The values of the blanks were subtracted and the relative absorbance was converted to pg of LT-B4 formed in 1 min of incubation per 1 mL of sample by an interpolation in a correspondent standard curve. The values of LT-B4 formed in each samples incubated without LT-A4 (endogenous LT-B4) were subtracted from the values of LT-B4 in the same samples incubated with LT-A4 thus representing the value of LT-B4 formed *in vitro*. The LT-A4-H activity was expressed as pg of LT-B4 formed *in vitro*/min/mL sample.

2.9. Data Analysis

Data are shown as mean ± standard error of the mean (S.E.M) and were analyzed statistically using the Graph-Pad Instat™ software package. Regression analysis was performed to obtain standard curve of LT-B4. To compare values among the control, arthritic and resistant groups one-way analysis of variance (ANOVA) was performed, followed by Student-Newman-Keuls multiple comparisons test when differences were detected. In all the calculations a minimum critical level of $P < 0.05$ was set.

3. Results

3.1. Classification of Experimental Animals Based on the Formation of Edema, Erythema and Cyanosis

The swelling (in mm; n = number of animals, two-tailed unpaired Student's t-test p < 0.0017), erythema and cyanosis were the main macroscopic characteristics of the hind paws of arthritic animals. Severe swelling (5.899 ± 0.037, n = 10) was found in 60% of animals treated with CII. Compared to controls (4.745 ± 0.052, n = 10), 30% of the animals treated with CII showed no erythema, cyanosis or edema (4.762 ± 0.309, n = 10). These data agree with the differential detection of serum TNF-α levels and histopathological alterations of the tibio-tarsal joint in the CII treated animals that develop severe edema (CIA-arthritic), which can be thus confidentially distinguished from CIA-resistant (without edema) [28,29]. Based on the macroscopic classification of edema formation, preconized by Erlandsson Harris *et al.* [39], all arthritic animals selected here had the maximum score in hind paws. 10% of CII treated animals were discarded because they did not reach this level of arthritis.

3.2. Gene Expression of APB (EC 3.4.11.6) and LT-A4-H (EC 3.3.2.6)

Figure 1 shows that APB (EC 3.4.11.6) and LT-A4-H (EC 3.3.2.6) genes are expressed in ST of healthy control animals.

3.3. LT-A4-H Activity

Table 1 shows LT-A4-H activity in plasma, SF, and S

and M from ST and PBMCs. Compared to controls, this activity is higher in SF and in S from PBMCs and lower in M from PBMCs in CIA-arthritic and CIA-resistant, and higher in M from ST in CIA-resistant.

Table 2 illustrates altered LT-A4-H (present study) and APB [28] activities in CIA-arthritic and CIA-resistant compared to healthy control rats.

4. Discussion

The existence of the genes for EC 3.3.2.6 and EC 3.4.11.6 was confirmed in the synovial tissue of healthy controls rats. The synovial tissue and synovial fluid collected from animals under study contain infiltrating leukocytes. Therefore, the total content of both activities in plasma, synovial fluid and synovial tissue should be at least partially derived from these cells, particularly in arthritic animals.

The present work showed parallel changes in LT-A4-H

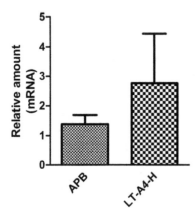

Figure 1. Relative gene expression of basic aminopeptidase (APB) (EC 3.4.11.6) and LT-A4 hydrolase (LT-A4-H) (EC 3.3.2.6) in synovial tissue of healthy control animals. Number of animals = 2.

Table 1. LT-A4-H activity[*].

Samples	Control	CIA-Arthritic	CIA-Resistant	*ANOVA* (p)
PLASMA	7.03 ± 0.26	9.73 ± 1.12	9.84 ± 1.27	$=0.1540$
SF	4.26 ± 0.29^a	7.12 ± 0.45^b	15.11 ± 1.01^c	<0.0001
S-ST	19.42 ± 2.76	13.06 ± 2.30	17.64 ± 1.55	$=0.2023$
M-ST	4.66 ± 0.01^a	0 ± 1.16^a	18.94 ± 5.08^b	$=0.0060$
S-PBMCs	0 ± 4.20^a	7.32 ± 3.37^b	253.60 ± 1.76^c	<0.0001
M-PBMCs	47.88 ± 10.66^a	19.32 ± 4.89^b	16.44 ± 0.21^b	$=0.0306$

[*]pg LT-B4 formed/min/mL of plasma, synovial fluid (SF) or soluble (S) and solubilized membrane-bound (M) fractions from synovial tissue (ST) and peripheral blood mononuclear cells (PBMCs) of control, arthritic and resistant rats. Values are means of duplicates ± SEM. Number of animals = 3. Comparison of the same samples among groups. Post hoc Student-Newman-Keuls (different letters indicate statistical differences: p < 0.05).

Table 2. Changes in LT-A4-H and APB activities in CIA-arthritic and CIA-resistant relatively to healthy control rats.

Samples	LT-A4-H activity		APB activity	
	CIA-Arthritic	CIA-Resistant	CIA-Arthritic	CIA-Resistant
PLASMA	=	=	=	↓
SF	↑	↑	=	↓
S-ST	=	=	↑	=
M-ST	=	↑	↑	=
S-PBMCs	↑	↑	↓	↓
M-PBMCs	↓	↓	=	↑

LT-A4-H activity assessed by EIA and APB activity assessed by fluorometry [28]. (=) No difference, (↓) decrease, (↑) increase.

activity in arthritic and resistant rats in relation to controls, although quantitative levels of these changes are distinct in some materials. Thus, regarding the LT-A4-H activity both, arthritic and resistant, are distinguishable from the controls, on the other hand they are distinct from each other only quantitatively. These features can be useful in further studies exploring the LT-A4-H activity as a diagnostic tool and the role of quantitative differences of this activity in the development and resistance to arthritis. The structural analysis of EC 3.3.2.6 and EC 3.4.11.6 showed that the differences in their distributions of electrostatic potential may reflect different interactions between protein-protein and/or the protein and the environment in which it is inserted, with EC 3.3.2.6 having less hydrophobic parts than EC 3.4.11.6 [15]. Different negative electrostatic potential in the catalytic site could explain the different specificities for their respective substrates [15], implying on the possibility that different catalytic activities do not interfere with each other. Another report shows that EC 3.4.11.6 from rat and human has no epoxy-hydrolase activity, suggesting that despite the great structural similarity between EC 3.3.2.6 and EC 3.4.11.6, the last one has another function [40]. The present study shows that changes in LT-A4-H and APB activities do not coincide in the plasma and membrane-bound fraction from the synovial tissue of resistant animals, as well as in soluble and membrane-bound fractions from synovial tissue, membrane-bound fraction from PBMCs and synovial fluid of arthritic animals. These results suggest the existence of differential modulation of catalytic specificity, efficiency and/or affinity of EC 3.3.2.6 and EC 3.4.11.6 enzymes on peptide and epoxy substrates, or that they act independently with a single catalytic action in these locations. However, in those situations where APB and LT-A4-H activities change concomitantly, such changes are inversely correlated, cor-

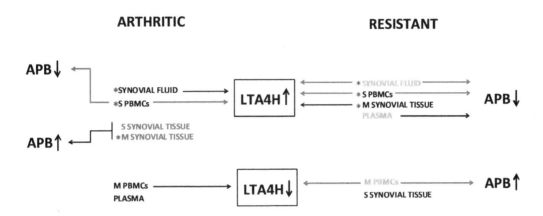

Figure 2. Schematic depicting the changes in LT-A4-H and APB activities in CIA-arthritic and CIA-resistant rats. Arrows ↑ and ↓ indicate, respectively, increased or decreased values relatively to healthy control rats. Locations where activity levels of APB are markers of arthritis or resistance [28] are respectively written in pink and green. The changes in the way and levels of LT-A4-H activity in any of examined locations underlined in yellow, except in plasma and S-ST of arthritic and resistant and in M-ST of arthritic, distinguish arthritic and/or resistant from controls and thus they have potential diagnostic use. The changes in the way of LT-A4-H activity in any of the examined locations, except in M-ST, do not distinguish between arthritic and resistant (see Table 2), but the changes in the levels of LT-A4-H activity in locations marked with blue asterisk (SF, M-ST and S-PBMCs) (see Table 1) may have implications for the resistance or development of arthritis in CIA model. The red solid lines indicate all the situations and locations where occur concomitant changes in activity levels of LT-A4-H and APB, showing that they are always inversely correlated.

roborating the existence of a bifunctional pattern currently described for EC 3.4.11.6 [15,25,27] and EC 3.3.2.6 [17,35,41].

Taken together, the results of the present study subsidize the scheme proposed in **Figure 2**, illustrating a hypothetical mechanism of interrelation between LT-A4-H and APB activities in CIA-arthritic and CIA-resistant in comparison with healthy control rats.

5. Conclusion

In summary, LT-A4-H (EC 3.3.2.6) and APB (EC 3.4.11.6) gene expressions were shown for the first time in joint-related samples from rats. Another interesting result is the fact that LT-A4-H and APB activities behave in a compartment-dependent manner. Moreover, these activities exhibit differential modulation of their specificity, efficiency and/or affinity or an inverse concurrent pattern. In this way, as previously observed for APB [28], changes in LT-A4-H activity also have implications in the development or resistance to arthritis in CIA model and deserve further investigation as a possible diagnostic tool.

6. Acknowledgements

This study was financially supported by a Research Grant 09/17613-0 from FAPESP (Fundação de Amparo à Pesquisa do Estado de São Paulo, Brazil). P.F.S was recipient of a Productivity Grant 302533/2011-7 from CNPq (Conselho Nacional de Desenvolvimento Cientifico e Tecnologico, Brazil). M.T.M. was recipient of a CAPES (Coordenacao de Aperfeicoamento de Pessoal de Nivel Superior, Brasil) fellowship. The authors thank all the staff at the Unit of Translational Endocrine Pharmacology and Physiology at Laboratory of Pharmacology for technical support.

REFERENCES

[1] R. Holmdahl, J. C. Lorentzen, S. Lu, P. Olofsson, L. Wester, J. Holmberg and U. Pettersson, "Arthritis Induced in Rats with Nonimmunogenic Adjuvants as Models for Rheumatoid Arthritis," *Immunological Reviews*, Vol. 184, No. 1, 2001, pp. 184-202.
http://dx.doi.org/10.1034/j.1600-065x.2001.1840117.x

[2] J. M. Stuart, A. S. Townes and A. H. Kang, "Collagen Autoimmune Arthritis," *Annual Reviews in Immunology*, Vol. 2, 1984, pp. 199-218.
http://dx.doi.org/10.1146/annurev.iy.02.040184.001215

[3] G. S. Panayi, "B Cells: A Fundamental Role in the Pathogenesis of Rheumatoid Arthritis?" *Rheumatology*, Vol. 44, No. S2, 2005, pp. ii3-ii7.
http://dx.doi.org/10.1093/rheumatology/keh616

[4] H. Kim, J. Bang, H. W. Chang, J. Y. Kim, K. U. Park, S. H. Kim, K. J. Lee, C. H. Cho, I. Hwang, S. D. Park, E. Ha and S. W. Jung, "Anti-Inflammatory Effect of Quetiapine on Collagen-Induced Arthritis of Mouse," *European Journal of Pharmacology*, Vol. 678, No. 1-3, 2012, pp. 55-60.
http://dx.doi.org/10.1016/j.ejphar.2011.12.017

[5] D. D. Brand, A. H. Kang and E. F. Rosloniec, "Immunopathogenesis of Collagen Arthritis," *Springer Seminars in Immunopathology*, Vol. 25, No. 1, 2003, pp. 3-18.

http://dx.doi.org/10.1007/s00281-003-0127-1

[6] L. K. Myers, E. F. Rosloniec, M. A. Cremer and A. H. Kang, "Collagen-Induced Arthritis, an Animal Model of Autoimmunity," *Life Sciences*, Vol. 61, No. 19, 1997, pp. 1861-1878. http://dx.doi.org/10.1016/S0024-3205(97)00480-3

[7] M. M. Griffiths, "Immunogenetics of Collagen-Induced Arthritis in Rats," *International Reviews of Immunology*, Vol. 4, No. 1, 1988, pp. 1-15. http://dx.doi.org/10.3109/08830188809044766

[8] J. M. Stuart, W. C. Watson and A. H. Kang, "Collagen Autoimmunity and Arthritis," *The FASEB Journal*, Vol. 2, No. 14, 1988, pp. 2950-2956.

[9] D. E. Trentham, A. S. Townes and A. H. Kang, "Autoimmunity to Type II Collagen an Experimental Model of Arthritis," *The Journal of Experimental Medicine*, Vol. 146, No. 3, 1977, pp. 857-868. http://dx.doi.org/10.1084/jem.146.3.857

[10] M. A. Cremer, E. F. Rosloniec and A. H. Kang, "The Cartilage Collagens: A Review of Their Structure, Organization, and Role in the Pathogenesis of Experimental Arthritis in Animals and in Human Rheumatic Disease," *Journal of Molecular Medicine*, Vol. 76, No. 3-4, 1998, pp. 275-288. http://dx.doi.org/10.1007/s001090050217

[11] M. A. Hietala, K. S. Nandakumar, L. Persson, S. Fahlén, R. Holmmahl and M. Pekna, "Complement Activation by Both Classical and Alternative Pathways Is Critical for the Effector Phase of Arthritis," *European Journal of Immunology*, Vol. 34, No. 4, 2004, pp. 1208-1216. http://dx.doi.org/10.1002/eji.200424895

[12] G. Tu, W. Xu, H. Huang and S. Li, "Progress in the Development of Matrix Metalloproteinase Inhibitors," *Current Medicinal Chemistry*, Vol. 15, No. 14, 2008, pp. 1388-1395. http://dx.doi.org/10.2174/092986708784567680

[13] M. Xue, L. March, P. N. Sambrook and C. J. Jackson, "Differential Regulation of Matrix Metalloproteinase 2 and Matrix Metalloproteinase 9 by Activated Protein C: Relevance to Inflammation in Rheumatoid Arthritis," *Arthritis & Rheumatism*, Vol. 56, No. 9, 2007, pp. 2864-2874. http://dx.doi.org/10.1002/art.22844

[14] M. H. Lee and G. Murphy, "What Are the Roles of Metalloproteinases in Cartilage and Bone Damage?" *Annals of the Rheumatic Diseases*, Vol. 64, No. S4, 2005, pp. iv44-iv47. http://dx.doi.org/10.1136/ard.2005.042465

[15] V. Pham, M. Cadel, C. Gouzy-Darmon, C. Hanquez, M. C. Beinfeld, P. Nicolas, C. Etchebest and T. Foulon, "Aminopeptidase B, a Glucagon-Processing Enzyme: Site Directed Mutagenesis of the Zn2+-Binding Motif and Molecular Modeling," *BMC Biochemistry*, Vol. 8, 2007, p. 21. http://dx.doi.org/10.1186/1471-2091-8-21

[16] T. D. Penning, M. A. Russell, B. B. Chen, H. Y. Chen, C. D. Liang, M. W. Mahoney, J. W. Malecha, J. M. Miyashiro, S. S. Yu, L. J. Askonas, J. K. Gierse, E. I. Harding, M. K. Highkin, J. F. Kachur, S. H. Kim, D. Villani-Price, E. Y. Pyla, N. S. Ghoreishi-Haack and W. G. Smith, "Synthesis of Potent Leukotriene A(4) Hydrolase Inhibitors. Identification of 3-[methyl[3-[4-(phenylmethyl)phenoxy]

propyl]amino] propanoic Acid," *Journal of Medicinal Chemistry*, Vol. 45, No. 16, 2002, pp. 3482-3490. http://dx.doi.org/10.1021/jm0200916

[17] T. Foulon, S. Cadel and P. Cohen, "Aminopeptidase B (EC 3.4.11.6)," *The International Journal of Biochemistry & Cell Biology*, Vol. 31, No. 7, 1999, pp. 747-750. http://dx.doi.org/10.1016/S1357-2725(99)00021-7

[18] M. J. Butler, "Metallopeptidases," In: A. J. Barrett, N. D. Rawlings and J. F. Woessner, Eds., *Handbook of Proteolytic Enzymes*, Academic Press, London, 1998, pp. 1022-1029.

[19] C. A. Grice, K. L. Tays, B. M. Savall, J. Wei, C. R. Butler, F. U. Axe, S. D. Bembenek, A. M. Fourie, P. J. Dunford, K. Lundeen, F. Coles, X. Xue, J. P. Riley, K. N. Williams, L. Karlsson and J. P. Edwards, "Identification of a Potent, Selective, and Orally Active Leukotriene A4 Hydrolase Inhibitor with Anti-Inflammatory Activity," *Journal of Medicinal Chemistry*, Vol. 51, No. 14, 2008, pp. 4150-4169. http://dx.doi.org/10.1021/jm701575k

[20] M. T. Mendes and P. F. Silveira, "Quantification of Leukotriene (LT) B4 and LT-A4-Hydrolase (LTA4H) by HPLC and Enzyme Immunoassay (EIA) in an Experimental Model of Arthritis," Abstracts of 14th International Congress on Antiphospholipid Antibodies & 4th Latin American Congress on Autoimmunity (APLA LACA 2013), Rio de Janeiro, 2013. http://www2.kenes.com/apla-laca/pages/home.aspx

[21] P. C. Rudberg, F. Tholander, M. M. Thunnissen, B. Samuelsson and J. Z. Haeggstrom, "Leukotriene A4 Hydrolase: Selective Abrogation of Leukotriene B4 Formation by Mutation of Aspartic Acid 375," *Proceedings of the National Academy of Sciences of the United States of America*, Vol. 99, No. 7, 2002, pp. 4215-4220. http://dx.doi.org/10.1073/pnas.072090099

[22] D. Mantle, G. Falkous and D. Walker, "Quantification of Protease Activities in Synovial Fluid from Rheumatoid and Osteoarthritis Cases: Comparison with Antioxidant and Free Radical Damage Markers," *Clinica Chimica Acta*, Vol. 284, No. 1, 1999, pp. 45-58. http://dx.doi.org/10.1016/S0009-8981(99)00055-8

[23] F. A. Fitzpatrick, R. Lepley, L. Orning and K. Duffin, "Suicide Inactivation of Leukotriene A4 Hydrolase/Aminopeptidase," *Annals of the New York Academy of Sciences*, Vol. 744, 1994, pp. 31-38. http://dx.doi.org/10.1111/j.1749-6632.1994.tb52721.x

[24] M. Hui and K. S. Hui, "A Novel Aminopeptidase with Highest Preference for Lysine," *Neurochemical Research*, Vol. 31, No. 1, 2006, pp. 95-102. http://dx.doi.org/10.1007/s11064-005-9234-9

[25] C. Piesse, S. Cadel, C. Gouzy-Darmona, J. C. Jeanny, V. Carrière, D. Goidin, L. Jonet, D. Gourdji, P. Cohen and T. Foulon, "Expression of Aminopeptidase B in the Developing and Adult Rat Retina," *Experimental Eye Research*, Vol. 79, No. 5, 2004, pp. 639-648. http://dx.doi.org/10.1016/j.exer.2004.06.030

[26] K. M. Fukasawa, J. Hirose, T. Hata and Y. Ono, "Aspartic Acid 405 Contributes to the Substrate Specificity of Aminopeptidase B," *Biochemistry*, Vol. 45, No. 38, 2006, pp. 11425-11431. http://dx.doi.org/10.1021/bi0604577

[27] S. Cadel, T. Foulon, A. Viron, A. Balogh, S. Midol-Monnet, N. Noël and P. Cohen, "Aminopeptidase B from the Rat Testis Is a Bifunctional Enzyme Structurally Related to Leukotriene-A4 Hydrolase," *Proceedings of the National Academy of Sciences of the United States of America*, Vol. 94, No. 7, 1997, pp. 2963-2968. http://dx.doi.org/10.1073/pnas.94.7.2963

[28] M. T. Mendes, S. Murari-do-Nascimento, I. R. Torrigo, R. F. Alponti, S. C. Yamasaki and P. F. Silveira, "Basic Aminopeptidase Activity Is an Emerging Biomarker in Collagen-Induced Rheumatoid Arthritis," *Regulatory Peptides*, Vol. 167, No. 2-3, 2011, pp. 215-221. http://dx.doi.org/10.1016/j.regpep.2011.02.012

[29] S. C. Yamasaki, S. Murari-do-Nascimento and P. F. Silveira, "Neutral Aminopeptidase and Dipeptidyl Peptidase IV in the Development of Collagen II-Induced Arthritis," *Regulatory Peptides*, Vol. 173, No. 1-3, 2012, pp. 47-54. http://dx.doi.org/10.1016/j.regpep.2011.09.004

[30] S. Hwanga and V. Hooka, "Zinc Regulation of Aminopeptidase B Involved in Neuropeptide Production," *FEBS Letters*, Vol. 582, No. 17, 2008, pp. 2527-2531. http://dx.doi.org/10.1016/j.febslet.2008.06.017

[31] M. Zaitsu, Y. Hamasaki, M. Matsuo, A. Kukita, K. Tsuji, M. Miyazaki, R. Hayasaki, E. Muro, S. Yamamoto, I. Kobayashi, T. Ichimaru, O. Kohashi and S. Miyazaki, "New Induction of Leukotriene A (4) Hydrolase by Interleukin-4 and Interleukin-13 in Human Polymorphonuclear Leukocytes," *Blood*, Vol. 96, No. 2, 2000, pp. 601-609.

[32] J. Gut, D. W. Goldman, G. C. Jamieson and J. R. Trudell, "Conversion of Leukotriene A4 to Leukotriene B4: Catalysis by Human Liver Microsomes under Anaerobic Conditions," *Archives of Biochemistry and Biophysics*, Vol. 259, No. 2, 1987, pp. 497-509. http://dx.doi.org/10.1016/0003-9861(87)90516-9

[33] G. D. Anderson, K. L. Keys, P. A. De Ciechi and J. L. Masferrer, "Combination Therapies That Inhibit Cyclooxygenase-2 and Leukotriene Synthesis Prevent Disease in Murine Collagen Induced Arthritis," *Inflammation Research*, Vol. 58, No. 2, 2009, pp. 109-117. http://dx.doi.org/10.1007/s00011-009-8149-3

[34] A. Ryan and C. Godson, "Lipoxins: Regulators of Resolution," *Current Opinion in Pharmacology*, Vol. 10, No. 2, 2010, pp. 166-172. http://dx.doi.org/10.1016/j.coph.2010.02.005

[35] J. Z. Haeggstrom, "Structure, Function, and Regulation of Leukotriene A4 Hydrolase," *American Journal of Respiratory and Critical Care Medicine*, Vol. 161, No. 2, 2000, pp. S25-S31. http://dx.doi.org/10.1164/ajrccm.161.supplement_1.ltta-6

[36] A. W. Ford-Hutchinson, "Leukotriene B4 in Inflammation," *Critical Reviews[TM] in Immunology*, Vol. 10, No. 1, 1990, pp. 1-12.

[37] B. Samuelsson, S. E. Dahlén, J. A. Lindgren, C. A. Rouzer and C. N. Serhan, "Leukotrienes and Lipoxins: Structures, Biosynthesis, and Biological Effects," *Science*, Vol. 237, No. 4819, 1987, pp. 1171-1176. http://dx.doi.org/10.1126/science.2820055

[38] E. Grage-Griebenow, J. Baran, H. Loppnow, M. Los, M. Ernst, H. D. Flad and J. Pryjma, "An Fcγ Receptor I (CD64)-Negative Subpopulation of Human Peripheral Blood Monocytes Is Resistant to Killing by Antigen-Activated CD4-Positive Cytotoxic T Cells," *European Journal of Immunology*, Vol. 27, No. 9, 1997, pp. 2358-2365. http://dx.doi.org/10.1002/eji.1830270934

[39] M. E. Harris, M. Liljestrom and L. Klareskog, "Characteristics of Synovial Fluid Effusion in Collagen-Induced Arthritis (CIA) in the DA Rat; a Comparison of Histology and Antibody Reactivity in an Experimental Chronic Arthritis Model and Rheumatoid Arthritis (RA)," *Clinical and Experimental Immunology*, Vol. 107, No. 3, 1997, pp. 480-484. http://dx.doi.org/10.1046/j.1365-2249.1997.3311221.x

[40] K. M. Fukasawa, K. Fukasawa, M. Harada, J. Hirose, T. Izumi and T. Shimizu, "Aminopeptidase B Is Structurally Related to Leukotriene-A4 Hydrolase but Is Not a Bifunctional Enzyme with Epoxide Hydrolase Activity," *Biochemical Journal*, Vol. 339, No. Pt 3, 1999, pp. 497-502.

[41] E. O. De Oliveira, K. Wanga, H. Kong, S. Kim, M. Miessau, R. J. Snelgrove, Y. M. Shim and M. Paige, "Effect of the Leukotriene A4 Hydrolase Aminopeptidase Augmentor 4-Methoxydiphenylmethane in a Pre-Clinical Model of Pulmonary Emphysema," *Bioorganic & Medicinal Chemistry Letters*, Vol. 21, No. 22, 2001, pp. 6746-6750. http://dx.doi.org/10.1016/j.bmcl.2011.09.048

22

Applying Item Response Theory Methods to Improve the Measurement of Fatigue in a Clinical Trial of Rheumatoid Arthritis Patients Treated with Secukinumab[*]

Mark Kosinski[1#], Jakob B. Bjorner[1], Ari Gnanasakthy[2], Usha Mallya[2], Shephard Mpofu[3]

[1]Quality Metric Incorporated, Lincoln, Rhode Island; [2]Novartis Pharmaceuticals Corporation, East Hanover, USA; [3]Novartis Pharma AG, Basel, Switzerland.
Email: [#]mkosinski@qualitymetric.com, jbjorner@qualitymetric.com, ari.gnanasakthy@novartis.com, usha.mallya@novartis.com, shephard.mpofu@novartis.com

ABSTRACT

Background: Many clinical trials include multiple patient-reported outcomes (PROs) to measure fatigue as secondary or exploratory endpoints of treatment effectiveness. Often, these instruments have overlapping content. The objective of this study was to compare the combined measurement properties of two fatigue scales, the Functional Assessment of Chronic Illness Therapy-Fatigue (FACIT-Fatigue) and SF-36 vitality (VT) scale using item response theory (IRT). **Methods:** The FACIT-Fatigue and SF-36v2 were administered at baseline and weeks 2, 4, 7, 12, and 16 to rheumatoid arthritis (RA) patients (n = 237) enrolled in a 52-week multicenter, randomized, double-blind, placebo-controlled, parallel-group, dose finding study to evaluate the efficacy and safety of subcutaneous secukinumab administered to patients with active RA. Confirmatory factor analysis (CFA) was used to investigate unidimensionality among FACIT-Fatigue and VT items. A generalized partial credit IRT model was used to cross-calibrate the FACIT-Fatigue and VT items and weighted maximum-likelihood estimation was used to score a composite fatigue index. Analysis of variance was used to compare the composite fatigue index with the original scales in responding to ACR improvement and treatment effects. **Results:** CFA found less than adequate fit to a unidimensional model. However, specifications of alternative multidimensional models were insufficient in explaining the common variance among items. An IRT model was successfully fitted and the composite fatigue index score was found to be more responsive than the original scales to ACR improvement and treatment effects. Effect sizes and significance tests for changes in scores on the composite index were generally larger than those observed with the original scales. **Conclusion:** IRT methods offer a promising approach to combining items from different scales measuring the same concept that could improve the detection of treatment effects in clinical studies of RA.

Keywords: Patient-Reported Outcomes; Fatigue; Rheumatoid Arthritis; Item Response Theory; Clinical Trial

1. Background

Rheumatoid arthritis (RA) is a systemic, chronic inflammatory disease characterized by joint pain, stiffness, and deformity in multiple regions, particularly the hands and feet. The disease affects approximately 0.5% - 1% of the population in developed countries [1-3]. The natural course of the disease is one of persistent symptoms, varying in intensity, with a progressive deterioration of joint structures leading to deformity and disability. The progression of the disease places an enormous burden on the patients, their families, and society as a whole. The annual direct costs of care attributable to RA from the societal perspective was estimated to be $3.6 billion [4] and increasing functional impairment due to RA often leads to work disability [5-8]. In addition, RA has a profound effect on

---

[*]Competing Interests: Mr. Gnanasakthy, Dr. Mallya, and Dr. Mpofu are employees of Novartis and own shares of stock from the company. Mr. Kosinski and Dr. Bjorner have no financial interests related to the work presented in this paper.
Authors' contributions: All authors were involved in the drafting of the article or reviewing it critically for important intellectual content. In addition, all authors approved the final draft to be published. Mr. Kosinski had full access to all of the data in the study and takes responsibility for the integrity of the data and the accuracy of the data analysis.
[#]Corresponding author.

health-related quality of life (HRQoL), impacting not only physical aspects, but psychological well-being, social and role functioning, and other areas as well [9-11]. Lastly, patients with RA are at a greater risk of early death [12]; it is estimated that RA reduces a patient's lifespan by anywhere from 3 to 12 years [13].

The disease course of RA varies greatly across individuals. Some experience mild short-term symptoms, but in most cases the disease is progressive for life. The goals of RA treatment include minimizing the clinical symptoms such as pain and swelling, preventing bone deformity and radiographic damage, and maintaining the individual's functional capacity and health-related quality of life [14]. With these treatment goals in mind, measuring the efficacy of RA treatment can be complex. Some of the clinical signs and symptoms of RA, such as swollen joints, elevated erythrocyte sedimentation rates (ESR), elevated C-reactive protein (CRP) levels, and radiographic damage, do not always correlate well with physical, social, or role functioning, fatigue, sense of well-being, or other long term outcomes [15,16]. Therefore, reductions in any one of the clinical indications of RA may not always translate into improved functioning and well-being for the patient. Because one of the primary goals of RA treatment is to maintain and improve functional capacity, it is vital that effectiveness of treatments is also measured by patient self-reports of functional ability and well-being.

Patient-reported outcome (PRO) measures of fatigue are recommended as core end points in clinical studies of rheumatoid arthritis [17]. Accordingly, many clinical trials include multiple PROs to measure fatigue as secondary or exploratory endpoints of treatment effectiveness. Often, these instruments have overlapping content. For example, the SF-36 Health Survey [18] and the FACIT-Fatigue [19] both measure energy and fatigue. Differences in item response options and scoring methods prevent investigators from simply combining the items of common content from these tools to score a composite index of fatigue. However, with the recent emergence of modern psychometric methods (Rasch and Item Response Theory) in constructing health status measures, it has been shown that items of similar content from different instruments can be successfully calibrated onto a single scale [20-24]. The advantages of a single cross-calibrated scale include extending the range of the concept being measured, allowing minimization of ceiling and floor effects, and improving the measurement precision over scales scored from the items scaled independently [25-27].

In this study, we employed methods of item-response theory (IRT) to evaluate the underlying measurement properties of two measures of fatigue (FACIT-Fatigue and SF-36 vitality scale) used in a randomized clinical

trial setting of secukinumab (Novartis Pharma AG, Basel, Switzerland) treatment for RA [28]. The goal of this research was to examine whether the two measures of fatigue can be calibrated on a common metric with IRT methods to yield one composite index of fatigue. As a practical test to this cross-calibration of items from different instruments, we compared the ability of the composite fatigue index to detect change over time against the original scoring of the fatigue scales of each instrument independently. Criteria for change over time included measures of change in disease status (ACR improvement criteria) and fatigue outcome comparisons between treatment and placebo groups.

2. Methods

Regulatory and ethical review board approvals from competent authorities in each country were obtained for the study protocol. All patients signed an informed consent document, and the study was conducted in accordance with the Declaration of Helsinki and followed good clinical practice guidelines.

2.1. Study Population

A total of 237 adults with RA participated in a 52-week, multi-center, double-blind, placebo-controlled, parallel group, dosing study to evaluate the efficacy, safety and tolerability of subcutaneous secukinumab as add-on therapy in patients with active RA despite stable treatment with methotrexate. Eligible patients met the ACR 1987 revised classification criteria for RA for at least 3 months and were required to present active RA defined by ≥ 6 out of 28 tender joints and ≥ 6 out of 28 swollen joints, and high sensitivity CRP ≥ 10 mg/L or ESR ≥ 28 mm/1st hour at the time of randomization. Eligible patients were also required to be on methotrexate for at least 3 months and treated with a stable weekly dose of ≥ 7.5 mg/week - ≤ 25 mg/week for at least 4 weeks.

2.2. Measures

2.2.1. Functional Assessment of Chronic Illness Therapy—Fatigue (FACIT-Fatigue)

The FACIT-Fatigue is part of the FACIT measurement system, a comprehensive compilation of questions that measure a range of health-related quality of life concepts with cancer and other chronic illnesses [29-31]. The FACIT-Fatigue consists of 13 items that assess self-reported fatigue and its impact upon daily activities and function over the past 7 days. Patients are asked to answer each of the following questions on a 5-point Likert-type scale (0 = not at all; 1 = a little bit; 2 = somewhat; 3 = quite a bit, and 4 = very much). The items are: 1) I feel fatigued; 2) I feel weak all over; 3) I feel listless (washed out); 4) I feel tired; 5) I have trouble starting things because I am tired; 6) I have trouble finishing things because I am tired; 7) I have energy; 8) I am able to do my usual activities; 9) I need to sleep during the day; 10) I am too tired to eat; 11) I need help doing my usual activities; 12) I am frustrated by being too tired to do the things I want to do; and 13) I have to limit my social activity because I am tired. After reverse coding all items but 7 and 8, a total score is computed by summing up the response values, with a higher score indicative of less fatigue. During the efficacy evaluation period of this study the FACIT-Fatigue was administered at baseline and weeks 2, 4, 8, 12 and 16.

2.2.2. SF-36 Health Survey Vitality Scale

The SF-36 Health Survey includes 4 items that are used to score the vitality (VT) scale [18,32]. The items of the VT scale are scored on a scale from 1 (all of the time) to 5 (none of the time). Patients are asked to give an answer that comes closest to the way they have been feeling in the past 4 weeks on the following questions: 1) did you feel full of life?; 2) Did you have a lot of energy?; 3) Did you feel worn out?; and 4) Did you feel tired? The SF-36 VT scale was scored using norm-based methods that standardize the scores to have a mean of 50 and standard deviation of 10 in the general US population, with higher scores indicating more energy, less fatigue [33]. During the efficacy evaluation period of this study the SF-36v2 was administered at baseline and weeks 2, 4, 8, 12 and 16.

2.3. Factor Analysis

A primary assumption underlying Item Response Theory (IRT) is that the items under evaluation are unidimensional. To examine whether the items from the SF-36 VT and FACIT-Fatigue scales measure one unidimensional construct of "fatigue," baseline data were analyzed using confirmatory factor analyses appropriate for categorical data and weighted least squares parameter estimation with the Mplus software [34]. The goodness of fit of the factor models was evaluated using the comparative fit index (CFI) [35] (suggested cut-off for acceptable fit > 0.9 [36]) and the root mean square error of approximation (RMSEA) (suggested cut-off for acceptable fit < 0.10 [37]), as well as an examination of residual correlations. Three different models were tested: 1) a one-factor model, 2) a two-factor model assuming that each form loaded on a separate factor, and 3) a model with several factors derived from theoretical considerations and results of previous models. The theoretical model for fatigue evaluated a separate factor for vitality (as opposed to fatigue) and a factor for fatigue impact (as opposed to the symptom fatigue). For models 2 and 3 we used a bifactor

model [38], which specifies both a global factor and specific factors, thus allowing a direct comparison of which factors explain more of the item variance.

2.4. IRT Analyses

Once it was confirmed that the items from the SF-36 VT and FACIT-Fatigue scales formed a unidimensional construct of fatigue, the next step consisted of fitting an IRT model for patients at baseline with complete responses to all items. The current analyses used the generalized partial credit (GPC) IRT model that can be defined in the following way:

$$\ln\left(\frac{P\left(X_{ij}=c\right)}{P\left(X_{ij}=c-1\right)}\right)=\alpha_i\left(\theta_j-\beta_{ic}\right)$$

where the item category parameters β_{ic} are the values where the category response functions for two adjacent categories intersect (point on latent scale where there is an equal likelihood of selecting two adjacent response categories), the slope parameter α_i (only one for each item) described the steepness of the curves, and θ_j is the IRT score for each person. The GPC model has previously been used in the analysis of health outcomes data [21]. The GPC model assumes that the item response categories have a rank order and was selected over other types of IRT models, such as the partial credit model [39] or the graded response model [40], based on previous successes in the analysis of patient-reported outcome instruments with the GPC model [20-22,25]. Using the item category and slope parameters estimated from the GPC model, IRT scores for the composite fatigue index were estimated using the expected a posteriori (EAP) approach [41]. Scores for the composite fatigue index was rescaled so that the "average" score in the trial population was 50, with a standard deviation of 10, at baseline.

2.5. Analysis of Discriminant Validity and Responsiveness to Change

Analyses were conducted to evaluate and compare the responsiveness of the composite fatigue index with the SF-36 VT and FACIT-Fatigue scales. First, mean changes in each scale from baseline to week 16 were compared between patients who did and did not meet the ACR 20, ACR 50, and ACR 70 response criteria. Student's t-tests were conducted to test the significance of differences in mean score changes between ACR responder groups. Since each scale was scored using different scaling methods, effect sizes (ES) were computed for each scale by dividing the difference in mean change scores by the baseline standard deviation (SD) of each scale. The ES provided a means to compare the relative magnitude of difference in mean score change between ACR responder groups across scales. Second, the responsiveness of each scale was evaluated by comparing mean changes in scale scores from baseline to week 16 within and between treatment groups. Student's t-tests were conducted to test the significance of mean changes in scale scores within treatment groups (change from zero) and between each treatment and placebo group. Effect sizes were computed for each scale by dividing the change in score within groups by the baseline SD and the difference in mean change scores between groups by the baseline SD.

Comparisons of the relative efficiency of each scale and index in responding to changes in disease status (ACR response) and treatment were conducted by computing relative validity (RV) coefficients. The RV is computed as a ratio of F-statistics in a given test. Each Student's t-test was transformed into an F-statistic by squaring the t-statistic. The F-statistic is a ratio of the amount of separation in scores between groups relative to the within-group variance (error). The F-statistic is larger when the separation between groups is larger or when the within-group error variance is smaller. The RV coefficient for each scale and index in each test indicates, in proportional terms, its empirical validity relative to the best measure in the test [42,43].

3. Results

3.1. Patient Characteristics

The average age of the RA trial patients was 55 years (ranging from 26 to 78); 77% of these patients were female and 74% were Caucasian. At baseline, patients showed elevated disease activity. The average number of swollen and tender joints was 11.2 and 14.6, respectively. The mean DAS28 score derived from CRP was 5.7 and the mean DAS28 score derived from ESR was 6.4.

3.2. Factor Analyses

Table 1 presents CFA results for the FACIT-Fatigue and SF-36 VT scale items. In a one-factor model for fatigue, most items loaded strongly on the global factor, except for two items with positive formulation (FACIT7 *I have energy* and FACIT8 *Able to do usual activities*). However, model fit was poor (CFI = 0.85, RMSEA = 0.21). A two-factor model improved fit, although not sufficiently (CFI = 0.93, RMSEA = 0.14). Also, items had strong loading on the global factor and some items had strong negative loadings on the form-specific factors (FACIT7, FACIT8, VT3, and VT4), again suggesting that the forms do not define different sub-domains. Acceptable fit (CFI = 0.97, RMSEA = 0.09) was achieved by a model that included two conceptual factors (fatigue impact and vitality) and further specified correlated error terms (local

dependence) between adjacent items with similar content (FACIT5/FACIT6, FACIT7/FACIT8, VT1/VT2, VT3/VT4). Loading on the global factor was strong for all items except FACIT7 and FACIT8, which had weak loadings on the global factor and loaded higher on the specific vitality factor. Based on these results, an IRT model was pursued for the combined set of items. The issue of local dependence was handled by fitting the IRT model in two steps, first excluding the first item from each pair of locally dependent items, then excluding the second item from each pair.

3.3. IRT Analyses

Table 2 presents the item threshold parameters and fit statistics for the generalized partial credit model for the FACIT-Fatigue and SF-36v2 VT items. The most discriminating items (highest slopes) were from the FACIT-Fatigue (FACIT4, FACIT5, and FACIT6). All three of these FACIT-Fatigue items measure the impact of tiredness on the individual's ability to function. As previously explained, item step parameters indicate the "location" at which each item response option falls on the latent scale, with the latent fatigue scale having a mean of 0 and SD of 1. As shown, the step parameters ranged from −4.53 (FACIT10 *Too tired to eat*) to 5.78 (FACIT8 *Able to do usual activities*). In looking at the location values, which is the mean of the step parameters of each item, the item indicative of the greatest impairment ("easiest item") is FACIT10 (−2.14, *Too tired to eat*) and the item indicative of the least impairment ("hardest item") is FACIT7 (1.72, *Have energy*). Lastly, only one item, VT03, showed significant misfit (Chi-square was 30.4, df = 15, p < 0.01), however the result was considered non-significant after controlling for multiple testing.

Table 3 presents mean changes in fatigue scale scores by ACR responder groups (ACR20, ACR50, and ACR70). As shown, mean changes in all fatigue scales differed significantly between the ACR responder groups in the hypothesized manner. Patients categorized as responders showed significantly greater improvement in fatigue scale scores than non-responders. As shown, the SF-36 VT scale had the largest effect size in tests involving the ACR50 and ACR70 response criteria, while the composite fatigue index had a slightly higher effect size in the test involving the ACR20 response criteria. The composite fatigue index was the most efficient at discriminating between responders and non-responders in tests involving the ACR20 and ACR50 response criteria. In these two tests, the SF-36 VT scale was 65% (ACR 20) and 91% (ACR 50) as efficient, and the FACIT-Fatigue was 95% (ACR 20) and 89% (ACR 50) as efficient. In the test involving the ACR70 response criteria, the SF-36 VT scale was most efficient at discriminating between re-

Table 1. Factor analysis of fatigue and vitality items.

Items	Content	1 factor model	2 factor model			2 factor model with correlated errors			
		Global	Global	Facit	VT	Global	Impact	Vitality	Correlated errors
FACIT1	I feel fatigued	0.83	0.63	0.58		0.85			
FACIT2	I feel week all over	0.82	0.64	0.55		0.85			
FACIT3	I feel listless	0.81	0.68	0.45		0.84			
FACIT4	I feel tired	0.89	0.70	0.58		0.93			
FACIT5	Trouble starting things	0.92	0.74	0.56		0.86	0.14		} 0.15
FACIT6	Trouble finishing things	0.90	0.74	0.53		0.82	0.26		
FACIT7	I have energy	0.30	0.43	−0.21		**0.28**		0.32[1]	} 0.30
FACIT8	Able to do usual activities	0.24	0.38	−0.27		**0.16**	0.25	0.32[1]	
FACIT9	Need to sleep during the day	0.53	0.46	0.29		0.55			
FACIT10	Too tired to eat	0.64	0.61	0.22		0.62	0.27		
FACIT11	Need help doing activities	0.71	0.69	0.22		0.63	0.48		
FACIT12	Frustrated by being too tired	0.80	0.75	0.29		0.77	0.31		
FACIT13	Limit my social activities	0.82	0.79	0.27		0.74	0.57		
VT1	Feel full of life	0.57	0.62		0.57	0.51		0.32[1]	} 0.29
VT2	Have a lot of energy	0.69	0.75		0.40	0.65		0.32[1]	
VT3	Feel worn out	0.75	0.80		−0.47	0.67			} 0.34
VT4	Feel tired	0.74	0.78		−0.31	0.67			
Model Fit									
CFI		0.850	0.929			0.969			
RMSEA		0.210	0.144			0.091			

[1]Loadings constrained to equality to identify the model.

Table 2. IRT parameter estimates and fit statistics for FACIT fatigue and SF-36 VT items.

Item	Abbreviated item text	Item Parameter Estimates						Item Fit Statistics		
		Slope	Step 1	Step 2	Step 3	Step 4	Location	Chi-Square	df	p-value
FACIT1	I feel fatigued	2.02	−1.71	−0.43	0.68	1.78	0.08	7.0	13	0.901
FACIT2	I feel week all over	1.86	−1.82	−0.71	0.56	1.32	−0.16	7.6	12	0.817
FACIT3	I feel listless	1.77	−1.84	−1.04	0.17	1.07	−0.41	7.0	11	0.797
FACIT4	I feel tired	2.83	−1.57	−0.28	0.57	2.07	0.20	6.4	11	0.842
FACIT5	Trouble starting things	2.41	−1.75	−0.66	0.29	1.35	−0.19	11.9	12	0.455
FACIT6	Trouble finishing things	2.00	−1.89	−0.78	0.38	1.12	−0.29	8.6	12	0.733
FACIT7	I have energy	0.40	−3.02	0.51	5.00	4.40	1.72	22.6	16	0.125
FACIT8	Able to do usual activities	0.27	−4.53	−1.45	2.77	5.78	0.64	17.7	17	0.411
FACIT9	Need to sleep during the day	0.63	−2.81	−0.66	−0.94	0.51	−0.98	7.8	13	0.859
FACIT10	Too tired to eat	0.89	−4.53	−2.28	−1.08	−0.67	−2.14	4.1	8	0.847
FACIT11	Need help doing activities	1.08	−2.86	−1.38	−0.35	0.72	−0.97	8.7	11	0.654
FACIT12	Frustrated by being too tired	1.63	−1.14	−0.06	0.48	1.02	0.07	12.2	12	0.430
FACIT13	Limit my social activities	1.51	−1.73	−0.43	0.02	0.74	−0.35	14.7	12	0.260
VT1	Feel full of life	0.65	−1.37	0.16	1.31	3.65	0.94	21.2	18	0.268
VT2	Have a lot of energy	0.94	−0.57	0.86	1.90	2.53	1.18	10.4	13	0.662
VT3	Feel worn out	0.99	−2.22	−0.68	1.07	1.92	0.02	30.4	15	0.010
VT4	Feel tired	1.08	−1.71	−0.14	1.76	3.12	0.75	22.7	16	0.123
Total								221.0	222	0.506

Table 3. Comparison of mean changes fatigue scale scores by ACR response categories.

Scales	ACR 20 Yes (n = 101)	No (n = 132)	Diff	ES	F	RV
SF-36 VT	6.68	0.62	6.06	0.65	26.3***	0.65
FACIT-F	6.77	0.47	6.30	0.63	38.8***	0.95
VT Index	7.21	0.55	6.66	0.66	41.0***	1.00
Scales	ACR 50 Yes (n = 36)	No (n = 197)	Diff	ES	F	RV
SF-36 VT	10.47	1.91	8.56	0.91	28.6***	0.91
FACIT-F	9.40	2.08	7.32	0.73	27.9***	0.89
VT Index	10.20	2.20	8.00	0.80	31.4***	1.00
Scales	ACR 70 Yes (n = 9)	No (n = 224)	Diff	ES	F	RV
SF-36 VT	14.30	2.80	11.50	1.22	13.8***	1.00
FACIT-F	11.33	2.90	8.43	0.84	9.8**	0.71
VT Index	12.63	3.09	9.54	0.95	11.4***	0.83

sponder and non-responder, followed by the composite fatigue index (83%) and the FACIT-Fatigue (71%).

Table 4 presents changes from baseline to week 16 for each of the fatigue scales by treatment group. From the within-groups analyses the composite fatigue index was found to be the most responsive to secukinumab treatment for all 4 secukinumab dose groups compared to the SF-36 VT and FACIT-F scales. Across secukinumab dose groups the effect size for the composite fatigue index was 11% - 93% larger than the effect sizes observed for the SF-36 VT and FACIT-F scales. In addition, the F-statistics testing the difference in change score from 0 within each of the secukinumab dose groups was largest for the composite fatigue index, indicating a greater response to treatment. In the between-groups analyses, both the 75 mg (mean difference of 3.4 points, F = 3.8, p < 0.05) and 150 mg (mean difference of 4.2 points, F = 4.8, p < 0.05) secukinumab groups showed significantly greater improvement in fatigue scores on the composite index compared to placebo. No significant differences in change scores between the 75 mg and 150 mg dose groups and placebo was observed with either the SF-36 VT or FACIT-F scales.

4. Discussion

In this study, we used factor analytic and IRT methods to evaluate the measurement properties of the FACIT-Fatigue and SF-36 VT scale in the context of an RA clinical trial setting. The purpose of these analyses was to evaluate the possibility of combining the items of the two fatigue measures to score one composite index. Additional

tests were conducted to determine whether combining the items from the two fatigue measures resulted in a scale that is more responsive to changes in disease status and treatment effects.

A requirement for combining items from different scales to score a composite index using IRT methods is evidence supporting unidimensionality, namely, evidence that shows all items to be defining one underlying construct. While a requirement for fitting an IRT model, the broader implication of items not fitting a unidimensional construct warrants further interpretation. Scales that combine items of various concepts into one scale are difficult to interpret as the item-content driving a difference in score between groups or a change in score over time is largely unknown. Furthermore, combining items that lack unidimensionality calls into question whether the scale validly measures the concept it was intended to measure. The results of factor analyses of the fatigue items of the FACIT-Fatigue and SF-36 VT scale did not point unequivocally to either a unidimensional or multidimensional structure underlying the items. Fit of the FACIT-Fatigue and SF-36 VT items to a unidimensional model was not ideal. Specification of survey-specific factors for the FACIT-Fatigue and SF-36v2 VT scale showed minimal improvement in model fit. Specification of models consisting of factors that were more conceptually based, such as fatigue impact and vitality for the fatigue index, showed the best overall model fit. However, all items showed sufficiently strong correlations on the global fatigue factor to warrant fitting a single IRT model. One potential source of the model fit problem may be

Table 4. Comparison of treatment outcomes (baseline to week 16) across the SF-36v2 vitality (VT) and FACIT-fatigue scales, and a composite fatigue (FT) index comprised of the cross calibration of items from both SF-36v2 VT and FACIT-fatigue items.

	Secukinumab 25 mg					Placebo					Between Treatment				
Scale	Mean Δ	SD	ES[1]	F	RV[2]	Mean Δ	SD	ES[1]	F	RV[2]	Diff	SD	ES[1]	F	RV[2]
SF-36 VT[4]	2.4	9.3	0.26	ns[3]	-	3.6	8.6	0.42	8.2[b]	1.00	−1.2	8.9	0.13	ns[3]	-
FACIT-F	2.3	7.9	0.29	4.0[a]	0.63	1.8	8.4	0.21	ns[3]	-	0.5	8.1	0.06	ns[3]	-
FT Index[4]	3.0	8.5	0.35	6.4[b]	1.00	1.6	8.6	0.18	ns[3]	-	1.4	8.5	0.16	ns[3]	-
	Secukinumab 75 mg					**Placebo**					**Between Treatment**				
Scale	Mean Δ	SD	ES[1]	F	RV[2]	Mean Δ	SD	ES[1]	F	RV[2]	Diff	SD	ES[1]	F	RV[2]
SF-36 VT	2.9	10.3	0.28	3.9[a]	0.22	3.6	8.6	0.42	8.2[b]	1.00	−0.7	9.4	0.07	ns[3]	-
FACIT-F	3.9	8.4	0.46	10.2[b]	0.56	1.8	8.4	0.21	ns[3]	-	2.1	8.4	0.25	ns[3]	-
FT Index	5.0	8.2	0.61	18.1[c]	1.00	1.6	8.6	0.18	ns[3]	-	3.4	8.5	0.40	3.8[a]	1.00
	Secukinumab 150 mg					**Placebo**					**Between Treatment**				
Scale	Mean Δ	SD	ES[1]	F	RV[2]	Mean Δ	SD	ES[1]	F	RV[2]	Diff	SD	ES[1]	F	RV[2]
SF-36 VT	5.4	11.0	0.49	10.2[a]	0.60	3.6	8.6	0.42	8.2[b]	1.00	1.8	9.8	0.18	ns[3]	-
FACIT-F	5.2	8.5	0.61	16.0[c]	0.94	1.8	8.4	0.21	ns[3]	-	3.4	8.7	0.39	ns[3]	-
FT Index	5.8	9.1	0.63	16.8[c]	1.00	1.6	8.6	0.18	ns[3]	-	4.2	9.1	0.46	4.8[a]	1.00
	Secukinumab 300 mg					**Placebo**					**Between Treatment**				
Scale	Mean Δ	SD	ES[1]	F	RV[2]	Mean Δ	SD	ES[1]	F	RV[2]	Diff	SD	ES[1]	F	RV[2]
SF-36 VT	2.0	6.9	0.29	ns[3]	-	3.6	8.6	0.42	8.2[b]	1.00	−1.6	7.8	0.21	ns[3]	-
FACIT-F	2.8	7.2	0.39	6.2[a]	0.46	1.8	8.4	0.21	ns[3]	-	1.0	8.3	0.12	ns[3]	-
FT Index	3.7	6.6	0.56	13.4[c]	1.00	1.6	8.6	0.18	ns[3]	-	2.1	7.7	0.27	ns[3]	-

[1]ES = Effect Size, mean change score divided by the SD; [2]RV = Relative Validity Coefficient, ratio of F-Statistics (1.00 representing best scale in a test); [3]ns = not statistically significant; [4]SF-36 VT scale and FT composite index are standardized scores, with a mean of 50 and SD of 10. [c]$p < 0.001$; [b]$p < 0.01$; [a]$p < 0.05$.

due to the use of baseline data from the trial. Inclusion and exclusion criteria in clinical trials are often designed to produce a fairly homogenous sample with respect to disease activity. This in turn can result in less variability in item response distributions, which can potentially pose a challenge in psychometric testing. In data not shown, fit of a unidimensional model improved significantly with data from post-treatment assessment periods for the fatigue items due in part to more variability in item response distributions.

Despite less than optimal fit to a unidimensional structure observed for fatigue items, the strength of the current study lies in comparing the composite fatigue index to the original scales in terms of responsiveness to changes in underlying clinical status, such as ACR improvement criteria. The results showed that the composite fatigue index was more responsive to changes in clinical disease activity than the FACIT-Fatigue and SF-36 VT scales in tests involving the ACR20 and ACR50. In tests of treatment response, the composite fatigue index showed larger effect sizes than the original scales with the

within-group evaluation of changes in scores for each dose group. Additionally, the composite fatigue index showed a greater response to treatment in comparisons of outcome scores between the 150 mg secukinumab dose group and placebo. These findings suggest that the deviation from unidimensionality detected with the psychometric tests had little impact on the ability of each index to respond in hypothesized ways to changes in underlying clinical status and treatment effects.

Previous studies investigating the implications of applying IRT methods to the scoring of a composite physical functioning index resulted in improved responsiveness to changes in disease status and treatment effects [27]. For example, item parameters estimated with IRT methods showed that the items of the Health Assessment Questionnaire (HAQ) and SF-36v2 physical functioning scale defined different ranges of physical functioning, with the HAQ items defining a very low range and the SF-36 defining a higher range of functioning [27,44]. The consequence of combining the items from both instruments extended the range of physical functioning measured and reduced problematic ceiling and floor effects, which resulted in improve responsiveness [27]. However, the explanation as to why the composite fatigue index performed relatively better than the original scales in this study seems less straightforward. Evaluating the IRT item parameters does not clearly indicate that either the FACIT-Fatigue or the SF-36 VT scale defines different ranges of the fatigue spectrum. In fact, both instruments conceptualize fatigue as a bipolar concept, including items that measure fatigue (lower range) and energy (upper range). Interestingly, the item parameters of "energy" (FACIT7, FACIT8, VT1, VT2) were less discriminating in both instruments as indicated by the magnitude of the slope parameters. This may be attributed to a greater number of items that measure fatigue. While further research is necessary to understand why the composite fatigue index performed better than the original scales, one possible explanation could be that the IRT item parameters provide better scaling of item responses by spreading them more appropriately throughout the continuum of fatigue as opposed to treating each item equally, as would the sum score approach. For example, the item FACIT12 (too tired to eat) has an item category parameter of -4.53, which defines a place on the continuum of fatigue that is almost 5 standard deviation units below the average of 0 in the trial sample, whereas the item category parameter of the item FACIT8 (able to do usual activities) has a value of $+5.78$, which is nearly 6 standard deviation units above the average of 0 in the trial sample. These parameter estimates are more than 9 standard deviations apart, yet the sum score approach would weight these items equally in the total score. This difference in the manner in which items are scored may explain the difference in the performance of the composite fatigue index over the original scales.

Several limitations of this study are recognized. First, this study included a relatively small sample size for IRT modeling. It is possible that the small sample size lacked the power to produce robust item parameter estimates as well as the ability to detect misfit or item bias among the items. Further studies with larger sample sizes are necessary to determine the underlying structures of both physical function and fatigue items from the instruments evaluated in this study. Another potential limitation concerns the use of multiple language versions of questionnaires in this trial. Coupled with the relatively small sample size, any chance of evaluating item bias as a result of differences in language was negligible. Such item bias tends to add noise in model testing of unidimensionality and parameter estimation. Additional studies in multinational settings with larger sample sizes is warranted to understand any differential item functioning that arises due to language or cultural differences.

5. Conclusion

In conclusion, IRT methods were useful in evaluating the underlying measurement properties of two widely used fatigue measures in RA treatment studies. Specifically, the use of IRT methods to cross calibrate the items from two different fatigue scales improved the measurement precision over a larger continuum on the latent physical fatigue measure, as compared to the original scales. Combining the best features of each instrument yielded a more powerful measure with greater sensitivity to clinical change and treatment response. As demonstrated in this study, a more precise measure may be important in deciding the optimal dose in treating patients with RA.

REFERENCES

[1] D. Symmons, G. Turner, R. Webb, et al., "The Prevalence of Rheumatoid Arthritis in the United Kingdom: New Estimates for a New Century," Rheumatology, Vol. 41, No. 7, 2002, pp. 793-800. http://dx.doi.org/10.1093/rheumatology/41.7.793

[2] K. Jordan, A. M. Clarke, D. P. Symmons, D. Fleming, M. Porcheret, U. T. Kadam, et al., "Measuring Disease Prevalence: A Comparison of Musculoskeletal Disease Using Four General Practice Consultation Databases," British Journal of General Practices, Vol. 57, No. 534, 2007, pp. 7-14.

[3] L. A. Rodriguez, L. B. Tolosa, A. Ruigomez, S. Johansson and M. A. Wallander, "Rheumatoid Arthritis in UK Primary Care: Incidence and Prior Morbidity," Scandinavia Journal of Rheumatology, Vol. 38, No. 3, 2009, pp. 173-177. http://dx.doi.org/10.1080/03009740802448825

[4] M. M. Ward, H. S. Javitz and E. H. Yelin, "The Direct Cost of Rheumatoid Arthritis," Value Health, Vol. 3, No. 4, 2000, pp. 243-252. http://dx.doi.org/10.1046/j.1524-4733.2000.34001.x

[5] R. C. Kessler, J. R. Maclean, M. Petukhova, C. A. Sarawate, L. Short, T. T. Li, et al., "The Effects of Rheumatoid Arthritis on Labor Force Participation, Work Performance, and Healthcare Costs in Two Workplace Samples," Journal of Occupational and Environmental Medicine, Vol. 50, No. 1, 2008, pp. 88-98. http://dx.doi.org/10.1097/JOM.0b013e31815bc1aa

[6] R. J. Ozminkowski, W. N. Burton, R. Z. Goetzel, R. Maclean and S. Wang, "The Impact of Rheumatoid Arthritis on Medical Expenditures, Absenteeism, and Short-Term Disability Benefits," Journal of Occupational and Environmental Medicine, Vol. 48, No. 2, 2006, pp. 135-148. http://dx.doi.org/10.1097/01.jom.0000194161.12923.52

[7] C. H. van Jaarsveld, J. W. Jacobs, A. J. Schrijvers, G. A. Albada-Kuipers, D. M. Hofman and J. W. Bijlsma, "Effects of Rheumatoid Arthritis on Employment and Social Participation during the First Years of Disease in The Netherlands," British Journal of Rheumatology, Vol. 37, No. 8, 1998, pp. 848-853. http://dx.doi.org/10.1093/rheumatology/37.8.848

[8] F. Wolfe, K. Michaud, H. K. Choi and R. Williams,

"Household Income and Earnings Losses among 6396 Persons with Rheumatoid Arthritis," *Journal of Rheumatology*, Vol. 32, No. 10, 2005, pp. 1875-1883.

[9]   M. Kosinski, S. C. Kujawski, R. Martin, L. A. Wanke, M. C. Buatti, J. E. Ware, *et al.*, "Health-Related Quality of Life in Early Rheumatoid Arthritis: Impact of Disease and Treatment Response," *American Journal of Managed Care*, Vol. 8, No. 3, 2002, pp. 231-240.

[10]   T. P. Suurmeijer, M. Waltz, T. Moum, F. Guillemin, F. L. van Sonderen, S. Briancon, *et al.*, "Quality of Life Profiles in the First Years of Rheumatoid Arthritis: Results from the EURIDISS Longitudinal Study," *Arthritis Rheum*, Vol. 45, No. 2, 2001, pp. 111-121. http://dx.doi.org/10.1002/1529-0131(200104)45:2<111:: AID-ANR162>3.0.CO;2-E

[11]   J. Talamo, A. Frater, S. Gallivan and A. Young, "Use of the Short Form 36 (SF36) for Health Status Measurement in Rheumatoid Arthritis," *British Journal of Rheumatology*, Vol. 36, No. 4, 1997, pp. 463-469. http://dx.doi.org/10.1093/rheumatology/36.4.463

[12]   T. Sokka, B. Abelson and T. Pincus, "Mortality in Rheumatoid Arthritis: 2008 Update," *Clinical and Experimental Rheumatology*, Vol. 26, No. 5, 2008, pp. S35-S61.

[13]   A. M. Wasserman, "Diagnosis and Management of Rheumatoid Arthritis," *American Family Physician*, Vol. 84, No. 11, 2011, pp. 1245-1252.

[14]   K. G. Saag, G. G. Teng, N. M. Patkar, J. Anuntiyo, C. Finney, J. R. Curtis, *et al.*, "American College of Rheumatology 2008 Recommendations for the Use of Nonbiologic and Biologic Disease-Modifying Antirheumatic Drugs in Rheumatoid Arthritis," *Arthritis Rheum*, Vol. 59, No. 6, 2008, pp. 762-784. http://dx.doi.org/10.1002/art.23721

[15]   R. B. Terry and G. Singh, "Quality of Life Measures in the Treatment of Arthritis in Clinical Practice," *New Standards in Arthiritis Care*, Vol. 5, No. 3, 2013, pp. 2-6.

[16]   T. Pincus, R. H. Brooks and L. F. Callahan, "Prediction of Long Term Mortality in Patients with Rheumatoid Arthritis According to Simple Questionnaire and Joint Count Measures," *Annals of Internal Medicine*, Vol. 120, No. 1, 1994, pp. 26-34. http://dx.doi.org/10.7326/0003-4819-120-1-199401010-0 0005

[17]   D. Aletaha, R. Landewe, T. Karonitsch, J. Bathon, M. Boers, C. Bombardier, *et al.*, "Reporting Disease Activity in Clinical Trials of Patients with Rheumatoid Arthritis: EULAR/ACR Collaborative Recommendations," *Annals of the Rheumatic Diseases*, Vol. 67, No. 10, 2008, pp. 1360-1364. http://dx.doi.org/10.1136/ard.2008.091454

[18]   J. E. Ware Jr. and C. D. Sherbourne, "The MOS 36-Item Short-Form Health Survey (SF-36). I. Conceptual Framework and Item Selection," *Medical Care*, Vol. 30, No. 6, 1992, pp. 473-483. http://dx.doi.org/10.1097/00005650-199206000-00002

[19]   D. Cella, S. Yount, M. Sorensen, E. Chartash, N. Sengupta and J. Grober, "Validation of the Functional Assessment of Chronic Illness Therapy Fatigue Scale Relative to Other Instrumentation in Patients with Rheumatoid

Arthritis," *Journal of Rheumatology*, Vol. 32, No. 5, 2005, pp. 811-819.

[20]   J. B. Bjorner, M. Kosinski, X. Sun and J. E. Ware Jr., "Calibration of Item Banks for Use in Improving Estimates of Eight SF-36 Health Constructs," 2006.

[21]   J. B. Bjorner, M. Kosinski and J. E. Ware Jr., "Using Item Response Theory to Calibrate the Headache Impact Test (HIT) to the Metric of Traditional Headache Scales," *Quality Life Research*, 2003, pp. 981-1002. http://dx.doi.org/10.1023/A:1026123400242

[22]   J. B. Bjorner, M. Kosinski and J. E. Ware Jr., "Calibration of an Item Pool for Assessing the Burden of Headaches: An Application of Item Response Theory to the Headache Impact Test (HIT™)," *Quality of Life Research*, Vol. 12, No. 8, 2003, pp. 887-902. http://dx.doi.org/10.1023/A:1026175112538

[23]   J. Fries, M. Rose and E. Krishnan, "The PROMIS of Better Outcome Assessment: Responsiveness, Floor and Ceiling Effects, and Internet Administration," *Journal of Rheumatology*, Vol. 38, No. 8, 2011, pp. 1759-1764. http://dx.doi.org/10.3899/jrheum.110402

[24]   M. Rose, J. B. Bjorner, J. Becker, J. F. Fries and J. E. Ware, "Evaluation of a Preliminary Physical Function Item Bank Supported the Expected Advantages of the Patient-Reported Outcomes Measurement Information System (PROMIS)," *Journal of Clinical Epidemiology*, Vol. 61, No. 1, 2008, pp. 17-33. http://dx.doi.org/10.1016/j.jclinepi.2006.06.025

[25]   J. B. Bjorner, M. Kosinski and J. E. Ware Jr., "The Feasibility of Applying Item Response Theory to Measures of Migraine Impact: A Reanalysis of Three Clinical Studies," *Quality Life Research*, Vol. 12, No. 8, 2003, pp. 887-902. http://dx.doi.org/10.1023/A:1026175112538

[26]   M. Kosinski, J. B. Bjorner, J. E. Ware Jr., A. Batenhorst and R. K. Cady, "The Responsiveness of Headache Impact Scales Scored Using 'Classical' and 'Modern' Psychometric Methods: A Re-Analysis of Three Clinical Trials," *Quality Life Research*, Vol. 12, No. 8, 2003, pp. 903-912. http://dx.doi.org/10.1023/A:1026111029376

[27]   M. Martin, M. Kosinski, J. B. Bjorner, J. E. Ware Jr., R. Maclean and T. Li, "Item Response Theory Methods Can Improve the Measurement of Physical Function by Combining the Modified Health Assessment Questionnaire and the SF-36 Physical Function Scale," *Quality Life Research*, Vol. 16, No. 4, 2007, pp. 647-660. http://dx.doi.org/10.1007/s11136-007-9193-5

[28]   M. Genovese, P. Durez, H. Richards, *et al.*, "Secukinumab Improves Signs and Symptoms in Patients with Active Rheumatoid Arthritis: Results of Dose-Finding, Double-Blind, Randomized, Placebo-Controlled, Phase II Studies," *World Psoriasis & Psoriatic Arthritis Conference*, 2012.

[29]   D. Cella, "The Functional Assessment of Cancer Therapy-Anemia (FACT-An) Scale: A New Tool for the Assessment of Outcomes in Cancer Anemia and Fatigue," *Seminars in Hematology*, Vol. 34, No. 3, 1997, pp. 13-19.

[30]   D. F. Cella, D. S. Tulsky, G. Gray, B. Sarafian, E. Linn, A. Bonomi, *et al.*, "The Functional Assessment of Cancer

Therapy Scale: Development and Validation of the General Measure," *Journal of Clinical Oncology*, Vol. 11, No. 3, 1993, pp. 570-579.

[31] K. Webster, D. Cella and K. Yost, "The Functional Assessment of Chronic Illness Therapy (FACIT) Measurement System: Properties, Applications, and Interpretation," *Health Quality Life Outcomes*, Vol. 1, 2003, p. 79. http://dx.doi.org/10.1186/1477-7525-1-79

[32] J. E. Ware Jr., K. K. Snow, M. Kosinski and B. Gandek, "SF-36 Health Survey Manual and Interpretation Guide," The Health Institite, New England Medical Center, Boston, 1993.

[33] J. E. Ware Jr., M. Kosinski and J. Dewey, "How to Score Version Two of the SF-36 Health Survey," Quality Metric Inc., Lincoln, 2000.

[34] "Mplus User's Guide [Computer Program]," Version 1. Muthén & Muthén, Los Angeles, 1998.

[35] P. M. Bentler, "Comparative Fit Indexes in Structural Models," *Psychological Bulletin*, Vol. 107, No. 2, 1990, pp. 238-246. http://dx.doi.org/10.1037/0033-2909.107.2.238

[36] L. Hu and P. M. Bentler, "Cutoff Criteria for Fit Indexes in Covariance Structure Analysis: Conventional Criteria versus New Alternatives," *Structural Equation Modeling*, Vol. 6, No. 1, 1999, pp. 1-55. http://dx.doi.org/10.1080/10705519909540118

[37] M. W. Browne and R. Cudeck, "Alternative Ways of Assessing Model Fit," *Sociological Methods and Research*, Vol. 21, No. 2, 1992, pp. 230-258. http://dx.doi.org/10.1177/0049124192021002005

[38] R. P. McDonald, "Test Theory: A Unified Treatment," Lawrence Erlbaum Associates, Hillsdale, 1999.

[39] G. N. Mastersm, "A Rasch Model for Partial Credit Scoring," *Psychometrika*, Vol. 47, No. 2, 1982, pp. 149-173. http://dx.doi.org/10.1007/BF02296272

[40] F. Samejima, "Graded Response Model," In: W. J. van der Linden and R. K. Hambleton, Eds., *Handbook of Modern Item Response Theory*, Springer, Berlin, 1997, pp. 85-100. http://dx.doi.org/10.1007/978-1-4757-2691-6_5

[41] R. D. Bock and R. J. Mislevy, "Adaptive EAP Estimation of Ability in a Microcomputer Environment," *Applied Psychological Measurement*, Vol. 6, No. 4, 1982, pp. 431-444. http://dx.doi.org/10.1177/014662168200600405

[42] C. A. McHorney, J. E. Ware Jr. and A. E. Raczek, "The MOS 36-Item Short-Form Health Survey (SF-36): II. Psychometric and Clinical Tests of Validity in Measuring Physical and Mental Health Constructs," *Medical Care*, Vol. 31, No. 3, 1993, pp. 247-263. http://dx.doi.org/10.1097/00005650-199303000-00006

[43] C. A. McHorney, S. M. Haley and J. E. Ware Jr., "Evaluation of the MOS SF-36 Physical Function Scale (PF-10): II. Comparison of Relative Precision Using Likert and Rasch Scoring Methods," *Journal of Clinical Epidemiology*, Vol. 50, No. 4, 1997, pp. 451-461. http://dx.doi.org/10.1016/S0895-4356(96)00424-6

[44] W. J. Taylor and K. M. McPherson, "Using Rasch Analysis to Compare the Psychometric Properties of the Short Form 36 Physical Function Score and the Health Assessment Questionnaire Disability Index in Patients with Psoriatic Arthritis and Rheumatoid Arthritis," *Arthritis Care & Research*, Vol. 57, No. 5, 2007, pp. 723-729. http://dx.doi.org/10.1002/art.22770

List of Abbreviations

CFI: Comparative Fit Index
CRP: C-Reactive Protein
EAP: Expected a Posteriori
ES: Effect Size
ESR: Erythrocyte Sedimentation Rate
FACIT: Functional Assessment of Chronic Illness Therapy
GPC: Generalized Partial Credit
HAQ: Health Assessment Questionnaire
HRQoL: Health Related Quality of Life
IRT: Item Response Theory
PRO: Patient Reported Outcome
RA: Rheumatoid Arthritis
RMSEA: Root Mean Square Error of Approximation
RV: Relative Validity

SD: Standard Deviation
VT: Vitality

23

Etiology of Arthritis in Lomé (Togo)

Owonayo Oniankitan, Prénam Houzou, Komi C. Tagbor, Eryam Fianyo, Viwalé E. S. Koffi-Tessio, Kodjo Kakpovi, Moustafa Mijiyawa

Department of Rheumatology, CHU Sylvanus Olympio, Lomé, Togo.
Email: Owonayo@yahoo.com

ABSTRACT

Aim: Determine the frequency and respective proportion of the various etiological forms of arthritis in Lomé (Togo). **Patients and Methods:** Transversal study carried out over 15 years on files of arthritis infected patients and submitted to rheumatologic consultation. **Results:** 1081 out of 13,517 patients examined (8%) were suffering from arthritis. Those 1081 patients (456 women, 42.2% and 625 men, 57.8%) were in average 38 years old and enjoyed an average duration of evolution of three years. The chronic inflammatory rheumatisms (CIR) (602 cases, 56.9%), the metabolic arthropathies (233 cases, 22%) and the infections (198 cases, 16.6%), were the main etiologies that were observed. The average age of 198 patients with infectious arthritis was 36 years and the average duration of 9 months. Infectious arthritis was preferably located at the knee (34.3%), and was essentially caused by a banal germ (157 patients; 79.3%) and associated with HIV in 25 patients (15.9%). The remaining 233 patients (9 women, and 224 men) suffering from metabolic arthritis were in average 52 years old and enjoyed an average duration of evolution of five years. The chronic inflammatory rheumatisms were mainly represented by spondyloarthropathies (90 cases, 14.9%) and the arthritis rheumatoid (64 cases, 10.6%). 399 out of 602 cases of the CIR were not classified while 52 cases were associated with HIV. The connective tissue diseases were dominated by the polymyositis (9 cases, 18.7%). **Conclusion:** The chronic inflammatory rheumatisms were the first causal form of arthritis in rheumatologic consultation in Lomé.

Keywords: Black Africa; Arthritis; Etiology of Arthritis

1. Introduction

Arthritis is a common reason for consultation in rheumatology [1-3]. In the Sub-Saharan Africa, little epidemiological research has been devoted to arthritis [2,4,5]. The infectious disease is still common in sub-Saharan Africa because of the underdevelopment and poor hygiene. The reputation of the extreme rarity of gout in sub-Saharan Africa was contradicted by the work undertaken over the last 30 years [6]. The Spondyloarthropathies (SPA), in particular ankylosing spondylitis is rare in Africa and the link between HIV and the SPA in this region seems now well known [7]. Rheumatoid arthritis (RA) is frequent in Eastern and Southern Africa while in West and Central Africa it seems rare [8]. Systemic lupus erythematosus (SLE) is deemed rare in black Africa unlike scleroderma which seems frequent [8]. The studies conducted in hospitals focused on relatively small samples [4,5,9,10]. The aim assigned to this study was to determine in a large population suffering from rheumatism, the respective proportion of the different etiological forms of arthritis during a rheumatologic consultation in Lomé (Togo).

2. Patients and Methods

It has been a transversal study conducted from October 1989 to December 2005 of which the subject matter was to focus on the files of the patients suffering from arthritis and seen in clinical consultation of rheumatology. This springs from the study of a series of case records of patients admitted in the Department of Rheumatology, University Hospital Sylvanus Olympio, of Lomé, Togo's capital. The patients suffering from congestive osteoarthritis were not part of the sample study. The demographic (sex, age of the patient at diagnosis), clinical (arthritis characteristics, systemic manifestations associated), and paraclinical (radiographic, biologic, immunologic) data of patients were collected from their records. The patients suffering from gout perfectly answered to the criteria of ARA [11]. The spondyloarthropathies answered the criteria of Amor [12] and the rheumatoid arthritis patients on their side answered to the criteria of ACR [13]. The connective tissue diseases on their part answered to the various diagnostic criteria. The positive diagnosis of the infectious arthritis has essentially been radio-clinical. The infection has been considered as certain in case of isolation of the causal germ in the organism or due to the underlining of evocative historical lesions in the suspected site. Otherwise, it was probable. Each patient has been the subject of a radiographic test of the infected part, of a hemogram, of a measurement of the speed of sedimentation, creatinine, and of a retroactive serology. A plasma creatinine greater than 115 μmol/L was considered as evidence of renal failure. The overweight has been defined as a corporal mass index (CMI) higher than 25 kg/m^2 while obesity is defined as a CMI higher than 30 kg/m^2. The immunologic tests undertaken had not been systematically conducted because of economic and technical limitations.

3. Results

3.1. General Characteristics of the Patients

One thousand and eighty one of the 13.517 patients examined (8%) were suffering from arthritis. Those 1081 patients (made up of 456 women, 42.2%; and 625 men, 57.8%) were about 38 years old at the beginning of the disease and enjoyed an average duration of evolution of three years. The chronic inflammatory rheumatism (602 cases, 55.7%) and the metabolic arthropathies (233 cases, 21.6%), were the main etiologies of arthritis observed in Lomé (**Table 1**).

3.2. Chronic Inflammatory Rheumatisms (CIR)

The average age of the patients suffering from chronic inflammatory rheumatisms was 34.6 year old while the average duration of evolution is 2.2 year. The chronic inflammatory rheumatisms were essentially represented by: the spondyloarthropathies (90 cases, 14.9%), the rheumatoid arthritis (64 cases, 10.6%), and the juvenile chronic arthritis (10 cases, 1.66%) (**Table 2**). Out of the 602 cases of CIR 399 cases were not classified. The 399 cases of CIR Unclassified fell into 295 cases (73.9%)

Table 1. Distribution of arthritis according to different clinical forms of arthritis.

	Number of cases	Percentage
Chronic inflammatory rheumatisms	602	55.7
Metabolic arthropathies	233	21.6
Arthritis infectious	198	18.3
Connective tissue diseases	48	4.4
Total	1081	100

Table 2. Demographic data of the patients infected with inflammatory rheumatisms and the connective tissue diseases according to the diagnosis.

	Number (%)	Sex W/M[*]	Age (years) m ± ET[**]
Unclassified CIR[***]	399 (63.7)	226/173	36.9 ± 14.5
Rheumatoid arthritis	62 (9.9)	52/10	41.8 ± 18.2
Unclassified spondyloarthropathies	53 (8.5)	7/46	34.4 ± 10.1
Unclassified connective tissue	26 (4.2)	23/03	34.9 ± 15.3
Ankylosing spondylitis	22 (3.5)	0/22	32.5 ± 7.6
Reactional arthritis	17 (2.7)	08/09	34.7 ± 10.2
Polymyositis	09 (1.4)	07/02	39.4 ± 09.5
Chronic juvenil arthritis	07 (1.1)	02/05	08.8 ± 04.9
SLE[****]	07 (1,1)	07/00	42.6 ± 08.2
Scleroderma	06 (0.9)	04/02	40.8 ± 13.5
Horton disease	05 (0,8)	04/01	63.5 ± 20.1
Dermatomyositis	04 (0.6)	02/02	35.3 ± 12.7
Still disease	03 (0,5)	02/01	29.0 ± 18.7
Unclassified vascularitis	03 (0.5)	01/02	39.0 ± 32.5
Rheumatic fever	02 (0.3)	01/01	18.0 ± 14.1
Psoriasic rheumatism	01 (0.1)	00/01	45.0 ± 00.0
Total	626 (100)	346/280	36.9 ± 14.9

[*]Women/Men, [**]average ± standard deviation, [***]unclassified chronic inflammatory rheumatisms, [****]Systemic lupus erythematosus.

of chronic polyarthritis, 80 cases (20.1%) of isolated oligoarthritis and 24 cases (6%) of isolated mono-arthritis. These 295 patients with chronic polyarthritis had an average age of 37.2 years and the average duration of the disease was 3 years. The chronic polyarthritis were characterized by the absence of deformation, joint destruction and systemic manifestations. The isolated oligoarthritis was sensitive to anti-inflammatory non-steroidal and had no radiological destruction. The 62 patients with rheumatoid arthritis had an age between 27 and 70 years. The average duration of evolution ranged from 3 months to 23 years. A distal joints location was observed in all patients (**Table 3**). The most frequent clinical forms of spondyloarthropathies were the ankylosing spondylitis (22 cases) and the reactional arthritis (17 cases). The chronic inflammatory rheumatisms were associated with HIV in 52 patients (spondyloarthropathies: 22 cases of which 17 cases of reactional arthritis, not classified inflammatory rheumatisms: 22 cases and rheumatoid arthritis: two cases).

The connective tissue diseases were dominated by the polymyositis (9 cases, 18.7%), the systemic lupus erythematosus (7 cases, 14.6%), and the scleroderma (6 cases,

Table 3. Clinical and paraclinical manifestations observed in 62 patients with rheumatoid arthritis.

	Number	Percentage
Distal joint location	62	100
Coxitis	4	6.5
Cervical spine affected	5	8.1
Erythrocyte sedimentation rate ≥ 20 mm (ranged from 25 to 131 mm in the first hour)	62	100
Present of a rheumatoid factor in 40 patients explored	25	40.3
Present of bilateral carpitis	43	69.3
Present of a demineralization in band of the hands and wrists	19	30.6

12.5%). The symptomatology of 13 patients with po-lymyositis-dermatomyositis was dominated by muscle weakness (13 cases), myalgia (10 cases), arthralgia and swelling of the face (8 cases). The erythrocyte sedimentation rate was between 40 and 121 mm in the first hour. Creatinine phosphokinase was increased in 10 patients explored with a value between 1300 and 4500 IU/L (normal range 15 - 110 IU/L). The most frequent clinical manifestations of systemic lupus erythematosus were alteration of general condition (five cases), polyarthralgia (seven cases), discoid lupus (six cases), malar rash (four cases), alopecia (three cases), and seritis (three cases). Laboratory findings included haemolytic anemia (five cases), and leucocytopenia (three cases), Antinuclear and anti-DNA antibodies were detected in three patients explored.

3.3. Metabolic Arthritis

Among the 233 patients (9 women and 224 men) with metabolic arthritis, 229 were suffering from gout (98.3%) and the four others suffered from chondrocalcinosis (1.7%). The average age of the patients suffering from metabolic arthritis was 52 years old and the average duration of evolution five years. The average age of the 229 patients (six women, 223 men) suffering from gout was 52 years. The average duration of evolution of gout upon diagnostic was five years. Fifty patients (21.8%) had tophus; one patient had a nephritic colic. No risk factor has been found with eight patients (3.5 %). Each of the 221 other patients (96.5 %) had at least one risk factor (**Table 4**).

3.4. Arthritis Infectious

The 198 patients (100 women and 98 men) suffering from infectious arthritis had an average age of 36.26 ± 17.47 years and an average duration of evolution of 9.28 ± 9.84 months. The knee (34.3%) was the most affected joint. The reach was essentially mono-articular (159 pa-

tients: 80.3%). Clinical signs were associated with a joint stiffness (180 patients, 90.9%) together with local inflammatory signs (97 patients, 49%) (**Table 5**). The infectious gate was essentially cutaneous (30 patients, 15.2%), uro-genital (23 patients, 11.6%), and pleuro-pulmonary (18 patients, 9.1%). The arthritis was caused by a banal germ in 157 cases (34 certain cases, and 123 probable cases) and by bacillus of Koch in 41 other cases (10 confirmed cases and 31 probable cases). The causal germ of the infection has been isolated in 39 of the 198 patients (19.7%). The *staphylococcus aureus* has been for most of the time the cause (42.5%). Apart from the weak economic level and the insufficiency of hygiene that has been observed in 172 patients (86.9%), the other risk factors that have been identified were the HIV infection source (28 cases), alcoholism (10 cases), Sickle-cell anemia (eight cases), a malignant tumor (three cases), and the diabetes (two cases).

Table 4. Risk factors for gout and co-morbid conditions in 229 patients with gout.

	Number of patients	Percentage
Alcoholism	193	84.3
Overweight/obesity	96	41.9
Arterial high blood pressure	65	28.4
Family history of gout	27	11.8
Renal failure	21	9.2
Hypertriglyceridemia	18	7.9
Hypercholesterolemia	12	5.2
Diabetes mellitus	5	2.3

Table 5. Clinical and paraclinical manifestations observed in 198 patients with infectious arthritis.

	Banal germ arthritis (157 cases) Number (%)	Tuberculous arthritis (41 cases) Number (%)
Inflammatory pain	157 (100)	18 (43.9)
Monoarticular infectious	121 (77.1)	38 (92.7)
Olygoarticular infectious	34 (21.6)	3 (7.3)
Joint stiffness	157 (100)	23 (56.1)
High fever	79 (50.3)	0 (0.0)
Leucocytosis	106 (67.5)	11 (26.8)
Erythrocyte sedimentation rate ≥ 20 mm	146 (92.9)	35 (85.4)
Infectious arthritis associated with HIV	25 (15.9)	3 (7.3)
Radiological signs of joint infection	118 (75.1)	41 (100)

4. Discussion

This study shows the crucial importance of arthritis in rheumatologic consultation in Lomé. Arthritis has, for 15 years, motivated the study of the consultation of 8% of the patients suffering from rheumatism. Despite the fact that there are insufficiencies (hospital recruiting, narrowness of the technical scale), this study, like those conducted in other countries, testifies the importance of the CIR in spite of the weight of the infectious pathology in Africa [11,12]. The importance of the CIR is the reflection of the epidemiologic transition that is observable on the African continent. The unclassified chronic inflammatory rheumatism has been identified as the first cause of arthritis. This high frequency can be explained by the insufficiency of the facilities of investigation; contrary to other countries where this rate in decrease is probably linked to the progress of the diagnostic refinement [5]. Like in Congo, the retroviral infection seems to be the first cause of reactional arthritis [14,15]. The rheumatoid arthritis seems less frequent in the black race and unevenly apportioned from one area to another [16,17]. The scarcity of the connective tissue diseases observed in this series seems to reinforce previous researches. [18-20].

The gout represents the second etiologic form of arthritis in our study. The high frequency of this affection in the black patients is henceforth established [3,6,9,10,]. The scarceness of renal colic seems to perpetuate the unique clinical particularity in this part of the world [6].

The demographic and semiologic characteristics of the patients suffering from infectious arthritis are comparables to those found with other African studies [21-24]. The risk factors found with our patients superpose themselves to those obtained by other researchers [22,23]. The high susceptibility at joint infections in HIV infected patients has not been found in our series. The same goes with the HIV-tuberculosis co-infection. Prospective researches with rigorous statistic analysis will allow establishing the existence of an eventual link of causality between the frequency of this affection in our countries, the conditions of life of the populations and the increase of the infection by the HIV.

5. Conclusion

The chronic inflammatory rheumatisms were the first causal form of arthritis in rheumatologic consultation in Lomé. This study demonstrates the importance of chronic inflammatory rheumatisms despite the weight of the infectious disease in Africa and reflects the scarcity of the connective tissue diseases in black Africa.

REFERENCES

[1] B. K. Rooney and A. J. Silman, "Epidemiology of the Rheumatic Diseases," *Current Opinion in Rheumatology*, Vol. 11, No. 2, 1999, pp. 91-97. doi:10.1097/00002281-199903000-00002

[2] A. Adebajo and P. Davis, "Rheumatic Diseases in African Blacks," *Seminars in Arthritis and Rheumatism*, Vol. 24, No. 2, 1994, pp. 139-153. doi:10.1016/S0049-0172(05)80007-1

[3] J. A. Singh, "Racial and Gender Disparities among Patients with Gout," *Current Rheumatology Reports*, Vol. 15, No. 2, 2013, p. 307. doi:10.1007/s11926-012-0307-x

[4] M. Mijiyawa, K. Etey and M. D. Amédegnato, "Chronic Inflammatory Rheumatic Diseases in Hospital Consultation in LOME (TOGO)," *Rhumatologie (Aix-les-Bains) A*, Vol. 45, No. 2, 1993, pp. 45-49.

[5] J. C. Daboiko, E. Eti, Y. I. Dollo, B. Ouali, B. Ouattara and N. M. Kouakou, "Inflammatory Rheumatic Diseases at Cocody University Medical Center (Abidjan) from March 1998 to March 2000," *Joint Bone Spine*, Vol. 71, No. 6, 2004, pp. 598-599. doi:10.1016/j.jbspin.2004.04.011

[6] M. Mijiyawa, "Gout in Black Africa," *La Revue de Médicine Interne*, Vol. 15, No. 12, 1994, pp. 797-799.

[7] M. Mijiyawa, O. Oniankitan and M. A. Khan, "Spondyloarthropathies in Sub-Saharan Africa," *Current Opinion in Rheumatology*, Vol. 12, No. 4, 2000, pp. 281-286. doi:10.1097/00002281-200007000-00008

[8] G. M. Mody, "Rheumatoid Arthritis and Connective Tissue Disorders," *Baillière's Clinical Rheumatology*, Vol. 9, No. 1, 1995, pp. 31-44. doi:10.1016/S0950-3579(05)80141-4

[9] J. R. Nzenzé, E. Belembaogo, C. Magne, A. S. Sanou, S. Coniquet, J. R. Moussavou-Kombila and J. B. Boguikouma, "Panorama des Arthropathies Inflammatoires à Libreville," *Analyse d'une Série de 57 Observations, Médecine d'Afrique Noire*, Vol. 48, No. 10, 2001, pp. 399-402.

[10] R. Bileckot, G. Koubemba, J. L. Nkoua, R. Bileckot, G. Koubemba and J. L. Nkoua, "Etiology of Oligoarthritis in Equatorial Africa. A Retrospective Study of 80 Cases in Brazzaville, Congo," *La Revue de Médecine Interne*, Vol. 20, No. 5, 1999, pp. 408-411. doi:10.1016/S0248-8663(99)83092-6

[11] S. I. Wallace, H. Robinson, A. T. Masi, H. Decker, D. J. McCarty and T. F. Yü, "Preliminary Criteria for the Classification of the Acute Arthritis of Primary Gout," *Arthritis and Rheumatism*, Vol. 20, No. 3, 1977, pp. 895-900. doi:10.1002/art.1780200320

[12] B. Amor, M. Dougados and M. Mijiyawa, "Criteria of the Classification of Spondylarthropathies," *Revue du Rhumatisme et des Maladies Ostéo-Articulaires*, Vol. 57, No. 2, 1990, pp. 85-89.

[13] F. C. Arnett, S. M. Edworthy, D. A. Bloch, D. J. McShane, J. F. Fries, N. S. Cooper, L. A. Healey, S. R. Kaplan, M. H. Liang, H. S. Luthra, et al., "The American Rheumatism Association 1978 Revised Criteria for the Classification of Rheumatoid Arthritis," *Arthritis and Rheumatism*, Vol. 31, No. 3, 1988, pp. 315-324.

[14] R. Bileckot, A. Mouaya and M. Makuwa, "Prevalence

and Clinical Presentations in HIV-Positive Patients Seen at a Rheumatology Department in Congo-Brazzaville," *Revue du rhumatisme (English Edition)*, Vol. 65, No. 10, 1998, pp. 549-554.

[15] H. Ntsiba, M. Ngandeu-Singwé, C. Makita-Bagamboula and F. Yala, "Human Immunodeficiency Virus Associated Arthritis in Congo Brazzaville," *Médecine et Maladies Infectieuses*, Vol. 37, No. 11, 2007, pp. 758-761. doi:10.1016/j.medmal.2006.09.004

[16] A. J. MacGregor, L. K. Riste, J. M. Hazes and A. J. Silman, "Low Prevalence of Rheumatoid Arthritis in Black-Caribbeans Compared with Whites in Inner City Manchester," *Annals of Rheumatic Diseases*, Vol. 53, No. 5, 1994, pp. 293-297. doi:10.1136/ard.53.5.293

[17] M. Mijiyawa, "Epidemiology and Semiology of Rheumatoid Arthritis in Third World Countries," *Revue du Rhumatisme (English Edition)*, Vol. 62, No. 2, 1995, pp. 121-126.

[18] K. Kombate, B. Saka, O. I. Oniankitan, P. Sodonougbo, A. Mouhari-Toure, K. Tchangai-Walla and P. Pitche, "Systemic Lupus Erythematosus in Lomé, Togo," *Médecine Tropicale: Revue du Corps de Santé Colonial*, Vol. 68, No. 3, 2008, pp. 283-286.

[19] P. Pitche, K. Amanga, K. Koumouvi, O. Oniankitan, M. Mijiyawa and K. Tchangaï-Walla, "Dermatomyositis and Polymyositis in Lomé (Togo)," *Annales de Dermatologie et de Vénéréologie*, Vol. 125, No. 6-7, 1998, pp. 429-430.

[20] P. Pitche, Y. Amanga, K. Koumouvi, O. Oniankitan, M. Mijiyawa and K. Tchangaï-Walla, "Scleroderma in a Hospital Setting in Togo," *Médecine Tropicale: Revue du Corps de Santé Colonial*, Vol. 58, No. 1, 1998, pp. 65-68.

[21] O. Oniankitan, Y. Bagayogo, E. Fianyo, V. Koffi-Tessio, K. Kakpovi, K. C. Tagbor, P. Houzou and M. Mijiyawa, "Infectious Arthritis in Hospital Patients in Lomé, Togo," *Médecine Tropicale: Revue du Corps de Santé Colonial*, Vol. 71, No. 1, 2011, pp. 61-62.

[22] H. Ntsiba, E. Makosso, M. Ngandeu-Singwé and F. Yala, "Septic Arthritis in Tropical Environment. 176 Cases Report in Brazzaville," *Le Mali Medical*, Vol. 21, No. 1, 2006, pp. 49-53.

[23] E. Eti, J. C. Daboiko, S. Debauly, B. Ouali, B. Ouattara and N. Yao, "Pyogenic Arthritis of the Member at Cocody Hospital: A Report of 79 Cases," *Rhumatologie (Aix-les-Bains) A*, Vol. 52, No. 4, 2000, pp. 18-21.

[24] C. Ben Taarit, S. Turki and H. Ben Maiz, "Infectious Spondylitis. Study of a Series of 151 Cases," *Acta Orthopaedica Belgica*, Vol. 68, No. 4, 2002, pp. 381-387.

24

Tuberculin Skin Reaction among Healthy People and Patients with Arthritis in the Southern Israeli Region[*]

Tatiana Reitblat[1#], Zeev Weiler[2], Lea Djin[1], Nelly Polyakov[2], Galina Reifman[1], Alexander Reitblat[3]

[1]Rheumatology, Barsilai Medical Center, Ashkelon, Israel; [2]Pulmonology, Barsilai Medical Center, Ashkelon, Israel; [3]Medical Physics, Barsilai Medical Center, Ashkelon, Israel.
Email: [#]reitblat@barzi.health.gov.il, weil@barzi.health.gov.ill, lerajin@walla.co.il, nelpolyakov@yahoo.co.uk, galinar@barzi.health.gov.il, alexry@barzi.health.gov.il

ABSTRACT

Introduction: Reactivation of latent tuberculosis is a major complication of tumor necrosis factor alpha (TNF-alpha) inhibitors. Therefore, screening for latent TB is recommended before initiation of this treatment. The aim of the study was to compare Tuberculosis skin test (TST) size reaction between healthy people and patients, with Rheumatoid arthritis (RA), Ankylosising spondylitis (AnS) and Psoriatic arthritis (PsA). **Patients and Methods:** Results of TST of 133 healthy subjects were compared with the results of TST of 79 patients, suffering from RA, AnS and PsA. A χ^2 test was used to compare the difference between the groups. A value of $p < 0.05$ was considered significant. Active tuberculosis (TB) was excluded by chest X-ray and through patient's history. The results of TST reaction were grouped according to the CDC's (Centers for Disease Control and prevention) recommendation, e.g. 0 - 4 mm, 5 - 9 mm, 10 - 15 mm and >15 mm. **Results:** Among RA patients 80% received Methotrexate (MTX), 50% Prednisone and 20% other DMARDs. 20% of patients suffering from AnS received MTX, 80%—NSAIDs, and among patients with PsA 70% received MTX, 30%—Salazopirin. There was no significant difference in history of bacilli Calmette-Guerine vaccination between the groups. There was no significant difference in TST reaction distribution between healthy subjects and patients with RA—$p > 0.5$. TST reaction distribution differed significantly between healthy people and AnS ($p < 0.05$) and PsA ($p < 0.001$) patients. The overall tendency in these two patients' groups was towards high positive TST, especially among PsA patients. **Conclusion:** Our results showed that RA patients may present TST reaction as healthy people. The high percent of our AnS and PsA patients that showed TST reaction above 15 mm need further exploration. We conclude that it may be not appropriate to use TST to recognize LTBI in our population.

Keywords: Latent Tuberculosis Infection; Tuberculosis Skin Test; Rheumatoid Arthritis; Ankylosing Spondylitis; Psoriatic Arthritis

1. Introduction

Tuberculosis (TB) remains a major cause of morbidity and mortality in the world. Almost 8 million new cases of TB infections occur annually, only 10% of these go on to develop an active disease [1]. The human immune response is highly effective in controlling primary infection resulting from exposure to Mycobacterium tubercu-

losis. However, all viable organisms might not be eliminated in some individuals. Thus, latency is established, a period during which the infected individual is asymptomatic, but harbors Mycobacterium organisms, which are capable of causing disease under special circumstances.

Tumor necrosis factor alpha (TNF-alpha) plays an important role in host defence against mycobacterium tuberculosis [2]. TNF-alpha is involved in the killing of mycobacteria by activating macrophages [3] and preventing the dissemination of infection by stimulation granuloma formation [4].

The introduction of tumor necrosis factor alpha inhibitors (TNF-i) in the treatment of Rheumatoid arthrtitis (RA), and other inflammatory arthritides such as Anky-

[*]Competing interests: The authors declare that they have no competing interests.
Author's contributions: All authors have contributed to study concept and design, acquisition of data, and critical revision of the manuscript. TR, ZW drafted the manuscript, AR performed statistical analysis of data, and all authors have read and approved the final manuscript.
[#]Corresponding author.

losing Spondylitis (AnSp) and Psoriatic arthritis (PsA) represents a major advance of science in this area. However, an increase in active TB disease has been reported in association with this therapy [5].

Until the last 10 years, the tuberculin skin test (TST) was the only available test for the detection of LTBI.

According to Centers for Disease Control (CDC) and Prevention guidelines, an induration of >= 5 mm is classified as positive in the following groups: patients, who have HIV infection, patients, who have recent close contact with persons, who have TB, patients with organ transplants or immunosuppression (including immunosuppressive drugs such as TNF-i, methotrexate, prednisone, ciclosporin), and patients with fibrotic changes on chest radiographs consiostent with previous TB [6].

The poor specificity of the test, in presence of previous Bacille Calmette-Guerin vaccination, exposure to nontuberculous mycobacteria, or altered immune state among patients with rheumatic disease lead to difficulties in TST interpretation in these patients, with a growing number of reports demonstrating the low positive predictive values and low negative values of this test among patients with rheumatic disease [7,8].

The aim of the study is to compare the distribution of TST reaction sizes among healthy people and patients, who suffer from Rheumatoid arthritis (RA), Ankylosisng spondylitis (AnS) and Psoriatic arthritis (PsA), who are candidates for TNF-i treatment and receiving the conventional treatment.

The primary end point of this study is to compare TST results distribution in the groups between healthy people and patients. The terms as "positive" or "negative" results were not considered.

2. Patients and Methods

The retrospective study was performed at the Rheumatology Unit in collaboration with Pulmonolgy Department, at the Barzilai Medical Centre, Israel. The study underwent institutional review board, for retrospective studies, approval. There was no need to obtain informed consent, because of design of the study.

Inclusion criteria were: results of TST of every consecutive patient, who underwent TST during the period of one year in 2010, were analyzed.

Overall exclusion criteria were active TB, known history of active TB, and recent immigrants (less then 5 years in Israel).

The results of TST of 133 healthy subjects (HS) were compared with the results of TST of 79 patients suffering from RA, PsA, AnS.

The TST was performed according to Mantoux method, using 5 tuberculin Units (TU) of Purified protein deprivate and maximal size of induration was measured

after 72 hours, as recommended[9].

The results of TST reaction were grouped according CDC recommendations, e.g. 0 - 4 mm, 5 - 9 mm, 10 - 15 mm, and >15 mm.

Anergy was excluded by repeating the TST within two weeks for all subjects with TST = 0 mm on the first test and considering the second record results as definitive.

The socio-demographic and TB screening questionaires were obtained from medical charts and, current medical treatment was recorded.

All subjects underwent a chest radiograph, as a method to rule out active pulmonary TB as well as thorough medical history.

A χ^2 or Fisher's exact test was used to compare the difference between groups. A value of $p < 0.05$ was considered significant.

3. Results

133 healthy subjects and 79 patients were enrolled into the study.

The mean age in the healthy control subject group was 35.3 years, while mean age of study group was 53.4 years ($p < 0.05$).

The study group had a gender distribution of 2 females: 1 male while the control group had a gender distribution of 5:3 male/female, and among the study group there were 41 patients with RA, 17 with AnS and 21 with PSA.

80% of the patients with RA were treated with Methotrexate (MTX), while 50% received Prednisone, and 20% other DMARDs.

19% of patients who suffered from AnS received MTX, 81%—NSAIDs, and among patients with PsA 71% received MTX, 29%—Salazopirin.

None of the patients were treated with TNF-i previously.

TST Assay

TST reaction < 5 mm was found in 60.9 % of healthy subjects, 61.0% among RA patients, 41.2% among AnS patients and 23.8% among PsA patients.TST reaction 5 - 9 mm was found in 19.5% of healthy subject, 17.1% RA patients, 23.5% AnS patients and 9.5% PsA patients.

TST reaction 10 - 14 mm was observed in 8.3% of healthy subjects, 3% of RA patients, 0% of AnS patients and 19% PsA patients

TST reaction > 15 mm was in 11.3% healthy subjects, 14.6% of RA patients, 35.3% AnS patients and 47.6% PsA patients.

There was no significant difference in TST reaction distribution between healthy subjects and patients with RA (RAxHS: $\chi^2 = 0.42$; $p > 0.5$). TST reaction distribution differed significantly between healthy people and AnS patients (AnSxHS: $\chi^2 = 8.7$; $p < 0.05$) and PsA

(PsAxHS: χ^2 = 22.4; p < 0.001). The overall tendency in these two patient's group was towards high positive TST, especially among PsA patients.

4. Discussion

An accurate diagnosis of LTBI in patients before starting TNF-i treatment as well as the prophylactic treatment anti-TB treatment is crucial to prevent TB reactivation. The current screening strategy is based onTST, chest X-Ray and risk stratification questionnaire.

This accepted strategy has significantly reduced the rate of TB reactivation under TNF-i therapy [9]. Despite this success, the correct approach to LTBI diagnosis is still under discussion, and the main issue is correct interpretation of TST among patients with inflammatory arthritis [10].

The TST is recall response to soluble antigens previously encountered during tuberculosis infection. After intradermal injection of purifed protein derivate (PPD), a crude mixture of more than 200 M. tuberculosis proteins, a sensitized individual antigen specific T cells are activated to secrete cytokines that mediate a hypersensitivity reaction. TST is classic delayed type hypersensitivity (DTH) reaction [11]. This reaction has been shown to be absolutely dependent on the presence of memory T cells. Both the CD4+ and CD8+ fractions of cells have been shown to modulate a response. Contemporary debate regarding the reaction is focused on the role of the Th1 and Th2 cells, originally discovered by Mosmann. It has been postulated that the Th1 cell is the "inducer" of a DTH response since it secretes interferon gamma (IFN-gamma), a potent stimulator of macrophages, while the Th2 cell is either not involved or acts as a downregulator of the cell mediated immune response [12].

In immune modulated inflammatory disease (IMID) immune disregulation is observed rather than immune deficiency. In Rheumatoid Arthritis patients, a type 1 cytokine predominance (IFN-gamma) is found in synovial membrane, synovial fluid and blood [13], in patients with psoriasis a type 1 cytokine reaction activity even is more prominent with IFN-gamma high production and up regulation of keratinocytes [14].

The data presented in this study, indicate, that patients with IMID have different TST response within the different disease groups, while in comparison with healthy people the TST reaction size distribution may be the same, or even more pronounced toward larger size of induration reaction.

Our RA patients showed the same distribution of TST reaction as healthy people, although most were receiving immune-supression treatment such as Methotrexate and Prednisone.

The results of TST reaction among RA patients in lit-erature are contradictory. The current accepted opinion is that RA patients have an attenuated test reaction, as was shown in several studies [8,15], while other studies documented the same TST reaction in RA patients as among healthy pupulation [16,17].

PsA patients in our study showed more prominent TST reaction in comparison to healthy pupulation, despite the fact, that most PsA patients treated with immunosuppressive treatment. The results are in accordance with other studies, among patients with PsA and also with psoriasis [18-20]. The phenomenon may be explained by the specific skin reaction to antigens among patients with psoriasis, that is an augmented type 1 cytokine activity with prominent IFN-gamma production, explaining the prominent TST reaction.

Patients with AnS showed a tendency to higher TST reaction in comparison to healthy controls and RA patients, although no significant statistical difference was observed. The same results among patients with AS were shown in another work. Thus, in the work of Pamik *et al.* the mean size of induration of TST reaction was 12.1 mm, which is higher than in their RA patients and Lupus Erythematosus patients [21]. Inanc N *et al.*, while analysing agreement between Quantiferon test and TST, showed, that 82% of AS patients had induration more, than 10 mm [22]. These interesting results confirm the similarities in the immune processes in the whole group of spondyloarthropaties, which may differ from those in RA patients.

In conclusion, the evidence presented here suggests that adherence to the accepted TST-based recommendations for the diagnosis of LTBI, may lead to overestimation of positive results and, overdiagnosis of LTBI.

The presented data raise the suggestion of revision of algoritms of LTBI, particulary among non-endemic population.

Our study has obvious limitations. First, it included a small number of subjects, paticulary in AnS group, which may have influence on our capacity to approach to statistical significance. Second, we did not analyse correlation between TST results and disease activity, and could not provide the BCG status, although the age of all examined persons suggested their previous vaccination.

Our group of patients was significantly older, than group of health controls, which may lead to lower results of TST in the patient group compared with health control.

REFERENCES

[1]   M. C. Raviglione, D. E. Snider Jr. and A. Kochi, "Global Epidemiology of Tuberculosis. Morbidity and Mortality of a Worldwide Epidemic," *Journal of the American Medical Association*, Vol. 273, No. 3, 1995, pp. 220-226. doi:10.1001/jama.1995.03520270054031

[2]   G. Kaplan and V. H. Freedman, "The Role of Cytokines in the Immune Response to Tuberculosis," *Research in Immunology*, Vol. 147, 1996, pp. 565-572. doi:10.1016/S0923-2494(97)85223-6

[3]   M. Denis, "Tumor Necrosis Factor and Granulocyte Macrophage-Colony Stimulating Factor Stimulate Human Macrophages to Restrict Growth of Virulent *Mycobacterium avium* and to Kill a Virulent *M. avium*: Killing Effector Mechanism Depends on the Generation of Reactive Nitrogen Intermediates," *Journal of Leukocyte Biology*, Vol. 49, No. 4, 1991, pp. 380-387.

[4]   V. Kindler, A.-P. Sappino, G. E. Grau, *et al.*, "The Inducing Role of Tumor Necrosis Factor in the Development of Bactericidal Granulomas during BCG Infection," *Cell*, Vol. 56, No. 5, 1989, pp. 731-740. doi:10.1016/0092-8674(89)90676-4

[5]   T. Ellerin, R. H. Rubin and M. E. Weinblatt, "Infections and Anti-Tumor Necrosis Factor Alpha Therapy," *Arthritis & Rheumatism*, Vol. 48, No. 11, 2003, pp. 3013-3022. doi:10.1002/art.11301

[6]   Targeted Tuberculin Testing and Treatment of Latent Tuberculosis Infection, MMWR ATS/CDC Statement Committee on Latent Tuberculosis Infection, June 2000.

[7]   E. C. Keystone, K. A. Papp and W. Wobeser, "Challenges in Diagnosing Latent Tuberculosis Infection in Patients Treated with Tumor Necrosis Factor Antagonists," *The Journal of Rheumatology*, Vol. 38, No. 7, 2011, pp. 1234-1243. doi:10.3899/jrheum.100623

[8]   D. Ponce de León, E. Acevedo-Vásquez, A. Sánchez-Torres, *et al.*, "Attenuated Response to Purified Protein Derivative in Patients with Rheumatoid Arthritis: Study in a Population with a High Prevalence of Tuberculosis," *Annals of the Rheumatic Diseases*, Vol. 64, No. 9, 2005, pp. 1360-1361. doi:10.1136/ard.2004.029041

[9]   J. Keane and B. Bresnihan, "Tuberculosis Reactivation during Immunosuppressive Therapy in Rheumatic Diseases: Diagnostic and Therapeutic Strategies," *Current Opinion in Rheumatology*, Vol. 20, No. 4, 2008, pp. 443-449. doi:10.1097/BOR.0b013e3283025ec2

[10] G. Matulis, P. Jüni, P. M. Villiger and S. D. Gadola, "Detection of Latent Tuberculosis in Immunosuppressed Patients with Autoimmune Diseases: Performance of a Mycobacterium Tuberculosis Antigen-Specific Interferon Gamma Assay," *Annals of the Rheumatic Diseases*, Vol. 67, No. 1, 2008, pp. 84-90. doi:10.1136/ard.2007.070789

[11] I. Roitt, J. Brostoff and D. Male, "Hypersensitivity Type IV," In: L. Cook, Ed., *Immunology*, 4th Edition, Mosby, Barcelona, 1998, p. 255.

[12] C. A. Black, "Delayed Type Hypersensitivity: Current Theories with an Historic Perspective," *Dermatology Online Journal*, Vol. 5, No. 1, 1999, p. 7.

[13] A. J. Quayle, P. Chomarat, P. Miossec, *et al.*, "Rheumatoid inflammatory T-cell clones express mostly Th1 but also Th2 and mixed (Th0-like) cytokine patterns," *Scandinavian Journal of Immunology*, Vol. 38, No. 1, 1993, pp. 75-82. doi:10.1111/j.1365-3083.1993.tb01696.x

[14] J. F. Schlaak, M. Buslau, W. Jochum, *et al.*, "T Cells Involved in Psoriasis Vulgaris Belong to the Th1 Subset," *Journal of Investigative Dermatology*, Vol. 102, No. 2, 1994, pp. 145-149. doi:10.1111/1523-1747.ep12371752

[15] I. Sezer, H. Kocabas, M. A. Melikoglu, *et al.*, "Positiveness of Purified Protein Derivatives in Rheumatoid Arthritis Patients Who Are Not Receiving Immunosuppressive Therapy," *Clinical Rheumatology*, Vol. 28, No. 1, 2009, pp. 53-57. doi:10.1007/s10067-008-0982-1

[16] K. H. Lee, S. Y. Jung, Y. J. Ha, *et al.*, "Tuberculin Reaction Is Not Attenuated in Patients with Rheumatoid Arthritis Living in a Region with Intermediate Burden of Tuberculosis," *Rheumatology International*, Vol. 32, No. 5, 2012, pp. 1421-1424. doi:10.1007/s00296-011-1889-8

[17] J. D. Greenberg, S. M. Reddy, S. G. Schloss, *et al.*, "Comparison of an *in Vitro* Tuberculosis Interferon-Gamma Assay with Delayed-Type Hypersensitivity Testing for Detection of Latent *Mycobacterium tuberculosis*: A Pilot Study in Rheumatoid Arthritis," *The Journal of Rheumatology*, Vol. 35, No. 5, 2008, pp. 770-775.

[18] I. D. Bassukas, M. Kosmidou, G. Gaitanis, *et al.*, "Patients with Psoriasis Are More Likely to Be Treated for Latent Tuberculosis Infection Prior to Biologics than Patients with Inflammatory Bowel Disease," *Acta Dermato-Venereologica*, Vol. 91, No. 4, 2011, pp. 444-446. doi:10.2340/00015555-1106

[19] G. Tsiouri, G. Gaitanis, D. Kiorpelidou, *et al.*, "Tuberculin Skin Test Overestimates Tuberculosis Hypersensitivity in Adult Patients with Psoriasis," *Dermatology*, Vol. 219, No. 2, 2009, pp. 119-125. doi:10.1159/000222431

[20] C. A. Nobre, M. R. Callado, J. R. Lima, *et al.*, "Tuberculosis Infection in Rheumatic Patients with Infliximab Therapy: Experience with 157 Patients," *Rheumatology International*, Vol. 32, No. 9, 2012, pp. 2769-2775. doi:10.1007/s00296-011-2017-5

[21] O. N. Pamuk, Y. Yesil, S. Donmez, *et al.*, "The Results of Purified Protein Derivative Test in Ankylosing Spondylitis Patients: Clinical Features, HRCT Results and Relationship with TNF-Blocker Usage," *Rheumatology International*, Vol. 29, No. 2, 2008, pp. 179-183. doi:10.1007/s00296-008-0665-x

[22] N. Inanc, S. Z. Aydin, S. Karakurt, *et al.*, "Agreement between Quantiferon-TB Gold Test and Tuberculin Skin Test in the Identification of Latent Tuberculosis Infection in Patients with Rheumatoid Arthritis and Ankylosing Spondylitis," *The Journal of Rheumatology*, Vol. 36, No. 12, 2009, pp. 2675-2681. doi:10.3899/jrheum.090268

List of Abbreviations

TST—Tuberculosis skin test
TNF-alpha—Tumor necrosis factor alpha
TNF-I—Tumor necrosis factor alpha-inhibitors

RA—Rheumatoid Arthritis
AnS—Ankylosing Spondylitis
LTBI—Latent Tuberculosis Infection
MTX—Methotrexate

25

TNF-α Antagonist and Infection in Rheumatoid Arthritis

Julia F. Simard[1,2*], Murray A. Mittleman[1], Nancy A. Shadick[3], Elizabeth W. Karlson[3]

[1]Department of Epidemiology, Harvard School of Public Health, Boston, USA; [2]Clinical Epidemiology Unit, Karolinska Institutet, Stockholm, Sweden; [3]Department of Medicine, Division of Rheumatology, Immunology, and Allergy, Brigham and Women's Hospital, Boston, USA.
Email: *julia.simard@post.harvard.edu

ABSTRACT

Background: Anti-TNF treatment may increase infection risk, although this has been difficult to study because the timing of anti-TNF treatment is driven by disease activity, which may influence infection susceptibility leading to confounding that varies over time. We evaluated the association between anti-TNF initiation in rheumatoid arthritis (RA) patients on disease modifying anti-rheumatic drugs (DMARD) and infection using multiple approaches adjusting for time-varying confounding. **Methods:** 383 anti-TNF-naïve RA patients on ≥1 non-biologic-DMARD at enrollment from the Brigham and Women's Rheumatoid Arthritis Sequential Study (BRASS) were followed up to two years. Pooled logistic regressions estimated the association between anti-TNF and infection by including time-varying covariates in the adjusted models and inverse probability treatment weighting (IPTW). **Results:** Adjustment for time-varying disease activity and other suspected confounders yielded non-statistically significant positive associations between anti-TNF start and infection regardless of analytic approach (RR_{mvar_adj} = 2.1, 95% CI: 0.8 - 5.8). **Conclusions:** Incorporating changing clinical status, and treatment indications and consequences, yielded consistently (though not significantly) elevated relative risks of infection associated with anti-TNF initiation. Due to limited statistical power, we cannot draw firm conclusions. However, we have illustrated multiple approaches adjusting for potential time-varying confounding in longitudinal studies and hope to replicate the approaches in larger studies.

Keywords: Inverse Probability Weighting; Anti-TNF; Infection; Rheumatoid Arthritis

1. Introduction

Until recently the treatment for rheumatoid arthritis (RA) centered on symptom management and medications to reduce inflammation, consisting of non-steroidal anti-inflammatory drugs, corticosteroids and non-biologic disease modifying anti-rheumatic drugs (DMARDs) such as hydroxychloroquine and methotrexate (MTX). Biologic agents, such as tumor necrosis factor alpha antagonists (anti-TNFs), were introduced in 1999 initially targeting patients with more severe disease and, in whom, the risks of infection with use of immunosuppressive drugs is of concern.

Bacterial and mycobacterial infections have been associated with TNF-α suppression [1-3], but some studies found that patients with RA also have an elevated incidence of infections [4-8]. Disease activity and measures of severity have been associated with higher risk of infection [9], even before the biologics era [4]. Furthermore, common immunosuppresive treatments [3,10-14] have also been associated with infection [15-17]. Therefore, it is unclear whether the observed risk of infection in RA is a product of disease-related activity, pharmacologically-induced immunosuppression, common co-morbid conditions, or a combination of these factors.

Early on, anti-TNF therapies were reserved for patients with active disease, poorly controlled by non-biologic DMARD therapy. This treated population was placed on anti-TNF treatment to manage increased levels of disease activity, both factors associated with infection. By focusing on prevalent non-biologic DMARD users at enrollment, our goal was to investigate the clinically-relevant question of what is the risk of infection associated with introducing an anti-TNF treatment to patients with RA on background non-biologic DMARDs at study start? In addition to this, we wanted to demonstrate alternate analytic approaches to account for the potential time-varying effects of changes in treatment indication and consequences of treatment such as changing disease activity. We, therefore, evaluated the effect of anti-TNF use on the occurrence of infection in a prospective cohort study of patients with confirmed RA in the Brigham and Women's RA Sequential Study (BRASS). The hypothesis was that the addition of anti-TNF treatment to patients

*Corresponding author.

treated with non-biologic-DMARDs would increase the risk of infection in subjects with RA.

2. Patients and Methods

2.1. Study Population

BRASS is an ongoing prospective cohort of patients with RA started in September 2003. Subjects had to be current confirmed RA patients treated at the Brigham and Women's Hospital in Boston, MA, English-speaking, at least 18 years of age, and have no diagnosis of lupus or psoriatic arthritis. Subjects provided signed, informed consent. Nearly 1000 patients with RA were recruited by May 2007. We restricted the study population to anti-TNF-naïve subjects who reported current non-biologic DMARD treatment at enrollment, did not have an infection in the prior month, and were followed for at least six months leaving 383 BRASS participants.

2.2. Data Collection

Subjects completed structured questionnaires every six months that included a disease activity instrument, the RA Disease Activity Index (RADAI) [18] and were examined by study physicians annually (**Figure 1**). At enrollment and annually, blood and urine were collected and data were collected on demographic and lifestyle factors, current and past medication use, general health, function, and pain symptoms. Rheumatoid factor (RF) was measured by an immunoturbidimetric technique on the Cobas Integra 700 analyzer (Roche Diagnostics—Indianapolis, IN). Anti-cyclic citrullinated peptide antibody titer (CCP) was measured by a second generation anti-CCP ELISA assay (Inova Diagnostics, Inc.—San Diego, CA). From the patient questionnaires, medication use, co-morbid conditions, adverse events, use of complementary and alternative medicines, disease exacerbations, diet, health care utilization, and quality of life were also collected. Subjects could seek medical care from their rheumatologists and other health care providers outside of the

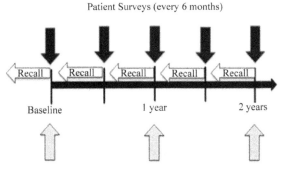

Figure 1. Structure of follow-up and data collection

BRASS follow-up protocol and the electronic inpatient and outpatient records were available for review for patients seen within the Partners HealthCare network.

2.3. Anti-TNF Treatment

Medication use including anti-TNF treatment was assessed at baseline and at 6, 12, 18 and 24 months. Physicians reported medication changes and reasons for changes. Subjects provided details about current medication use (dose, frequency, and duration), including etanercept, adalimumab and infliximab. There was excellent agreement between self-reported medication use and medical records in a sample of approximately 10% of the full BRASS cohort ($\kappa = 0.8$ to 0.95) [19]. For the present analysis exposure was defined as initiation of an anti-TNF drug between enrollment and the 18 month survey. Subjects were considered exposed when their first anti-TNF treatment was reported during follow-up and allowed to vary over time; to account for prolonged exposure we also evaluated the effect of current exposure while simultaneously adjusting for exposure in the previous survey period. During follow-up, however, nearly all patients remained on therapy once initiated. In a sensitivity analysis, we assumed once a subject was exposed, they were always exposed.

2.4. Documented Infection

Infections were reported by rheumatologists and subjects by survey (**Figure 1**). Study physicians annually reported data on infections and drug-related toxicities occurring since the previous assessment. Questionnaire items asked about infections requiring antibiotics or intravenous therapy, as well as any infections as reason for change in therapy. Subjects were asked to self-report infections every six months during follow-up; they were specifically asked about infections requiring antibiotics. Any report of infection during the follow-up was verified by medical record review using a previously published algorithm that incorporated serologic evidence, antimicrobial treatment, and clinical and radiologic findings [20,21].

2.5. Other Covariates

At enrollment, we collected data on age, sex, education (college graduate vs not), race/ethnicity, co-morbidities (diabetes, alcoholism/drug abuse, COPD), cigarette smoking, and disease duration. RA-related autoantibodies were measured at baseline to assess seropositivity, which was defined as either RF > 15 or CCP > 20. Baseline presence of extra-articular manifestations was reported by each patient's treating rheumatologist and included pericarditis, pulmonary nodule and neuropathy, among others.

Time-varying factors included disease activity, assessed by RADAI scores collected every 6 months [18]; high disease activity was defined as RADAI ≥ 4.9. Use of concomitant medications (corticosteroids, MTX, and other DMARDs) and frequency of physician visits was collected at each survey (baseline and during follow-up). Results from laboratory tests were collected from the electronic medical records on white blood cell count (WBC), albumin, and hematocrit for any time during participation in BRASS. Abnormal serology was defined as WBC > 10 × 109 cells per liter, albumin < 3.7 U/L, or hematocrit < 36%.

2.6. Follow-Up

Subjects were followed until first documented infection, loss to follow-up, two years of follow-up, or end of study period (May 2007), whichever came first. The structured survey and data collection resulted in interval censored data. Subjects initiating anti-TNF therapy between their first (baseline) and second (6 months) survey periods reported exposure on the 6 month survey and were therefore classified as having exposure start at month 6 (or the second survey period). Infection outcomes were included from the next survey period to ensure temporality.

2.7. Statistical Analysis

Cohort characteristics were summarized using descriptive statistics by initiation of anti-TNF treatment during follow-up and by whether an infection was documented during follow-up. These groups were compared using t-tests, chi-square tests and Fisher's exact test as appropriate. Pooled logistic regression models were used to estimate the relative risk (odds ratios) of infection associated with use of anti-TNF exposure. Subjects were followed to the end of each survey period and classified as having an event or not at that time. Covariates in the multivariable-adjusted models were selected a priori based on their hypothesized relationship to anti-TNF initiation, other exposures and risk of infection. In multivariable-adjusted models, we included time-invariant confounders measured at baseline including sex, age, education, race/ethnicity, co-morbid conditions, disease duration and seropositivity. We modeled disease activity, concomitant medications, and physician visit frequency as time-varying covariates. Logistic regression models were used to calculate each subject's probability of remaining uncensored as a function of age, sex, disease duration, race/ethnicity, seropositivity, disease activity, MTX treatment, doctor visit frequency, and extra-articular manifestations, and conducted analyses incorporating inverse probability of censoring weights (IPCW) to account for possible loss to follow-up related to disease status [22].

Finally, inverse probability treatment weighting (IPTW)

of pooled logistic regression models with robust variance to estimate 95% CI, was conducted to estimate the OR of infection [23]. We used standard methods to construct the IPW by logistic regression to include disease activity and other suspected determinants of treatment status (i.e. the time-varying confounders included in the unweighted, adjusted pooled logistic models). Time-invariant and baseline covariates were also included in the models to construct weights. Stabilized weights were calculated and their distribution examined to check for outliers and influential weights. We used simple diagnostics to identify overt violations to the positivity assumption such as examining contingency tables for zero cells and looking at the distribution of propensity of treatment and the above calculated weights. To account for potential informative censoring, IPCW were also incorporated into the stabilized weights [23].

3. Results

Of 383 BRASS subjects taking non-biologic DMARDs at baseline, 66 (17%) initiated anti-TNF treatment during follow-up; initiators were more likely to be female, younger, and have been treated with corticosteroids (**Table 1**). There were 56 subjects with at least one documented infection during follow-up. Seven subjects had documented infections after initiating anti-TNF therapy and the remaining 49 infections were among those had not initiated anti-TNF treatment. Women, corticosteroid users, those with extra-articular manifestations, and higher disease activity at enrollment had a higher incidence of documented infection (**Table 2**).

In the simplest models accounting for follow-up time, recent anti-TNF exposure was positively but not significantly associated with infection (RR = 2.3, 95% CI = 0.9 to 5.9) adjusting for anti-TNF exposure during the previous survey period as well. Results were similar in multivariable adjusted models adjusting for age, sex, extra-articular manifestations, corticosteroids and seropositivity (RR = 2.3, 95% CI: 0.9 to 6.0). Further adjustment for education, disease duration at baseline, race, smoking status at baseline, baseline disease activity, high MDHAQ, and presence of co-morbid conditions with potential contraindications for therapy did not materially alter the results, nor did using propensity score adjustment for multivariable adjustment. When adjusting for changing disease activity and treatment status, i.e. the time-varying confounders, the results were similar (RR = 2.1, 95% CI: 0.8, 5.8) (**Table 3**). When we applied IPCW to the above pooled logistic regression models, effect estimates and 95% CI were consistent with those obtained from IPTW models.

Most of the infections among the anti-TNF initiators occurred early; six of the seven anti-TNF exposed events

Table 1. Characteristics of BRASS participants by TNF-α treatment initiation in the first 18 months of follow-up (restricted to TNF-naïve, prevalent DMARD users).

	Anti-TNF initiation		
	yes	no	
	n = 66	n = 317	p
Female	57 (86.4)	257 (81.1)	0.31
Age*, yrs, mean (sd)	55 (14)	59 (14)	0.03
Age < 40	12 (18.2)	32 (10.1)	
40 - 59	30 (45.5)	122 (38.5)	
60 - 74	19 (28.8)	121 (38.2)	
75+	5 (7.6)	42 (13.3)	
Race (white)	63 (95.5)	286 (90.2)	0.24
BMI, mean (sd)	26.1 (4.6)	26.1 (4.8)	0.96
College graduate	39 (59.1)	153 (48.3)	0.11
Current smoker*	2 (3.0)	27 (8.5)	0.20
Seropositive RA	47 (71.2)	212 (66.9)	0.49
Extra-articular manifestations	18 (27.3)	95 (30.0)	0.66
High disease activity*	2 (3.0)	18 (5.7)	0.55
Disease duration, mean years (sd)	10.4 (10.4)	13.0 (11.9)	0.10
Disease duration < 5 years	29 (43.9)	102 (32.4)	0.07
Methotrexate*	42 (63.6)	187 (59.0)	0.48
Hydroxychloroquine*	17 (25.8)	110 (34.7)	0.16
Sulfasalazine*	9 (13.6)	39 (12.3)	0.77
Leflunomide*	9 (13.6)	47 (14.8)	0.80
Corticosteroid*	25 (37.9)	76 (24.0)	0.02
No. co-morbid conditions			0.94
0	53 (80.3)	251 (79.2)	
1	11 (16.7)	56 (17.7)	
2	2 (3.0)	8 (2.5)	
3	0 (0)	2 (0.6)	
Diabetes	3 (4.6)	17 (5.4)	1.0
COPD	0 (0)	4 (1.3)	1.0

Presented as n (%) unless otherwise notes; * at enrollment.

occurred in the first 6 month period following anti-TNF treatment initiation.

4. Discussion

Using different analytic techniques to explore the association between anti-TNF treatment and documented infection in subjects with RA, we found that initiating anti-TNF therapy in subjects on non-biologic DMARDs at enrollment may increase the risk of infection although we did not have sufficient statistical power in this study with only seven infections occurring after anti-TNF initiation. However, the magnitude of our observed associations between anti-TNF exposure and infection were

Table 2. Clinical predictors of documented infection during follow-up of 383 patients with rheumatoid arthritis.

	Documented Infection during follow-up		
	yes	no	
	n = 56	n = 327	p
Age*, yrs, mean (sd)	58 (14.9)	58 (14.2)	0.99
Female	52 (92.9)	262 (80.1)	0.02
Race (white)	51 (91.1)	298 (91.1)	0.99
College graduate	26 (46.4)	166 (50.9)	0.55
Current smoker*	5 (8.9)	24 (7.3)	0.68
Seropositive RA	39 (69.6)	220 (67.3)	0.73
Extra-articular manifestations	25 (44.6)	88 (26.9)	0.007
Corticosteroid use	21 (37.5)	80 (24.5)	0.041
RADAI, mean (sd)	1.83 (1.8)	1.72 (1.6)	0.61
Disease duration < 5 y	16 (28.6)	115 (35.3)	0.32
Diabetes	2 (3.6)	18 (5.5)	0.75
COPD	1 (1.8)	3 (0.9)	0.47

Presented as n (%) unless otherwise notes; * at enrollment.

Table 3. Estimated effect of anti-TNF therapy on infection in RA under multiple modeling scenarios.

Model	OR	95% CI
Pooled logistic regression		
Crude	2.3	0.9 - 5.9
Multivariable model 1: *Baseline variables*	2.3	0.9 - 6.0
Multivarable model 2: *Time-varying adjustment*	2.1	0.8 - 5.8
Inverse probability of treatment weighting		
Crude	2.4	0.6 – 9.2
+ additional adjustment for baseline confounders	4.2	0.9 - 19.0

1) Adjusted for age, gender corticosteroid use at baseline, presence of extra-articular manifestations, and seropositivity; 2) Model 1 plus time-varying factors: corticosteroids, methotrexate, disease activity (RADAI), high medical care and hospital utilization.

consistent with some previously published results [24,25]. As we demonstrated in our analyses, the highest risk of infection associated with anti-TNF initiation was observed in the period following initiation, which suggests a higher risk is in the early period following treatment start [8,26].

Over the past decade numerous investigators have studied the link between infection and anti-TNF medications [25] but not all studies have agreed. Differences in patient populations, outcome ascertainment and validation, follow-up, and study design may explain the differences between the studies. One ongoing discussion in this area is the prevalent vs. incident user design [26,27]. Briefly, the debate focuses on whether it is appropriate to compare a new user of a therapy (incident user) to a current or ongoing user (prevalent user) because those most susceptible to the adverse reactions or outcomes of interest may no longer be included in the prevalent pool because they discontinued the medication. Those susceptible to the outcomes associated with treatment initiation, such as infection, may be depleted from the study population and those remaining exposed (prevalent users) have survived without the outcome.

The present study evaluates start of anti-TNF therapy (*i.e.* incident user) compared to no anti-TNF exposure, in a study population that was restricted to anti-TNF-naïve patients with RA on at least one non-biologic DMARD therapy at start of follow-up. Thus, our study addresses the clinical question: what is the risk of infection associated with initiation of anti-TNF therapy in patients on background non-biologic DMARDs? We believe that this research question is clinically relevant because prescription of anti-TNF therapy, since its introduction is common for patients with RA following non-biologic DMARDs [28].

A number of other studies have made the comparison between initiators of an anti-TNF therapy and prevalent users of non-biologic DMARDs or specifically, methotrexate [24,29]. Unlike some of these studies, we did not require that the non-initiators maintain their non-biologic DMARD therapy for an extended period of time. Among both the anti-TNF initiators and non-initiators, longitudinal changes in methotrexate and corticosteroid treatment were modeled as time-varying confounders. Similar to analysis from the National Data Bank for Rheumatic Diseases, users of a treatment were compared to non-users, conditional on other therapies [30].

Several studies before the introduction of anti-TNF medications in RA management have reported conflicting results regarding the risk of infections in RA patients. Higher infection incidence rates were found in one study of RA patients compared to subjects free of RA, suggesting that either RA or its management might be associated with infections [4,6,31]. These, and other similar findings, highlighted the need to consider possible bias due to changes in susceptibility to infection related to disease activity that may lead to changes in treatment choice over time. In other studies [32,33] results from employing alternative modeling strategies have yielded significantly different results, both statistically and clinically. Choi and colleagues found a dramatically reduced mortality associated with methotrexate in RA using IPTW [32]. In this study we showed that using IPTW to adjust for time-varying confounders did not alter the results as compared to the conventional modeling approach where these potential confounders were included as time-varying covariates in the model. Whether residual confounding, power limitations, unmeasured confounders, or limited time-varying confounding in the data explain this is

unknown. When the baseline confounders were added to the IPTW model to further reduce potential residual confounding, the magnitude of the association increased but was not statistically significant.

Conventional regression models with time-varying covariates in the models do not fully account for time-varying confounding; ignoring confounders may result in bias from residual confounding, but statistical adjustment may lead to other biases [23,32,34]. Inverse probability weighting tries to circumvent this bias by reweighting the observed population to answer our counterfactual question: "What would happen if everyone in our study population were treated as compared to if everyone were not treated?". The unweighted approach evaluated asks instead whether those who were treated were more likely to have an infection compared to those who were untreated. While the difference is subtle, it has led to different results in previous studies [33]. Similarly, the primary regression analysis here evaluated the risk of infection in those exposed to anti-TNF treatment versus those who did not receive treatment. Using the IPTW approach, we answered the question: "What is the risk of infection if everyone in our study population had been exposed to anti-TNF treatment versus if everyone had not?". The statistical method employed changes the scientific question answered, as does how the study population is defined and what comparator is used [26]. Therefore, special attention should be paid when interpreting the results of the present study into the context of what has been published.

Our study has some limitations. Despite the plethora of clinical data and patient-reported measures, we had limited follow-up of a maximum of two years for each subject, during which time only 66 patients started anti-TNF treatment, and only seven of whom also had an infection. Also, we may have missed infections treated outside of the network by another physician for which we had no documentation. We found no overt violation of the positivity assumption for the IPW method, however due to the sparsity of the data, results must be interpreted cautiously. As such we had limited statistical power and were unable to explore possible effect modification, subtypes of infection or type of anti-TNF, or investigate seropositive and seronegative RA separately. Protocol required only annual examination by physicians and semi-annual reporting by the participants, possibly resulting in residual confounding by a number of potential confounders. Further we relied upon self-report of treatment, for exposure and concomitant therapies, which was previously shown to be reliable [19].

Despite these limitations, our study explores alternative methods to address potential bias due to time-varying confounding. Incorporating changing clinical status and strong indications for treatments, and also the consequences of treatment, we found generally consistent results using a variety of statistical approaches. This study sought to illustrate the use of these methods to address the common analytic problem of time-varying confounding in a context familiar to clinical researchers. Although we are limited from drawing any significant conclusions from this underpowered study, we have illustrated the use of alternative statistical models that may be of use in the presence of time-varying confounding in longitudinal studies and hope to replicate the approaches herein in larger, longer term studies.

5. Acknowledgements

We would like to extend a sincere thanks to the staff, clinicians, and participants of BRASS. In addition, we thank Dr. Daniel H. Solomon for his critical feedback on study design and analysis.

6. Statement of Funding

JFS was supported by the Arthritis Foundation Doctoral Dissertation Award and the NIH training grant, T32-A1007535-07: Ruth L. Kirschstein National Research Service Award (NRSA) Institutional Research Training Grants (T32) Epidemiology of Infectious Disease and Biodefense Training Program. Additional support includes NIH grants AR0524, AR47782, AR049880 for EWK. NAS receives additional grant funding from AMGEN and Abbott pharmaceuticals. BRASS is funded by Biogen Idec and Crescendo Biosciences.

REFERENCES

[1] V. P. Mohan, C. A. Scanga, K. Yu, H. M. Scott, K. E. Tanaka, E. Tsang, et al., "Effects of Tumor Necrosis Factor Alpha on Host Immune Response in Chronic Persistent Tuberculosis: Possible Role for Limiting Pathology," Infection and Immunity, Vol. 69, No. 3, 2001, pp. 1847-1855. doi:10.1128/IAI.69.3.1847-1855.2001

[2] M. Nucci and K. A. Marr, "Emerging Fungal Diseases," Clinical Infectious Diseases, Vol. 41, No. 4, 2005, pp. 521-526. doi:10.1086/432060

[3] N. Wig, R. Handa, P. Aggarwal and J. P. Wali, "Rheumatoid Arthritis—Current Trends in Management," Indian Journal of Medical Sciences, Vol. 51, No. 8, 1997, pp. 255-264.

[4] M. F. Doran, C. S. Crowson, G. R. Pond, W. M. O'Fallon and S. E. Gabriel, "Predictors of Infection in Rheumatoid Arthritis," Arthritis and Rheumatism, Vol. 46, No. 9, 2002, pp. 2294-2300. doi:10.1002/art.10529

[5] M. F. Doran, C. S. Crowson, G. R. Pond, W. M. O'Fallon and S. E. Gabriel, "Frequency of Infection in Patients with Rheumatoid Arthritis Compared with Controls: A Population-Based Study," Arthritis and Rheumatism, Vol. 46, No. 9, 2002, pp. 2287-2293. doi:10.1002/art.10524

[6] G. A. Van Albada-Kuipers, J. Linthorst, E. A. Peeters, F. C. Breedveld, B. A. Dijkmans, J. Hermans, et al., "Frequency of Infection among Patients with Rheumatoid Arthritis versus Patients with Osteoarthritis or Soft Tissue Rheumatism," Arthritis and Rheumatism, Vol. 31, No. 5, 1988, pp. 667-671. doi:10.1002/art.1780310513

[7] J. P. Vandenbroucke, R. Kaaks, H. A. Valkenburg, J. W. Boersma, A. Cats, J. J. Festen, et al., "Frequency of Infections among Rheumatoid Arthritis Patients, before and after Disease Onset," Arthritis and Rheumatism, Vol. 30, No. 7, 1987, pp. 810-813. doi:10.1002/art.1780300711

[8] E. C. Keystone, "Does Anti-Tumor Necrosis Factor Alpha Therapy Affect Risk of Serious Infection and Cancer in Patients with Rheumatoid Arthritis?: A Review of Longterm Data," The Journal of Rheumatology, Vol. 38, No. 8, 2011, pp. 1552-1562. doi:10.3899/jrheum.100995

[9] K. Au, G. Reed, J. R. Curtis, J. M. Kremer, J. D. Greenberg, V. Strand, et al., "Extended Report: High Disease Activity Is Associated with an Increased Risk of Infection in Patients with Rheumatoid Arthritis," Annals of the Rheumatic Diseases, Vol. 70, No. 5, 2011, pp. 785-791. doi:10.1136/ard.2010.128637

[10] M. E. Weinblatt and A. L. Maier, "Treatment of Rheumatoid Arthritis," Arthritis and Rheumatism, Vol. 2, No. 3, 1989, pp. A23-A32. doi:10.1002/anr.1790020311

[11] M. E. Weinblatt and A. L. Maier, "Disease-Modifying Agents and Experimental Treatments of Rheumatoid Arthritis," Clinical Orthopaedics and Related Research, Vol. 265, 1991, pp. 103-115.

[12] G. Stucki and T. Langenegger, "Management of Rheumatoid Arthritis," Current Opinion in Rheumatology, Vol. 9, No. 3, 1997, pp. 229-235. doi:10.1097/00002281-199705000-00009

[13] S. Anuradha and N. P. Singh, "Recent Trends in the Management of Rheumatoid Arthritis," The Journal of the Indian Medical Association, Vol. 96, No. 11, 1998, pp. 345-348.

[14] P. Lamprecht, "TNF-α Inhibitors in Systemic Vasculitides and Connective Tissue Diseases," Autoimmunity Reviews, Vol. 4, No. 1, 2005, pp. 28-34. doi:10.1016/j.autrev.2004.06.001

[15] L. A. Witty, F. Steiner, M. Curfman, D. Webb and L. J. Wheat, "Disseminated Histoplasmosis in Patients Receiving Low-Dose Methotrexate Therapy for Psoriasis," Archives of Dermatology, Vol. 128, No. 1, 1992, pp. 91-93. doi:10.1001/archderm.1992.01680110101015

[16] G. P. LeMense and S. A. Sahn, "Opportunistic Infection during Treatment with Low Dose Methotrexate," American Journal of Respiratory and Critical Care Medicine, Vol. 150, No. 1, 1994, pp. 258-260.

[17] K. S. Kanik and J. M. Cash, "Does Methotrexate Increase the Risk of Infection or Malignancy?" Rheumatic Disease Clinics of North America, Vol. 23, No. 4, 1997, pp. 955-967. doi:10.1016/S0889-857X(05)70368-9

[18] G. Stucki, M. H. Liang, S. Stucki, P. Bruhlmann and B. A. Michel, "A Self-Administered Rheumatoid Arthritis Disease Activity Index (RADAI) for Epidemiologic Research. Psychometric Properties and Correlation with Parameters of Disease Activity," Arthritis and Rheumatism, Vol. 38, No. 6, 1995, pp. 795-798. doi:10.1002/art.1780380612

[19] D. H. Solomon, M. Stedman, A. Licari, M. E. Weinblatt, N. Maher and N. Shadick, "Agreement between Patient Report and Medical Record Review for Medications Used for Rheumatoid Arthritis: The Accuracy of Self-Reported Medication Information in Patient Registries," *Arthritis and Rheumatism*, Vol. 57, No. 2, 2007, pp. 234-239. doi:10.1002/art.22549

[20] S. Schneeweiss, A. Robicsek, R. Scranton, D. Zuckerman and D. H. Solomon, "Veteran's Affairs Hospital Discharge Databases Coded Serious Bacterial Infections Accurately," *Journal of Clinical Epidemiology*, Vol. 60, No. 4, 2007, pp. 397-409. doi:10.1016/j.jclinepi.2006.07.011

[21] J. F. Simard, M. L. Stoll, N. A. Shadick, E. W. Karlson and D. H. Solomon, "Validity of Self-Report of Infections in a Longitudinal Cohort of Patients with Rheumatoid Arthritis Differs by Source of Report and Infection Severity," *Journal of Clinical Epidemiology*, Vol. 63, No. 12, 2010, pp. 1358-1362. doi:10.1016/j.jclinepi.2010.01.014

[22] J. M. Robins and D. M. Finkelstein, "Correcting for Noncompliance and Dependent Censoring in an AIDS Clinical Trial with Inverse Probability of Censoring Weighted, (IPCW) Log-Rank Tests," *Biometrics*, Vol. 56, No. 3, 2000, pp. 779-788. doi:10.1111/j.0006-341X.2000.00779.x

[23] M. A. Hernan, B. A. Brumback and J. M. Robins, "Estimating the Causal Effect of Zidovudine on CD4 Count with a Marginal Structural Model for Repeated Measures," *Statistics in Medicine*, Vol. 21, No. 12, 2002, pp. 1689-1709. doi:10.1002/sim.1144

[24] J. R. Curtis, N. Patkar, A. Xie, C Martin, J. J. Allison, M. Saag, *et al.*, "Risk of Serious Bacterial Infections among Rheumatoid Arthritis Patients Exposed to Tumor Necrosis Factor Alpha Antagonists," *Arthritis and Rheumatism*, Vol. 56, No. 4, 2007, pp. 1125-1133. doi:10.1002/art.22504

[25] T. Bongartz, A. J. Sutton, M. J. Sweeting, I. Buchan, E. L. Matteson and V. Montori, "Anti-TNF Antibody Therapy in Rheumatoid Arthritis and the Risk of Serious Infections and Malignancies: Systematic Review and Meta-Analysis of Rare Harmful Effects in Randomized Controlled Trials," *The Journal of the American Medical Association*, Vol. 295, No. 19, 2006, pp. 2275-2285. doi:10.1001/jama.295.19.2275

[26] D. H. Solomon, M. Lunt and S. Schneeweiss, "The Risk of Infection Associated with Tumor Necrosis Factor Alpha Antagonists: Making Sense of Epidemiologic Evidence," *Arthritis and Rheumatism*, Vol. 58, No. 4, 2008, pp. 919-928. doi:10.1002/art.23396

[27] W. G. Dixon, L. Carmona, A. Finckh, M. L. Hetland, T. K. Kvien, R. Landewe, *et al.*, "EULAR Points to Consider When Establishing, Analysing and Reporting Safety Data of Biologics Registers in Rheumatology," *Annals of Rheumatic Diseases*, Vol. 69, No. 9, 2010, pp. 1596-1602. doi:10.1136/ard.2009.125526

[28] P. P. Sfikakis, "The First Decade of Biologic TNF Antagonists in Clinical Practice: Lessons Learned, Unresolved Issues and Future Directions," *Current Directions in Autoimmunity*, Vol. 11, 2010, pp. 180-210. doi:10.1159/000289205

[29] W. G. Dixon, K. Watson, M. Lunt, K. L. Hyrich, A. J. Silman and D. P. Symmons, "Rates of Serious Infection, Including Site-Specific and Bacterial Intracellular Infection, in Rheumatoid Arthritis Patients Receiving Anti-Tumor Necrosis Factor Therapy: Results from the British Society for Rheumatology Biologics Register," *Arthritis and Rheumatism*, Vol. 54, No. 8, 2006, pp. 2368-2376. doi:10.1002/art.21978

[30] F. Wolfe, L. Caplan and K. Michaud, "Treatment for Rheumatoid Arthritis and the Risk of Hospitalization for Pneumonia: Associations with Prednisone, Disease-Modifying Antirheumatic Drugs, and Anti-Tumor Necrosis Factor Therapy," *Arthritis and Rheumatism*, Vol. 54, No. 2, 2006, pp. 628-634. doi:10.1002/art.21568

[31] M. J. Van Der Veen, A. Van Der Heide, A. A. Kruize and J. W. Bijlsma, "Infection Rate and Use of Antibiotics in Patients with Rheumatoid Arthritis Treated with Methotrexate," *Annals of the Rheumatic Diseases*, Vol. 53, No. 4, 1994, pp. 224-228. doi:10.1136/ard.53.4.224

[32] H. K. Choi, M. A. Hernan, J. D. Seeger, J. M. Robins and F. Wolfe, "Methotrexate and Mortality in Patients with Rheumatoid Arthritis: A Prospective Study," *The Lancet*, Vol. 359, No. 9313, 2002, pp. 1173-1177. doi:10.1016/S0140-6736(02)08213-2

[33] T. Kurth, A. M. Walker, R. J. Glynn, K. A. Chan, J. M. Gaziano, K. Berger, *et al.*, "Results of Multivariable Logistic Regression, Propensity Matching, Propensity Adjustment, and Propensity-Based Weighting under Conditions of Nonuniform Effect," *American Journal of Epidemiology*, Vol. 163, No. 3, 2006, pp. 262-270. doi:10.1093/aje/kwj047

[34] M. A. Hernan, B. Brumback and J. M. Robins, "Marginal Structural Models to Estimate the Causal Effect of Zidovudine on the Survival of HIV-Positive Men," *Epidemiology*, Vol. 11, No. 5, 2000, pp. 561-570. doi:10.1097/00001648-200009000-00012

26

Dickkopf-1 Is Associated with Periarticular Bone Loss in Patients with Rheumatoid Arthritis[*]

Berit Grandaunet[1#], Silje Watterdal Syversen[2#], Mari Hoff[3,4], Glenn Haugeberg[3,5], Désirée van der Heijde[6], Tore K. Kvien[2], Therese Standal[1,7†]

[1]KG Jebsen Center for Myeloma Research and Department of Cancer Research and Molecular Medicine, Norwegian University of Science and Technology, Trondheim, Norway; [2]Department of Rheumatology, Diakonhjemmet Hospital, Oslo, Norway; [3]Department of Neuroscience, Norwegian University of Science and Technology, Trondheim, Norway; [4]Department of Rheumatology, St. Olavs Hospital, Trondheim, Norway; [5]Department of Rheumatology, Sørlandet Hospital, Kristiansand, Norway; [6]Department of Rheumatology, Leiden University Medical Centre, Leiden, The Netherlands; [7]Centre of Excellence for Molecular Inflammation Research, Trondheim, Norway.
Email: [†]therese.standal@ntnu.no

ABSTRACT

Objective: To examine whether cytokines shown to suppress osteoblasts, Dickkopf-1 (DKK1) and hepatocyte growth factor (HGF), are associated with periarticular bone loss in rheumatoid arthritis (RA). **Methods**: RA patients with short disease duration were prospectively followed and hand bone mineral density was assessed by digital X-ray radiogrammetry (DXR) at baseline and after 1, 2 and 5 years. Plasma samples collected at baseline from 136 of the included patients were analyzed for HGF and DKK1. Group comparisons, correlation analyses and multivariate analyses were performed to evaluate the relationship between baseline cytokine levels and DXR-BMD. **Results**: Patients with hand bone loss after 1 year had significantly higher baseline plasma levels of DKK1 than patients without bone loss. Patients with periarticular bone loss after 2 and 5 years had significantly higher baseline plasma levels of HGF. Baseline DKK1 but not HGF levels were independently associated with periarticular bone loss after 1 year. **Conclusion**: High serum levels of DKK1 are weakly but independently associated with periarticular bone loss in RA. The importance of DKK1 and HGF for loss of periarticular bone needs to be defined in future studies.

Keywords: Rheumatoid Arthritis; Osteoporosis; Osteoblast; DKK1; HGF

1. Introduction

Bone loss presents as focal joint erosions, periarticular bone loss and generalized osteoporosis in rheumatoid arthritis (RA). Periarticular bone loss occurs within the bone adjacent to inflamed joints and has been shown to precede and predict development of erosions [1]. Inflam-

[*]Competing interests: No competing interests to declare.
Funding: This study was supported by the Norwegian Research Council, Central Norway Regional Health Authority and the Norwegian Cancer Society.
Author's contributions: BG and SS acquired analysed and interpreted data and wrote the paper. MH, GH, AS, DvdH interpreted data and contributed to writing of the paper. TK designed the study, interpreted data and wrote the paper. TS designed the study, acquired and interpreted data and wrote the paper. All authors were involved in drafting the article or revising it critically for intellectual content.
[#]These two authors shared the first authorship.
[†]Corresponding authors.

matory cytokines involved in osteoclast differentiation and activation is thought to be the dominant mechanism behind the development of both erosions and periarticular bone loss [2]. Recent data, however, suggest that osteoblasts and their precursors are also influenced by RA inflammation, hypothesizing that lack of bone repair contribute to the development of erosions [3-5].

Osteoblast dysfunction in relation to the development of periarticular bone loss has not been thoroughly studied. Central signaling pathways in osteoblast differentiation are the wingless (Wnt)-signaling pathway and the bone morphogenetic protein (BMP) pathway. Inhibitors of these pathways, Dickkopf-1 (DKK1) and hepatocyte growth factor (HGF), respectively, inhibit osteoblast differentiation and are associated with bone destruction in RA and multiple myeloma [4-8].

Periarticular bone loss is assessed with digital X-ray

radiogrammetry (DXR) [1], whereas presence of focal erosions is commonly evaluated by scoring radiographs according to the Sharp Heijde method [9]. In a previous study on the same cohort we found that plasma level of HGF, but not DKK1, was an independent predictor of radiographic damage of joints both at short- and long-term follow-up [10]. In the present study we wanted to investigate if DKK1 and HGF were associated with periarticular hand bone loss assessed by DXR in RA.

2. Materials and Methods

2.1. Patients

The patients were recruited from the European Research on Incapacitating Disease and Social Support study (EURIDISS). The study enrolled 238 patients with RA of less than four years disease duration in 1992 [1,11,12]. The study was performed in compliance with Helsinki declaration and approved by regional ethics committee (REK Sør-Øst, number 2009/1770a). All patients had given informed consent. Patients were assessed at baseline and after 1, 2, 5 and 10 years. In total, 136 patients had both radiographs available for the 5-year follow-up and plasma samples stored at baseline. There were no significant differences between baseline characteristics of RA patients with or without available data (**Table 1**).

2.2. Plasma Samples and Laboratory Analyses

Samples were obtained at enrolment and stored at −70°C with no freezing and thawing. Levels of HGF, DKK1, Anti-CCP, rheumatoid factor (RF), C-reactive protein (CRP) and erythrocyte sedimentation rate (ESR) were measured as previously described [10,13].

Table 1. Baseline characteristics of the study population and the excluded patients in the cohort.

	Included patients N = 136	Excluded patients N = 102
Female %	76	71
Disease duration mean ± SD years	2.2 ± 1.2	2.4 ± 1.1
Age mean ± SD years	51.3 ± 12.1	52.8 ± 14.2
Anti CCP positive, %	62	59
RF IgM positive, %	48	48
Steroid treatment, %	26	29
DMARD treatment, %	54	49
CRP, mean ± SD mg/L	12 ± 17	13 ± 16
ESR, mean ± SD mm/hour	26.2 ± 20.8	25.5 ± 18.3
Baseline vdHeijde Sharp score, median (IQR)	2 (8)	3 (10) (n = 26)

2.3. Radiographs and DXR-BMD

Conventional hand radiographs were analyzed with the DXR Pronosco X-posure system, V. 2.0 (Sectra, Linköping, Sweden). DXR-BMD was calculated based on hand radiographs taken at baseline and after 1, 2 and 5 years of observation. Least significant change (LSC) was used as a cut-off to define loss in DXR-BMD exceeding the measurement error on the individual level and calculated as previously reported [1].

2.4. Statistics

Statistical analyses were performed using SPSS19 (IBM-SPSS, Chicago, Illinois, USA).

Variables were selected for multivariate analyses based on previous studies on the EURIDISS material and known prognostic factors for radiographic progression in RA: Baseline DXR BMD, gender, CRP, ESR, age at inclusion, disease duration, anti-CCP positivity, RF IgM positivity, current DMARD and corticosteroid dose. The factors with a p-value < 0.15 in univariate analyses were included in multivariate analyses.

3. Results

3.1. Radiographic Results

Mean (SD) DXR BMD was 0.547(0.088) at baseline, 0.532(0.092) at one year, 0.522(0.092) at two years, and 0.508(0.098) at 5 years' follow-up. The proportion of patients with DXR hand bone loss exceeding LSC was 67% at 1 year, 79% at 2 years and 89% after 5 years.

3.2. Associations between HGF and DKK1 Levels and Baseline Characteristics

The median baseline levels of HGF and DKK1 were 723 pg/mL (interquartile range (IQR) 255) and 1575 pg/mL (IQR 3230), respectively.

HGF levels at baseline were positively correlated to age (rho 0.50, p < 0.001) and markers of inflammation (CRP, rho 0.21, p < 0.05, ESR, rho 0.39, p < 0.001) whereas DKK1 levels did not correlate to these parameters. There was a slightly higher median HGF level in the anti-CCP positive group (742.0 pg/mL, IQR 282.5, p < 0.05) compared with the anti-CCP negative group (668.5 pg/mL, IQR 240) but no difference in the baseline DKK-1 level comparing these two groups.

3.3. Higher Levels of DKK1 in Patients Developing Periarticular Osteoporosis

DKK1 plasma levels at baseline were significantly higher (2010 pg/mL, IQR 3086) in patients developing periarticular bone loss after 1 year compared with patients without periarticular bone loss (1332.2 pg/mL, IQR 2094, p =

0.03), but this difference was not present at 2- and 5-years follow up (2104.9 pg/mL, IQR 3062.5 vs 1790.4 pg/mL, IQR 2782, p = 0.4 and 2087.1 pg/mL, IQR 3084.9 vs 1105.8 pg/mL, IQR 1885.9, p = 0.13, respectively).

3.4. Higher Levels of HGF in Patients Developing Periarticular Osteoporosis

Baseline HGF levels were borderline significantly higher in the group of patients who developed periarticular bone loss compared with patients who did not after one-year follow up (769 pg/mL, IQR 277 vs. 653 pg/mL, IQR 229, p = 0.056) and significantly higher in the group of patients who developed periarticular bone loss after 2 years (752 pg/mL, IQR 284) and 5 years (737 pg/mL, IQR 271) compared with patients who did not (676 pg/mL, IQR 199 and 622 pg/mL, IQR 303, p = 0.038, p = 0.045, respectively).

3.5. Associations between Cytokine Levels and Prospective Bone Loss

Levels of HGF were associated with percentage bone loss at 1, 2 and 5 years (p = 0.001, p = 0.001, p = 0.005). Levels of DKK1 were significantly associated with percentage bone loss at 1-year observation (p = 0.013), but not after 2 years (p = 0.094) or 5 (p = 0.714) (**Table 2**).

In multivariate regression analyses levels of DKK1 were found to be significantly associated with percentage bone loss at 1-year observation as were also CRP, ESR, and anti-CCP (**Table 3**). Baseline plasma levels of DKK1 were not associated with percentage bone loss after 2 and 5 years (β: 0.105, p = 0.193, β: 0.01, p = 0.907, respectively).

HGF was not associated with percentage bone loss in multivariate regression models at any time point (1 year:

Table 2. Associations with baseline plasma levels of cytokines and percentage bone loss.

Baseline cytokine levels	Standardized β	R^2	p-value
	Percentage bone loss after 1 year observation		
DKK1 pg/mL	0.214	0.046	0.013
HGF pg/mL	0.285	0.081	0.001
	Percentage bone loss after 2 years observation		
DKK1 pg/mL	0.148	0.022	0.094
HGF pg/mL	0.298	0.089	0.001
	Percentage bone loss after 5 years observation		
DKK1 pg/mL	0.034	0.001	0.714
HGF pg/mL	0.255	0.065	0.005

Table 3. Baseline predictors of percentage bone loss after 1-year observation.

	β	p	R^2 combined regression model
CRP	−0.280	0.008	
ESR	0.597	<0.001	0.355
Anti-CCP positive	0.232	0.008	
DKK1	0.178	0.022	

β: 0.092, p = 0.319, 2 year. β: 0.080, p = 0.405, 5 year. β: 0.083, p = 0.400).

4. Discussion

The main finding in this study is that high plasma levels of DKK1 at baseline are independently associated with short-term loss of periarticular bone-mass assessed by DXR-BMD. These findings support that, as for the development of focal erosions, osteoblast suppression may play a role in the development of periarticular bone loss.

In a previous study from the same cohort we found that levels of DKK1 at baseline were not associated with development of focal erosions assessed by Sharp Heijde score [10], while we here found DKK1 to weakly but independently predict periarticular bone loss at 1-year follow up. Even though such a conclusion cannot be made based on the present study, this raises the hypothesis of an even more important role for DKK1 in development of periarticular bone loss as compared to development of erosions.

Levels of HGF, on the other hand, was shown to be an independent predictor of radiographic damage of joints both at short- and long-term follow-up [10], but was not associated with periarticular bone loss in adjusted analyses at any time point. Although we and others have shown that HGF inhibits osteoblast differentiation [6,7] it seems clear that the effect of HGF on osteoblast differentiation is dependent on the concentration of the cytokine, and that HGF at low concentrations in fact may promote rather than inhibit osteoblastogenesis [14]. Plasma levels of HGF correlate to levels of HGF in synovial fluid, and levels of HGF are higher in synovial fluid than in serum obtained simultaneously from the same individuals [15,16]. Hence, HGF at high concentrations in the joints are more likely to act negatively on osteoblasts than HGF at the lower concentrations found in circulation. On the other hand, lack of an independent association of HGF with periarticular bone loss might also be due to confounding or methodological issues.

There are several important limitations to this study. First of all, the observed associations are rather weak and need to be confirmed in future studies. It is not possible to draw conclusions regarding mechanisms for patho-physiologic processes based on plasma levels of cytokines.

Periarticular bone loss was determined by examination of radiographs of the hands only, while cytokine levels measured in the circulation probably reflect the degree of inflammation and destruction in several joints. Preanalysis sources of variation (different treatment regimens, diurnal variation, comorbidity) as well as possible effects of sampling and storage can affect plasma levels of cytokines and must be taken into account in the interpretation of the data. Another important limitation is the small group of patients (n = 13) that were classified as not having a significant loss in DXR BMD at 5 years observation. Thus the group is probably too small to reveal any association between the measured cytokines and hand bone loss in a long-term perspective.

5. Conclusion

Our data suggest an independent association of plasma levels of DKK1 and loss of periarticular bone in RA. The relative importance of DKK1 and HGF in terms of loss of periarticular bone compared with development of erosions needs to be explored in future studies.

6. Acknowledgements

We thank Berit Størdal for technical assistance.

REFERENCES

[1] M. Hoff, G. Haugeberg, S. Odegard, S. Syversen, R. Landewe, H. D. van der and T. K. Kvien, "Cortical Hand Bone Loss after 1 Year in Early Rheumatoid Arthritis Predicts Radiographic Hand Joint Damage at 5-Year and 10-Year Follow-Up," *Annals of the Rheumatic Diseases*, Vol. 68, No. 3, 2009, pp. 324-329. http://dx.doi.org/10.1136/ard.2007.085985

[2] G. Schett, "Cells of the Synovium in Rheumatoid Arthritis. Osteoclasts," *Arthritis Research & Therapy*, Vol. 9, No. 1, 2007, p. 203. http://dx.doi.org/10.1186/ar2110

[3] N. C. Walsh and E. M. Gravallese, "Bone Remodeling in Rheumatic Disease: A Question of Balance," *Immunological Reviews*, Vol. 233, No. 1, 2010, pp. 301-312. http://dx.doi.org/10.1111/j.0105-2896.2009.00857.x

[4] D. Diarra, M. Stolina, K. Polzer, J. Zwerina, M. S. Ominsky, D. Dwyer, A. Korb, J. Smolen, M. Hoffmann, C. Scheinecker, H. D. van der, R. Landewe, D. Lacey, W. G. Richards and G. Schett, "Dickkopf-1 Is a Master Regulator of Joint Remodeling," *Nature Medicine*, Vol. 13, No. 2, 2007, pp. 156-163. http://dx.doi.org/10.1038/nm1538

[5] M. M. Matzelle, M. A. Gallant, K. W. Condon, N. C. Walsh, C. A. Manning, G. S. Stein, J. B. Lian, D. B. Burr and E. M. Gravallese, "Resolution of Inflammation Induces Osteoblast Function and Regulates the Wnt Signaling Pathway," *Arthritis and Rheumatism*, 2011.

[6] T. Standal, N. Abildgaard, U. M. Fagerli, B. Stordal, O. Hjertner, M. Borset and A. Sundan, "HGF Inhibits BMP-Induced Osteoblastogenesis: Possible Implications for the Bone Disease of Multiple Myeloma," *Blood*, Vol. 109, No. 7, 2007, pp. 3024-3030.

[7] T. Kawasaki, Y. Niki, T. Miyamoto, K. Horiuchi, M. Matsumoto, M. Aizawa and Y. Toyama, "The Effect of Timing in the Administration of Hepatocyte Growth Factor to Modulate BMP-2-Induced Osteoblast Differentiation," *Biomaterials*, Vol. 31, No. 6, 2010, pp. 1191-1198. http://dx.doi.org/10.1016/j.biomaterials.2009.10.048

[8] E. Tian, F. Zhan, R. Walker, E. Rasmussen, Y. Ma, B. Barlogie and J. D. Shaughnessy Jr., "The Role of the Wnt-Signaling Antagonist DKK1 in the Development of Osteolytic Lesions in Multiple Myeloma," *New England Journal of Medicine*, Vol. 349, No. 26, 2003, pp. 2483-2494. http://dx.doi.org/10.1056/NEJMoa030847

[9] D. M. van der Heijde, "Radiographic Imaging: The 'Gold Standard' for Assessment of Disease Progression in Rheumatoid Arthritis," *Rheumatology*, Vol. 39, No. S1, 2000, pp. 9-16. http://dx.doi.org/10.1093/oxfordjournals.rheumatology.a031496

[10] B. Grandaunet, S. W. Syversen, M. Hoff, A. Sundan, G. Haugeberg, H. D. van der, T. K. Kvien and T. Standal, "Association between High Plasma Levels of Hepatocyte Growth Factor and Progression of Radiographic Damage in the Joints of Patients with Rheumatoid Arthritis," *Arthritis and Rheumatism*, Vol. 63, No. 3, 2011, pp. 662-669. http://dx.doi.org/10.1002/art.30163

[11] L. M. Smedstad, T. K. Kvien, T. Moum and P. Vaglum, "Life Events, Psychosocial Factors, and Demographic Variables in Early Rheumatoid Arthritis: Relations to One-Year Changes in Functional Disability," *Journal of Rheumatology*, Vol. 22, No. 12, 1995, pp. 2218-2225.

[12] F. C. Arnett, S. M. Edworthy, D. A. Bloch, D. J. McShane, J. F. Fries, N. S. Cooper, L. A. Healey, S. R. Kaplan, M. H. Liang, H. S. Luthra, et al., "The American Rheumatism Association 1987 Revised Criteria for the Classification of Rheumatoid Arthritis," *Arthritis and Rheumatism*, Vol. 31, No. 3, 1988, pp. 315-324. http://dx.doi.org/10.1002/art.1780310302

[13] S. W. Syversen, P. I. Gaarder, G. L. Goll, S. Odegard, E. A. Haavardsholm, P. Mowinckel, D. van der Heijde, R. Landewe and T. K. Kvien, "High Anti-Cyclic Citrullinated Peptide Levels and an Algorithm of Four Variables Predict Radiographic Progression in Patients with Rheumatoid Arthritis: Results from a 10-Year Longitudinal Study," *Annals of the Rheumatic Diseases*, Vol. 67, No. 2, 2008, pp. 212-217. http://dx.doi.org/10.1136/ard.2006.068247

[14] Q. Wen, L. Zhou, C. Zhou, M. Zhou, W. Luo and L. Ma, "Change in Hepatocyte Growth Factor Concentration Promote Mesenchymal Stem Cell-Mediated Osteogenic Regeneration," *Journal of Cellular and Molecular Medicine*, 2011.

[15] K. Yukioka, M. Inaba, Y. Furumitsu, M. Yukioka, T. Nishino, H. Goto, Y. Nishizawa and H. Morii, "Levels of Hepatocyte Growth Factor in Synovial Fluid and Serum

of Patients with Rheumatoid Arthritis and Release of Hepatocyte Growth Factor by Rheumatoid Synovial Fluid Cells," *Journal of Rheumatology*, Vol. 21, No. 12, 1994, pp. 2184-2189.

[16] A. E. Koch, M. M. Halloran, S. Hosaka, M. R. Shah, C. J. Haskell, S. K. Baker, R. J. Panos, G. K. Haines, G. L. Ben-nett, R. M. Pope and N. Ferrara, "Hepatocyte Growth Factor. A Cytokine Mediating Endothelial Migration in Inflammatory Arthritis," *Arthritis and Rheumatism*, Vol. 39, No. 9, 1996, pp. 1566-1575.
http://dx.doi.org/10.1002/art.1780390917

27

The Effects of Sex on Patient Reported Outcomes in Inflammatory Arthritis and Connective Tissue Diseases[*]

Jason J. Lee[1], Janet E. Pope[2#]

[1]Schulich School of Medicine, Western University, London, Canada; [2]Schulich School of Medicine, Western University, St. Joseph's Health Care, London, Canada.
Email: [#]janet.pope@sjhc.london.on.ca

ABSTRACT

Background: It was thought that women report higher pain than men. We studied if there was a sex difference for several patient reported outcomes (PROs) in rheumatic diseases. **Materials and Methods:** Health Assessment Questionnaire disability index (HAQ-DI) as well as 100 mm Visual Analogue Scale (VAS) for pain, fatigue, sleep disturbance, and patient global assessment were compared cross-sectionally between the sexes for ankylosingspondylitis (AS), psoriatic arthritis (PsA), rheumatoid arthritis (RA), systemic lupus erythematosus (SLE) and systemic sclerosis (SSc). Data were collected using standardized forms administered during routine care. **Results:** The sample included 136 patients (97 males) with AS, 200 (83 males) with PsA, 232 (40 males) with RA, 199 (12 males) with SLE, and 113 (17 males) with SSc. There were no significant differences in AS. There were sex differences in PsA for HAQ (0.85 females, 0.57 males; $p < 0.003$), pain (45.2 females, 36.8 males; $p < 0.03$), sleep (42.1 females, 31.6 males; $p < 0.025$), and not significantly for fatigue and global scores (fatigue: 44.4 females, 36.0 males; $p < 0.07$. global: 40.1 females, 33.1 males; $p < 0.06$). There were similar non-significant differences observed in RA and SLE; whereas, in SSc, men had a higher global assessment (52.9 males, 38.1 females; $p < 0.03$). **Conclusions:** A significant sex difference was observed in PsA with females reporting worse symptoms. In SSc, global assessments were worse in males possibly due to proportionately more diffuse cutaneous SSc. Sex differences for PROs are not consistent between rheumatic inflammatory diseases in prevalent patients.

Keywords: Sex Differences; Patient Reported Outcomes; Inflammatory Arthritis; Connective Tissue Disease

1. Introduction

The effects of inflammatory arthritis and connective tissue diseases have high impact on patients including pain, fatigue, functional loss, and work loss [1-6]. As these groups of patients with chronic disease grow in incidence and prevalence, it is increasingly more important to better evaluate and understand these patients. A good example of such an initiative is a recent epidemiological study from the Mayo Clinic in Minnesota, USA, which concluded that the incidence of rheumatoid arthritis (RA), one of the most common forms of inflammatory arthritis, is increasing, particularly in women [7].

Several studies that have explored the effects of sex on patient reported outcomes (PROs) in inflammatory arthritis have focused on pain in RA [1,2,6,8]. Disease activity measured by Disease Activity Score 28 (DAS28) (which includes a patient global assessment), and self reported functional impairment as measured by the Health Assessment Questionnaire Disability Index (HAQ-DI) [9] were significantly higher in females compared to males. In ankylosing spondylitis (AS), there are sex differences in phenotype where females may present with less severe disease, but have more peripheral arthritis [4]. The authors in the 2007 study found that males with AS present with worse radiographic axial disease. However, females reported worse function despite less severe objective measures of disease. This could have been confounded perhaps by more peripheral arthritis.

The distributions of males compared to females vary between rheumatic diseases [1,2,4,6,7,10-14]. It is highest in AS with often 7 to 9 males to 1 female [4,10], to approximately equal in PsA [11], female predominance in RA [1,2,6] (approximately 75% to 80% female in RA

[*]There was no funding for this project. There are no conflicts of interest. Ethics approval was obtained for the chart audit.
[#]Corresponding author.

RCTs) and greater than 8:1 females to males in SSc [13] and SLE [14]. The differences in disease manifestations between males and females could potentially affect PROs.

PROs are often used in intervention studies so recognizing potential sex related differences may help in the interpretation of and generalizability to patients in rheumatologists' practices. Currently, it is widely believed that females suffer more pain from their arthritis. Data is sparse in the rheumatology literature for potential sex differences in other PROs such as fatigue or sleep disturbance. Sex differences in PROs in other inflammatory rheumatic conditions such as psoriatic arthritis (PsA), systemic lupus erythematosus (SLE) and systemic sclerosis (SSc) have not been as well studied.

We compared HAQ-DI, pain, fatigue, sleep disturbance, and patient reported global disease activity between sexes for AS, PsA, RA, SLE, and SSc to determine if each disease has sex effects on patient reported outcomes. We hypothesized that women would report worse outcomes across all inflammatory arthritis and CTDs.

2. Patients and Methods

Multiple data are collected routinely on patients seen at St. Joseph's Hospital Rheumatology clinic in London, Ontario, which is affiliated with Western University, and services a referral region of over one million. The clinic is heavily weighted towards seeing patients with inflammatory arthritis and CTDs. Patients are primarily English speaking, representing the full spectrum of disease severity, and are generally followed 1 - 4 times a year depending on disease severity and flare-ups. The databases from previous studies of minimally important differences (MID) were used in AS, PsA, RA, SLE and SSc where patients seen consecutively who completed their clinic forms and were seen in follow up in less than one year were included [10-14]. These publications had Ethics Approval from the University of Western Ontario Ethics Committee for studying RA, SLE, SSc, PsA, AS, and Sjogren's syndrome and this current project utilized the data collected under the approval which covered this project also.

The data are from patients seen serially by one rheumatologist (JP) who had been diagnosed with RA [15] and SLE [16] meeting the ACR criteria, diagnosed with PsA meeting the Moll and Wright criteria [17], and diagnosed with SSc by expert opinion, most of whom met the ACR criteria [18], or having the limited cutaneousSSc subset who did not meet criteria (as 12% of patients with SSc in the limited subset may not meet ACR criteria) [19]. The data for AS are from patients seen serially by five rheumatologists in the clinic who had been diagnosed with AS as per ACR criteria [20]. The patients

are referred from the community and patients with rare diseases such as scleroderma are often referred from a larger catchment area.

Mean and distribution of scores for consecutive patients with these diseases were recorded. Patient data were collected during routine visits, as part of usual patient care. For analysis, data points were collected for two consecutive visits that were 6 to 18 months apart. Patient global status was defined and measured with the following question: "How would you describe your overall status since your last visit: *much better, better, the same, worse, much worse*". HAQ-DI was scored as 0 (no disability) to 3 (severe disability/limitation in function), and VAS for pain, fatigue, sleep and global health (0 as no problem and 100 as worst). Changes of 10% or approximately 10% on a 100 mm visual analogue scale (VAS) correspond to MID for patient reported measures across many studies [21].

Data for each disease were extracted by a single trained data-extractor and entered into a common database. From these databases, one author (JL) extracted relevant clinical and demographic data using Microsoft Excel and performed the necessary statistical analyses. PROs from a cross sectional follow-up visit were used for analysis. Two-tailed distribution T-tests were done to determine if there were significant sex differences for PROs in each disease. Data were analyzed using SPSS v. 19.0. A two-tailed $p < 0.05$ was considered significant. Results were presented as mean (SD) unless if otherwise specified.

3. Results

A total of 880 patients were included for this observational study. Descriptive demographic statistics are summarized in **Table 1**. The breakdown of patient groups according to disease were as follows: 136 (29% female) with AS, 200 patients (59% female) with PsA, 232 patients (83% female) with RA, 199 patients (94% female) with SLE and 113 patients (85% female) with SSc. Patients' age and duration of disease were similar between men and women as well as across all diseases. The average age in years for men and women respectively were as follows: AS: 44 (11.5), 45 (12.2); PsA: 51 (14.7), 51 (13.5); RA: 62 (11.3), 58 (14.7); SLE: 56 (10.1), 52 (14.3); and SSc: 53 (10.2), 58 (11.6). The average duration of disease was long (10 to 16 years) (**Table 1**).

There were no significant differences for PROs in AS. There were differences in PsA for HAQ (0.85 females, 0.57 males; $p < 0.003$), pain (45.2 females, 36.8 males; $p < 0.034$), and sleep (42.1 females, 31.6 males; $p < 0.025$) where females had worse scores. There were non-significant higher scores observed in women with RA and SLE, except in HAQ-DI within SLE where there was a significant difference (0.65 females, 0.20 males; $p < 0.001$).

Table 1. Study patient demographics.

Patient Demographics	Ankylosing Spondylitis (N = 136)		Psoriatic Arthritis (N = 200)		Rheumatoid Arthritis (N = 232)		Systemic Lupus Erythematosus (N = 199)		Systemic Sclerosis (N = 113)	
	Male	Female	Male	Female	Male	Female	Male	Female	Male	Female
N (%)	97 (71%)	39 (29%)	83 (41%)	117 (59%)	40 (17%)	192 (83%)	12 (6%)	187 (94%)	17 (15%)	96 (85%)
Mean Age (SD)	44.2 (11.5)	44.6 (12.2)	50.8 (14.7)	51.2 (13.5)	62.9 (12.0)	59.7 (13.8)	56.0 (10.1)	51.7 (14.3)	53.1 (10.2)	57.7 (11.6)
Mean Disease Duration (SD)	15.8 (10.7)	14.6 (10.3)	12.3 (9.2)	10.4 (6.7)	10.6 (11.2)	11.8 (10.5)	12.6 (8.9)	10.0 (7.2)	9.8 (7.1)	9.9 (6.5)
Median Duration (min, max)	12 (1, 45)	13 (1, 35)	11 (1, 60)	10 (1, 36)	6 (1, 45)	8 (1, 57)	10 (1, 30)	8 (1, 40)	7 (1, 29)	10 (1, 35)

Age and disease duration in years; SD = Standard Deviation.

The opposite occurred between males and females within SSc where men scored higher, but only the global assessment was significantly different (52.9 males, 38.1 females; p < 0.035). The PROs are shown in **Figure 1**.

4. Discussion

The incidence and prevalence of inflammatory arthritis and connective tissue diseases may be increasing [7]. The evolving epidemiology of the diseases may include changes in prognosis and can influence treatment [1,2,4,6,7]. One important, but under-explored, observation is the effects of sex on disease symptom severity and associated clinical impact. Understanding PROs are important because they are widely used and can influence treatment decisions.

Earlier studies in the 1980s, before the discovery modern disease modifying anti-rheumatic drugs (DMARDs), reported poor outcomes in many patients without appreciable sex differences [3,5]. However, more recent studies in the 1990s and 2000s with more effective therapeutic agents and early aggressive treatment strategies have discovered major differences between sexes with respect to various disease outcomes [1,2,6]. Currently, it is widely believed that there are significant sex differences in objective measures of disease such as remission rates, age of onset, and production of biologic markers for common rheumatic diseases, particularly in RA [2,6]. There is evidence of worse pain and associated disability in women with RA and PsA [1,2,6,11].

Contrary to these recent findings, in our patient cohort, consistent sex differences were not observed for patient reported outcome measures. Only females with PsA reported marginally significant worse symptoms compared to males. Of note, in our RA patients, the PROs differed from other RA cohorts reported in literature [1,2,6]. There was lower pain compared to Ahlmen et al. [1] who reported pain VAS of approximately 47in men over a 5-year span, and approximately 43 in women during the same time interval. In comparison, pain VAS scores were 38.5 and 38.7 for men and women in our patients. It is

possible that, while women and men may respond to therapies differently, contemporary DMARD treatment with early intervention and use of combination therapies may alter sex differences for PROs in RA. Interestingly, in the most recent meta-analysis by Barnabe et al. [2], only 3 of 16 cohorts of patients with RA reported mean pain VAS of less than 40mm for both men and women. Of these three cohorts, 2 of 3 did not find significance in the difference between men and women.

In SSc males numerically had higher scores, although not statically significant for most of the PROs that were studied. We believe that this is likely due to males having proportionately more diffused subset of SSc (dcSSc) with worse disease severity than localized scleroderma (lcSSc) [13], but we did not have the power to divide the subsets for this study.

The study has limitations. It consists of patients with long disease duration seen cross-sectionally and there could have been differences in disease activity and treatment as objective disease measures were not studied. However, it is unlikely that treatment would be biased by gender. The study could have been underpowered; especially where there were small numbers for certain subsets by sex within a disease. For instance, some p-values may have been significant if numbers were larger. The proportion of males in each group, with the exception of AS, was smaller than females, which is consistent with epidemiological studies [2,4,6,8,10-14,19]. The different proportions of males in each disease could also impact on comorbidities that may have different proportions between the sexes and comorbidities can affect patient reported outcomes. For instance, fibromyalgia is a common comorbidity in women with SLE. We did not take co-morbidities into account in this study. The patients were from a single clinic and, with exception of the AS group, from a single rheumatologist. The patient population was somewhat homogeneous with most patients being Caucasian, able to read English. Also, the long disease duration (mean 10 - 16 years) would affect patient scores (adaptation over time and more damage over time) so the results

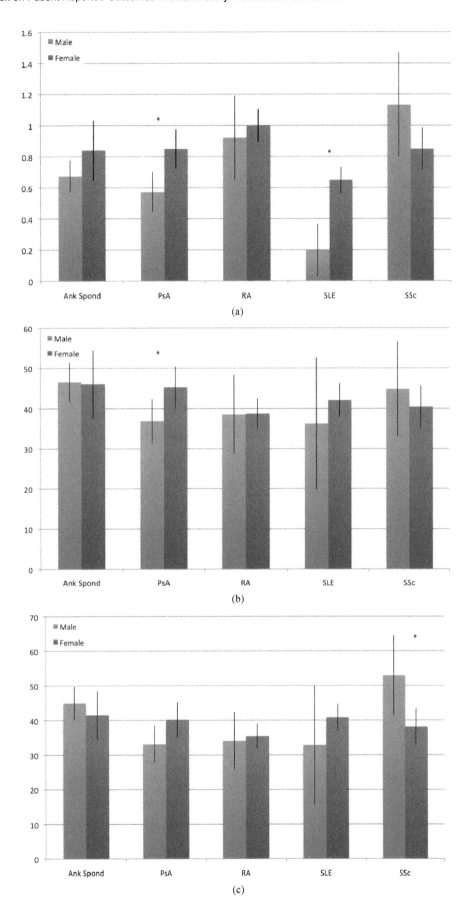

(a)

(b)

(c)

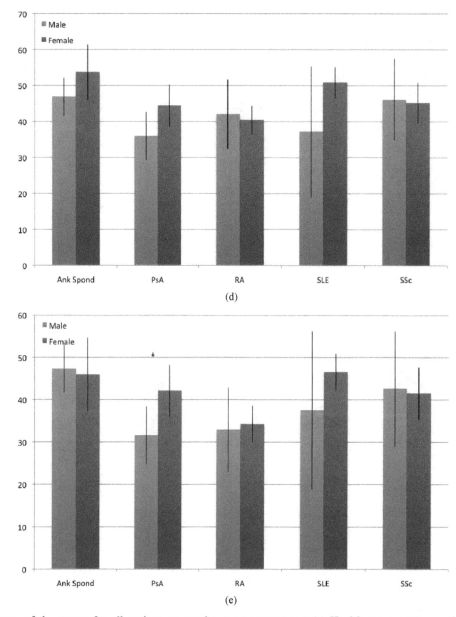

Figure 1. Summary of the means for all patient reported outcome measures: (a) Health assessment questionnaire disability index; (b) Pain visual analog scale in mm; (c) Global visual analog scale in mm; (d) Fatigue visual analog scale in mm; (e) Sleep visual analog scale in mm. The error bars represent 95% confidence intervals and *Indicates significance with $p < 0.05$.

may not be generalizable to early disease. The data presented here were collected at a single visit. Although this has the potential for bias, data analyzed within the same patients from a subsequent follow-up usually within 6 to 12 months were similar (data not shown). Multiple statistical testing was not corrected using Bonferroni's as the entire study was a secondary hypothesis as data were used from previous MCID studies. It may be that disease activity is affecting the differences in PROs more than gender but we did not have all variables for disease activity consistently collected on the patients included in this study. It may be that sex affects treatment which then would influence the PROs (such as a disparity between

use of biologics in inflammatory arthritis).

5. Conclusion

In summary, this is the first study to comprehensively characterize sex differences for several inflammatory rheumatologic diseases for many PROs. Mostly there were no sex differences. However, a significant sex difference was observed in PsA, with females reporting worse symptoms. In SSc patient global assessment was worse in males. Sex differences for patient reported outcomes are not consistent between rheumatic inflammatory diseases.

REFERENCES

[1]   M. Ahlmen, B. Svensson, K. Albertsson, K. Forslind and I. Hafström, "Influence of Gender on Assessments of Disease Activity and Function in Early Rheumatoid Arthritis in Relation to Radiographic Joint Damage," *Annals of the Rheumatic Diseases*, Vol. 69, No. 1, 2010, pp. 230-233.

[2]   C. Barnabe, L. Bessette, C. Flanagan, S. Leclercq, A. Steiman, F. Kalache, *et al.*, "Sex Differences in Pain Scores and Localization in Inflammatory Arthritis: A Systematic Review and Metaanalysis," *The Journal of Rheumatology*, Vol. 39, No. 6, 2012, pp. 1221-1230. doi:10.3899/jrheum.111393

[3]   K. Kaarela, "Prognostic Factors and Diagnostic Criteria in Early Rheumatoid Arthritis," *Scandinavian Journal of Rheumatology*, Vol. 14, No. s57, 1985, pp. 1-54. doi:10.3109/03009748509104317

[4]   W. Lee, J. D. Reveille, J. C. J. Davis, T. J. Learch, M. M. Ward and M. H. Weisman, "Are There Gender Differences in Severity of Ankylosing Spondylitis? Results from the PSOAS Cohort," *Annals of Rheumatic Diseases*, Vol. 66, No. 5, 2007, pp. 633-638. doi:10.1136/ard.2006.060293

[5]   G. Makisara and P. Makisara, "Prognosis of Functional Capacity and Work Capacity in Rheumatoid Arthritis," *Clinical Rheumatology*, Vol. 1, No. 2, 1982, pp. 117-125. doi:10.1007/BF02275601

[6]   T. Sokka, S. Toloza, M. Cutolo, H. Kautiainen, H. Makinen, F. Gogus, *et al.*, "Women, Men, and Rheumatoid Arthritis: Analyses of Disease Activity, Disease Characteristics, and Treatments in the QUEST-RA Study," *Arthritis Research & Therapy*, Vol. 11, No. 1, 2009, p. R7.

[7]   E. Myasoedova, C. S. Crowson, H. M. Kremers, T. M. Therneau and S. E. Gabriel, "Is the Incidence of Rheumatoid Arthritis Rising? Results from Olmsted County, Minnesota, 1955-2007," *Arthritis & Rheumatism*, Vol. 62, No. 6, 2010, pp. 1576-1582. doi:10.1002/art.27425

[8]   D. Khanna, J. E. Pope, P. P. Khanna, M. Maloney, N. Samedi, D. Norrie, *et al.*, "The Minimally Important Difference for the Fatigue Visual Analog Scale in Patients with Rheumatoid Arthritis Followed in an Academic Clinical Practice," *The Journal of Rheumatology*, Vol. 35, No. 12, 2008, pp. 2339-2343. doi:10.3899/jrheum.080375

[9]   J. Fries, P. Spitz, R. Kraines and H. Holman, "Measurement of Patient Outcome in Arthritis," *Arthritis & Rheumatism*, Vol. 23, No. 2, 1980, pp. 137-145. doi:10.1002/art.1780230202

[10]   L. Wheaton and J. Pope, "The Minimally Important Difference for Patient-Reported Outcomes in Spondyloarthropathies Including Pain, Fatigue, Sleep, and Health Assessment Questionnaire," *The Journal of Rheumatology*, Vol. 37, No. 4, 2010, pp. 816-822. doi:10.3899/jrheum.090086

[11]   T. Kwok and J. E. Pope, "Minimally Important Difference for Patient-Reported Outcomes in Psoriatic Arthritis: Health Assessment Questionnaire and Pain, Fatigue, and Global Visual Analog Scales," *The Journal of Rheumatology*, Vol. 37, No. 5, 2010, pp. 1024-1028. doi:10.3899/jrheum.090832

[12]   J. Pope, D. Khanna, D. Norrie and J. M. Ouimet, "The Minimally Important Difference for the Health Assessment Questionnaire in Rheumatoid Arthritis Clinical Practice Is Smaller than in Randomized Controlled Trials," *The Journal of Rheumatology*, Vol. 36, No. 2, 2009, pp. 254-259. doi:10.3899/jrheum.080479

[13]   S. Sekhon, J. Pope, Canadian Scleroderma Research Group and M. Baron, "The Minimally Important Difference in Clinical Practice for Patient-Centered Outcomes Including Health Assessment Questionnaire, Fatigue, Pain, Sleep, Global Visual Analog Scale, and SF-36 in Scleroderma," *The Journal of Rheumatology*, Vol. 37, No. 3, 2010, pp. 591-598. doi:10.3899/jrheum.090375

[14]   K. J. Colangelo, J. Pope and C. Peschken, "The Minimally Important Difference for Patient Reported Outcomes in Systemic Lupus Erythematosus Including the HAQ-DI, Pain, Fatigue, and SF-36," *The Journal of Rheumatology*, Vol. 36, No. 10, 2009, pp. 2231-2237. doi:10.3899/jrheum.090193

[15]   F. C. Arnett, S. M. Edworthy, D. A. Bloch, D. J. McShane, J. F. Fries, N. S. Cooper, *et al.*, "The American Rheumatism Association 1987 Revised Criteria for the Classification of Rheumatoid Arthritis," *Arthritis & Rheumatism*, Vol. 31, No. 3, 1988, pp. 315-324. doi:10.1002/art.1780310302

[16]   M. C. Hochberg, "Updating the American College of Rheumatology Revised Criteria for the Classification of Systemic Lupus Erythematosus," *Arthritis & Rheumatism*, Vol. 40, No. 9, 1997, p. 1725. doi:10.1002/art.1780400928

[17]   J. M. Moll and V. Wright, "Psoriatic Arthritis," *Seminars in Arthritis and Rheumatism*, Vol. 3, No. 1, 1973, pp. 55-78. doi:10.1016/0049-0172(73)90035-8

[18]   T. Alfonse, "Preliminary Criteria for the Classification of Systemic Sclerosis (Scleroderma)," *Arthritis & Rheumatism*, Vol. 23, No. 5, 1980, pp. 581-590. doi:10.1002/art.1780230510

[19]   E. C. LeRoy, C. M. Black, R. Fleischmajer, *et al.*, "Scleroderma (Systemic Sclerosis): Classification, Subsets and Pathogenesis," *The Journal of Rheumatology*, Vol. 15, No. 2, 1988, pp. 202-205.

[20]   S. Van der Linden, H. A. Valkenburg and A. Cats, "Evaluation of Diagnostic Criteria for Ankylosing Spondylitis: A Proposal for Modification of the New York Criteria," *Arthritis & Rheumatism*, Vol. 27, No. 4, 1984, pp. 361-368. doi:10.1002/art.1780270401

[21]   G. R. Norman, J. A. Sloane and K. W. Wyrwich, "Interpretation of Changes in Health-Related Quality of Life: The Remarkable Universality of Half a Standard Deviation," *Medical Care*, Vol. 41, No. 5, 2003, pp. 582-592. doi:10.1097/01.MLR.0000062554.74615.4C

28

Changes in mRNA Expression and Activity of Xenobiotic Metabolizing Enzymes in Livers from Adjuvant-Induced Arthritis Rats

Atsushi Kawase, Syoko Wada, Masahiro Iwaki[*]

Department of Pharmacy, School of Pharmacy, Kinki University, Osaka, Japan.
Email: *iwaki@phar.kindai.ac.jp

ABSTRACT

Pathophysiological changes in human patients and in animal models of infection or inflammation are associated with alterations in the production of numerous liver-derived proteins including metabolizing enzymes. In this study, the effects of adjuvant-induced arthritis (AA) in rats on the levels of mRNA and activity of hepatic xenobiotic metabolizing enzymes were determined during the inflammatory response. The mRNA levels of cytochrome P450 (CYP) 1A2, CYP2C12, CYP2D1, CYP2D2, and CYP3A1 were significantly decreased compared with control levels in almost all phases of inflammation. A reduction in the activity of CYP2C and CYP3A, which are abundantly expressed in the liver, was also observed. For phase II metabolizing enzymes, mRNA levels of uridine 5'-diphospho-glucuronosyltransferase (UGT) 1A1, UGT1A6, sulfotransferase (SULT) 2A1, and glutathione S-transferase 2 were significantly decreased compared with control levels. However, the mRNA levels of UGT2B and SULT1A1 returned to control levels during the subacute (7 d after adjuvant treatment) and chronic (21 d after adjuvant treatment) phases although these levels decreased during the acute (3 d after adjuvant treatment) phase. These results suggest that the effects of inflammation on the expression of xenobiotic metabolizing enzymes differ depending on the isoform of the enzyme and could affect the pharmacokinetics of each substrate.

Keywords: Inflammation; Arthritis; Enzyme; Cytochrome; Metabolism

1. Introduction

Pathophysiological changes in human patients and in animal models of infection or inflammation are associated with immediate and often dramatic alterations in the production of numerous liver-derived proteins, including metabolizing enzymes such as cytochrome P450s (CYP), UDP-glucuronosyltransferases (UGT), sulfotransferases (SULT), and glutathione S-transferases (GST) [1,2]. Inflammatory conditions such as rheumatoid arthritis and Crohn's disease have been shown to reduce hepatic clearance of several highly cleared drugs [3-5]. Adjuvant-induced arthritis (AA) in rats has been used as an animal model for rheumatoid arthritis in the development of new anti-inflammatory medicines because rats exhibit a systemic inflammatory disease with similar bone and cartilage alterations to those observed in rheumatoid arthritis on day 3 (acute), day 7 (subacute) and day 21

(chronic) after adjuvant treatment [6]. Changes in the pharmacokinetics and pharmacological effects of several drugs via altered CYP activities and serum protein binding have been reported in AA rats, including elevated plasma concentrations of cyclosporine A, acebutolol and propranolol [4,7], and prolongation of sleeping time with pentobarbital [8]. We also demonstrated that flurbiprofen glucuronidation activity and CYP content in liver microsomes were reduced [9] and intestinal CYP3A activity was decreased in AA rats [10]. Inflammatory cytokines, for example, tumor necrosis factor (TNF)-α, interleukin (IL)-6, and IL-1 could be involved in the decrease of metabolizing enzymes [11-13]. The nuclear receptor NR1I2, which is a pregnane X receptor (PXR) and NR1I3, which is a constitutive androstane receptor (CAR), is involved in the regulation of CYP transcription by interacting with xenobiotics and endogenous toxins [14-16].

However, a comprehensive understanding of the changing profile of xenobiotic metabolizing enzymes in acute

---

*Corresponding author.

(3 d after adjuvant treatment), subacute (7 d after adjuvant treatment) and chronic (21 d after adjuvant treatment) phases of inflammation remains elusive, despite their importance on the pharmacokinetics of drug-related substrates. In this study, we examined the influence that the inflammatory response in an AA rat model has on hepatic enzymes involved in phase I (CYP1A2, CYP2C11, CYP2D1, CYP2D2, and CYP3A1) and phase II (SULT1A1, SULT2A1, UGT1A1, UGT1A6, UGT2B, and GSTP2) metabolism.

2. Materials and Methods

2.1. Preparation of AA Rats

Female Sprague-Dawley rats (seven weeks old), weighing 180 - 240 g, were purchased from CLEA Japan, Inc. (Tokyo, Japan). The animals were housed in a temperature-controlled room with free access to standard laboratory chow and water. Adjuvant was prepared from 100 mg heat-killed *Mycobacterium butyricum* (Difco Laboratories, Detroit, MI, USA) suspended in 10 mL of Bayol F oil. Hindpaw volumes were measured by liquid plethysmometry. Animals were studied 5, 10, 24 and 3 d (acute phase), 7 d (subacute phase), and 14 and 21 d (chronic phase) after the injection of adjuvant or Bayol F. AA rats in the acute phase exhibit local inflammation at the treated site. In the chronic phase, severe inflammation was observed in local and systemic sites. The experiments were approved by the Committee for the Care and Use of Laboratory Animals at Kinki University School of Pharmacy.

2.2. Measurement of mRNA

After the animals were anesthetized with diethyl ether, the liver was perfused with ice-cold saline and then removed. After flash freezing in liquid nitrogen, each sample was preserved at $-80°C$ until used for RNA extraction.

Determination of mRNA levels was performed using real-time reverse transcriptase polymerase chain reaction (RT-PCR) as previously described [17]. Total RNA (500 ng) was extracted from each liver and reverse-transcribed to complementary DNA (cDNA) using a PrimeScript-RT reagent Kit (TaKaRa, Shiga, Japan). Reactions were incubated for 15 min at $37°C$ and 5 sec at $85°C$. The reverse-transcribed cDNA was used as a template for real-time RT-PCR. Amplification was performed in 50 μL reaction mixtures containing 2 × SYBR Premix Ex Taq (TaKaRa) and 0.2 mM of each primer set shown in **Table 1**. PCRs were incubated at $95°C$ for 10 sec, and then amplified at $95°C$ for 5 sec, $55°C$ for 20 sec, and $72°C$ for 31 sec for 40 cycles. Data was normalized to the amount of 18S rRNA in each sample. The data were analyzed

Table 1. Primer sequences used in PCR assays.

Gene		Primer sequence (5'-3')
CYP1A2	Forward:	ACGTGAGCAAAGAGGCTAACCA
	Reverse:	ATTAGCCACCGATTCCACCAC
CYP2C11	Forward:	CGCACGGAGCTGTTTTTGTT
	Reverse:	GCAAATGGCCAAATCCACTG
CYP2D1	Forward:	GCAAAGTCTTCCCCAAGCTCA
	Reverse:	GGAAGGCATCAGTCATGTCTCG
CYP3A1	Forward:	GCCTTTTTTTGGCACTGTGCT
	Reverse:	GCATTTGACCATCAAACAACCC
SULT1A1	Forward:	GCCCGAAATGCAAAGGATG
	Reverse:	TGCAGCTTGGCCATGTTGT
SULT2A1	Forward:	CAGTAGCCCAAGCTGAAGCCTT
	Reverse:	CGGCCATTTTCTCCTGGAAA
UGT1A1	Forward:	CGGAGTTATTCAGCAGCTCCAG
	Reverse:	GGTGCTATGACCACCACTTCGT
UGT1A6	Forward:	AACCTAGAAGAGTTGCGGACCC
	Reverse:	CAGCAAAGTGGTTGTTCCCAA
UGT2B	Forward:	TCCCCACCCAACATTACCAA
	Reverse:	AGCAGGTTTGCAATGGAGTCC
GSTP2	Forward:	GCAGCTCCCCAAGTTTGAAGA
	Reverse:	GGTGCCTCAAGATGGCATTAGA
18S rRNA	Forward:	CGCCGCTAGAGGTGAAATTC
	Reverse:	CCAGTCGGCATCGTTTATGG

with ABI Prism 7000 SDS Software (Applied Biosystems) using the multiplex comparative method.

2.3. Preparation of Hepatic Microsomes

Livers were perfused with ice-cold saline and chopped into small pieces. A 25% (w/v) homogenate was made in ice-cold 1.15% KCl solution using a Physcotron homogenizer. The homogenate was centrifuged at 12,000 g for 20 min, and the supernatant was further centrifuged at 105,000 g for 60 min to obtain a microsomal pellet. The microsomal pellet was washed by resuspending it in 3 mL of 1.15% KCl, and the suspension was centrifuged at 105,000 g for 30 min to obtain the final microsomal pellet, which was resuspended in 1.5 mL of 1.15% KCl and stored at $-80°C$ until use. All procedures were carried out at $4°C$. Protein concentrations were determined using a BCA protein assay kit (Pierce Biotechnology, Rockford, IL, USA).

2.4. CYP Activity Measurements

CYP3A activity was determined using a P450-Glo CYP3A4 assay (Promega, Madison, WI, USA). P450-Glo CYP3A4 was used to determine CYP3A1 and

CYP3A2 activities in rats and CYP3A4 activity in humans as per the manufacturer's instructions. In brief, CYP3A reactions were performed in a 96-well plate (OptiPlate-96 (PerkinElmer, Waltham, MA, USA)). An incubation mixture (50 µL total volume) was prepared, containing 200 mM potassium phosphate buffer (pH 7.4), NADPH regeneration system (Promega), 20 µg rat liver microsomes and 50 µM of luciferin 6' benzyl ether (luciferin-BE) as a substrate for CYP3A1 and CYP3A2. The concentrations of luciferin-BE were around the K_m values (50 µM). After preincubation for 10 min at 37°C, the reaction was initiated by addition of the NADPH regeneration system and then incubated for 30 min at 37°C with constant shaking. The reconstituted luciferin detection reagent (50 µL) was then added to stop the reaction and to generate chemiluminescence. CYP3A converts luciferin-BE to luciferin by a debenzylation reaction and the production of luciferin by CYP3A1 and CYP3A2 was determined using a luciferase assay. Luminescence was measured using the FLUOstar Optima (Moritex, Tokyo, Japan). CYP2C9 activity was determined using a P450-Glo CYP2C9 assay (Promega). 100 µM of 6'-deoxyluciferin (luciferin-H) was used as a substrate for CYP2C9. All other conditions were the same as for the CYP3A assay. CYP2C9 converts 6'-deoxyluciferin (luciferin-H) to luciferin and the production of luciferin by CYP2C9 was determined using a luciferase assay. All CYP isoform activity determinations were performed in duplicate.

2.5. Statistical Analysis

Separate control groups were made for acute, subacute and chronic phases. The differences between the AA and control groups for (each of) the three phases were estimated using the Student's unpaired t-test.

3. Results and Discussion

Changes in mRNA levels of various xenobiotic metabolizing enzymes from the CYP, UGT and SULT families and GSTP during each response phase of inflammation were determined. CYP1A2, CYP2C12, CYP2D1, CYP2-D2, and CYP3A1 mRNA levels are shown in **Figure 1**. The mRNA level of all examined CYPs exhibited significant decreases 24 h after adjuvant treatment. Sanada *et al.* demonstrated that the hepatic mRNA and protein levels of inflammatory cytokines such as TNF-α, IL-6, and IL-1 significantly increased by 24 h after adjuvant treatment in rats [18]. The increased cytokines in the early stage of inflammation could cause a reduction in CYP mRNA levels. It is reported that IL-1β inhibits the expression of various hepatic CYP isoforms [19]. The recovery of CYP1A2, CYP2C12, and CYP2D1 mRNA occurred by day 3. All examined CYP mRNAs were re-

duced to approximately half of control levels by day 21 (chronic phase).

These results showed that almost all examined CYP isoforms significantly decreased in the acute, and subacute and the chronic phases in the arthritic (rats) compared with control rats. In particular, CYP3A1 mRNA decreased to low levels 24 h after adjuvant treatment. It is possible that the diminished expression of CYP3A1 could affect the pharmacokinetics of substrates because CYP3A participates mainly in the metabolism of various drugs. **Figure 2** shows the alterations in the activities of CYP2C and CYP3A, which have relatively high protein content in the liver in each phase of inflammation. The activity of CYP2C decreased going from the acute to the chronic phase of inflammation and was less than 10% of control levels in the subacute and chronic phases of inflammation. The activity of CYP3A also significantly decreased at 3, 14 and 21 d, suggesting that both protein and mRNA levels had decreased. Total CYP2C metabolizing activity showed a further decrease compared with the mRNA level of CYP2C12 in AA rats. It could be that the changes in expression of these other CYP2C isoforms, such as CYP2C6 and CYP2C7, accounted for this difference between activity and mRNA level.

These results could be interpreted to mean that the expression of all examined CYP isoforms were suppressed during inflammation and this decreased activity could affect the pharmacokinetics of various drugs. The transcription of CYPs is regulated by nuclear receptors such as PXR and CAR. For example, the transcription of CYP2B and CYP3A is known to be regulated through CAR and PXR, respectively [20,21]. CAR and PXR show overlapping regulation of transcription of CYPs and transporters [22]. The effects of the phases of inflammation on the expression of nuclear receptors are unclear but warrant examination.

To further clarify the effects of AA on other metabolizing enzymes, we examined the alterations of SULTs, UGTs and GSTP involved in the phase II metabolic pathway. The changes in mRNA of three isoforms of UGTs (UGT1A1, UGT1A6, and UGT2B) are shown in **Figure 3**. UGT1A1 and UGT1A6 mRNAs exhibited significant decreases in the acute, subacute, and chronic phases of inflammation. On the other hand, UGT2B showed little change from control levels except on day one (acute phase). Interestingly, the distinct effects of AA on the mRNA levels of UGT unlike CYP isoforms were presented. The UGT1 locus is located on chromosome 2q37 and the UGT2 family is located on chromosome 4q13. UGT1A participates in the metabolism of endobiotic substrates such as bilirubin and estrogens and drug substrates such as irinotecan, imipramine and cyproheptadine [23]. It is possible that the metabolism of substrates by UGT1A was affected by the inflammatory

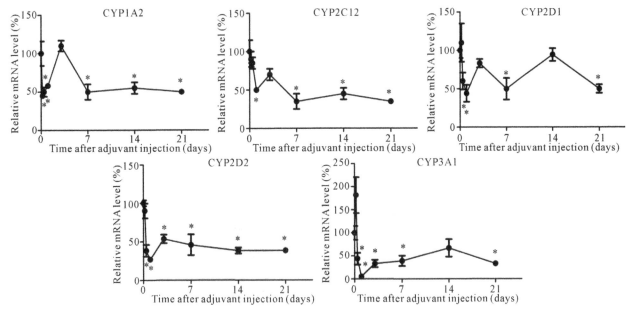

Figure 1. Changes in relative mRNA levels of CYP1A2, 2C12, 2D1, 2D2, and 3A1 in the liver of AA rats. The results are expressed as the mean ± S.D. (n = 4). There were significant differences between control and AA rats ($^*p < 0.05$).

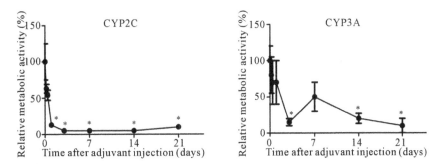

Figure 2. Changes in relative metabolic activities of CYP2C and 3A in the liver of AA rats. The results are expressed as the mean ± S.D. (n = 4). There were significant differences between control and AA rats ($^*p < 0.05$).

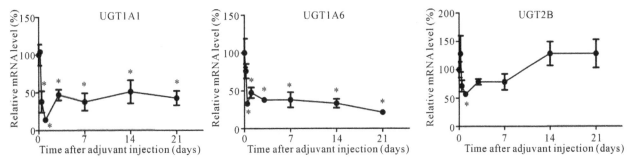

Figure 3. Changes in relative mRNA levels of UGT1A1, 1A6, and 2B in the liver of AA rats. The results are expressed as the mean ± S.D. (n = 4). There were significant differences between control and AA rats ($^*p < 0.05$).

response in AA rats. It has been reported that UGT1A and UGT2B are regulated by the aryl hydrocarbon receptor and NF-E2-related factor 2, respectively [24,25]. These different mechanisms in transcriptional regulation could lead to differences in the expression of UGT isoforms. Our future research will be focused on investigat-

ing alterations between UGTs and transcription factors.

The changes in mRNA of SULT1A1, SULT2A1 and GSTP2 are shown in **Figure 4**. The SULTs are categorized into two major groups, the arylsulfotransferases (SULT1 family) and the hydroxysteroid sulfotransferases (SULT2 family) [26]. Although both SULT1A1 and

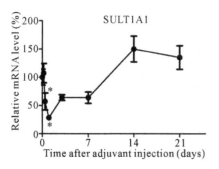 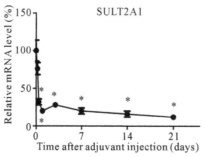 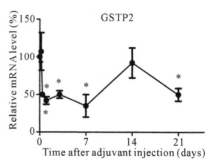

Figure 4. Changes in relative mRNA levels of SULT1A1, 2A1, and GSTP2 in the liver of AA rats. The results are expressed as the mean ± S.D. (n = 4). There were significant differences between control and AA rats ($^*p < 0.05$).

SULT2A1 mRNAs decreased in the acute phase, the mRNA level of SULT1A1 but not SULT2A1 recovered to control levels in the subacute and chronic phases. It has been reported that SULT2A1 is predominantly regulated by PXR [27,28]. In our previous report, we demonstrated that the mRNA level of PXR but not CAR was significantly decreased in AA rats [29]. Therefore, it is possible that the inflammatory response could lead to the inhibition of transcription of SULT2A1 through regulation of PXR levels. Further research is needed to better understand the differences in regulation between SULT1-A1 and SULT2A1. The mRNA level of GSTP2 decreased by close to 50% in all phases. These results suggest that phase II enzymes could have more distinct patterns of changes in mRNA for each isoform compared with CYPs.

In conclusion, the mRNA level of almost all metabolizing enzymes examined were decreased in all three response phases in AA rats, suggesting that the inflammatory condition could affect the pharmacokinetics of substrates used by these enzymes, most likely as a result of decreased protein expression. However, some enzymes such as UGT2B and SULT1A1 showed a relatively quick recovery to control mRNA levels, indicating that the effects of inflammation on mRNA levels of metabolizing enzymes differ depending on the isoform.

4. Acknowledgements

This work was supported in part by the "High-Tech Research Center" Project for Private Universities: matching fund subsidy from MEXT (Ministry of Education, Culture, Sports, Science and Technology), 2007-2011.

REFERENCES

[1] A. E. Aitken, T. A. Richardson and E. T. Morgan, "Regulation of Drug-Metabolizing Enzymes and Transporters in Inflammation," *Pharmacology and Toxicology*, Vol. 46, 2006, pp. 123-149. doi:10.1146/annurev.pharmtox.46.120604.141059

[2] K. W. Renton, "Cytochrome P450 Regulation and Drug Biotransformation during Inflammation and Infection," *Current Drug Metabolism*, Vol. 5, No. 3, 2004, pp. 235-243. doi:10.2174/1389200043335559

[3] F. M. Belpaire, F. D. Smet, B. F. Chidavijak, N. Fraeyman and M. G. Bogaert, "Effect of Turpentine-Induced Inflammation on the Disposition Kinetics of Propranolol, Metoprolol, and Antipyrine in the Rat," *Fundamental & Clinical Pharmacology*, Vol. 3, No. 2, 1989, pp. 79-88. doi:10.1111/j.1472-8206.1989.tb00667.x

[4] M. Piquette-Miller and F. Jamali, "Selective Effect of Adjuvant Arthritis on the Disposition of Propranolol Enantiomers in Rats Detected Using a Stereospecific HPLC Assay," *Pharmaceutical Research*, Vol. 10, No. 2, 1993, pp. 294-299. doi:10.1023/A:1018907431893

[5] M. E. Laethem, F. M. Belpaire, P. Wijnant, M. T. Rosseel and M. G. Bogaert, "Influence of Endotoxin on the Stereoselective Pharmacokinetics of Oxprenolol, Propranolol, and Verapamil in the Rat," *Chirality*, Vol. 6, No. 5, 1994, pp. 405-410. doi:10.1002/chir.530060508

[6] R. O. Williams, M. Feldmann and R. N. Maini, "Anti-Tumor Necrosis Factor Ameliorates Joint Disease in Murine Collagen-Induced Arthritis," *Proceedings of the National Academy of Sciences of the United States of America*, Vol. 89, No. 20, 1992, pp. 9784-9788. doi:10.1073/pnas.89.20.9784

[7] N. Shibata, H. Shimakawa, T. Minouchi and A. Yamaji, "Pharmacokinetics of Cyclosporin A after Intravenous Administration to Rats in Various Disease States," *Biological & Pharmaceutical Bulletin*, Vol. 16, No. 11, 1993, pp. 1130-1135. doi:10.1248/bpb.16.1130

[8] G. Dipasquale, P. Welaj and C. L. Rassaert, "Prolonged Pentobarbital Sleeping Time in Adjuvant-Induced Polyarthritic Rats," *Research Communications in Chemical Pathology and Pharmacology*, Vol. 9, No. 2, 1974, pp. 253-264.

[9] T. Nagao, T. Tanino and M. Iwaki, "Stereoselective Pharmacokinetics of Flurbiprofen and Formation of Covalent Adducts with Plasma Protein in Adjuvant-Induced Arthritic Rats," *Chirality*, Vol. 15, No. 5, 2003, pp. 423-428. doi:10.1002/chir.10227

[10] S. Uno, A. Kawase, A. Tsuji, T. Tanino and M. Iwaki, "Decreased Intestinal CYP3A and P-Glycoprotein Activities in Rats with Adjuvant Arthritis," *Drug Metabolism and Pharmacokinetics*, Vol. 22, No. 4, 2007, pp. 313-321.

doi:10.2133/dmpk.22.313

[11] G. W. Warren, S. M. Poloyac, D. S. Gary, M. P. Mattson and R. A. Blouin, "Hepatic Cytochrome P-450 Expression in Tumor Necrosis Factor-Alpha Receptor (p55/p75) Knockout Mice after Endotoxin Administration," *Journal of Pharmacology and Experimental Therapeutics*, Vol. 288, No. 3, 1999, pp. 945-950.

[12] E. Siewert, R. Bort, R. Kluge, P. C. Heinrich, J. Castell and R. Jover, "Hepatic Cytochrome P450 Down-Regulation during Aseptic Inflammation in the Mouse Is Interleukin 6 Dependent," *Hepatology*, Vol. 32, No. 1, 2000, pp. 49-55. doi:10.1053/jhep.2000.8532

[13] E. T. Morgan, "Regulation of Cytochrome P450 by Inflammatory Mediators: Why and How?" *Drug Metabolism and Disposition*, Vol. 29, No. 3, 2001, pp. 207-212.

[14] P. Honkakoski, I. Zelko, T. Sueyoshi and M. Negishi, "The Nuclear Orphan Receptor CAR-Retinoid X Receptor Heterodimer Activates the Phenobarbital-Responsive Enhancer Module of the CYP2B Gene," *Molecular and Cellular Biology*, Vol. 18, No. 10, 1998, pp. 5652-5658.

[15] S. A. Kliewer, J. T. Moore, L. Wade, J. L. Staudinger, M. A. Watson, S. A. Jones, D. D. McKee, B. B. Oliver, T. M. Willson, R. H. Zetterstrom, T. Perlmann and J. M. Lehmann, "An Orphan Nuclear Receptor Activated by Pregnanes Defines a Novel Steroid Signaling Pathway," *Cell*, Vol. 92, No. 1, 1998, pp. 73-82. doi:10.1016/S0092-8674(00)80900-9

[16] D. J. Waxman, "P450 Gene Induction by Structurally Diverse Xenochemicals: Central Role of Nuclear Receptors CAR, PXR, and PPAR," *Archives of Biochemistry and Biophysics*, Vol. 369, No. 1, 1999, pp. 11-23. doi:10.1006/abbi.1999.1351

[17] A. Kawase, A. Fujii, M. Negoro, R. Akai, M. Ishikubo, H. Komura and M. Iwaki, "Differences in Cytochrome P450 and Nuclear Receptor mRNA Levels in Liver and Small Intestine between SD and DA Rats," *Drug Metabolism and Pharmacokinetics*, Vol. 23, No. 3, 2008, pp. 196-206. doi:10.2133/dmpk.23.196

[18] H. Sanada, M. Sekimoto, A. Kamoshita and M. Degawa, "Changes in Expression of Hepatic Cytochrome P450 Subfamily Enzymes during Development of Adjuvant-Induced Arthritis in Rats," *Journal of Toxicological Sciences*, Vol. 36, No. 2, 2011, pp. 181-190. doi:10.2131/jts.36.181

[19] E. Assenat, S. Gerbal-Chaloin, D. Larrey, J. Saric, J. M. Fabre, P. Maurel, M. J. Vilarem and J. M. Pascussi, "Interleukin 1β Inhibits CAR-Induced Expression of Hepatic Genes Involved in Drug and Bilirubin Clearance," *Hepatology*, Vol. 40, No. 4, 2009, pp. 951-960.

[20] S. A. Kliewer, J. T. Moore, L. Wade, J. L. Staudinger, M. A. Watson, S. A. Jones, D. D. McKee, B. B. Oliver, T. M. Willson, R. H. Zetterstrom, T. Perlmann and J. M. Lehmann, "An Orphan Nuclear Receptor Activated by Pregnanes Defines a Novel Steroid Signaling Pathway," *Cell*, Vol. 92, No. 1, 1998, pp. 73-82.

doi:10.1016/S0092-8674(00)80900-9

[21] B. Goodwin, E. Hodgson and C. Liddle, "The Orphan Human Pregnane X Receptor Mediates the Transcriptional Activation of CYP3A4 by Rifampicin through a Distal Enhancer Module," *Molecular Pharmacology*, Vol. 56, No. 6, 1999, pp. 1329-1339.

[22] J. M. Maglich, C. M. Stoltz, B. Goodwin, D. Hawkins-Brown, J. T. Moore and S. A. Kliewer, "Nuclear Pregnane x Receptor and Constitutive Androstane Receptor Regulate Overlapping but Distinct Sets of Genes Involved in Xenobiotic Detoxification," *Molecular Pharmacology*, Vol. 62, No. 3, 2002, pp. 638-646. doi:10.1124/mol.62.3.638

[23] T. Izukawa, M. Nakajima, R. Fujiwara, H. Yamanaka, T. Fukami, M. Takamiya, Y. Aoki, S. Ikushiro, T. Sakaki and T. Yokoi, "Quantitative Analysis of UDP-Glucuronosyltransferase (UGT) 1A and UGT2B Expression Levels in Human Livers," *Drug Metabolism and Disposition*, Vol. 37, No. 8, 2009, pp. 1759-1768. doi:10.1124/dmd.109.027227

[24] R. L. Yeager, S. A. Reisman, L. M. Aleksunes and C. D. Klaassen, "Introducing the TCDD-Inducible AhR-Nrf2 Gene Battery," *Toxicological Sciences*, Vol. 111, No. 2, 2009, pp. 238-246. doi:10.1093/toxsci/kfp115

[25] S. Chen, D. Beaton, N. Nguyen, K. Seneko-Effenberger, E. Brace-Sinnokrak, U. Argikar, R. P. Remmel, J. Trottier, O. Barbier, J. K. Ritter and R. H. Tukey, "Tissue-Specific, Inducible, and Hormonal Control of the Human UDP-Glucuronosyltransferase-1 (UGT1) Locus," *Journal of Biological Chemistry*, Vol. 280, 2005, pp. 37547-37557. doi:10.1074/jbc.M506683200

[26] T. P. Dooley, R. Haldeman-Cahill, J. Joiner and T. W. Wilborn, "Expression Profiling of Human Sulfotransferase and Sulfatase Gene Superfamilies in Epithelial Tissues and Cultured Cells," *Biochemical and Biophysical Research Communications*, Vol. 277, No. 1, 2000, pp. 236-245. doi:10.1006/bbrc.2000.3643

[27] M. Runge-Morris, W. Wu and T. A. Kocarek, "Regulation of Rat Hepatic Hydroxysteroid Sulfotransferase (SULT2-40/41) Gene Expression by Glucocorticoids: Evidence for a Dual Mechanism of Transcriptional Control," *Molecular Pharmacology*, Vol. 56, No. 6, 1999, pp. 1198-1206.

[28] J. Sonoda, W. Xie, J. M. Rosenfeld, J. L. Barwick, P. S. Guzelian and R. M. Evans, "Regulation of a Xenobiotic Sulfonation Cascade by Nuclear Pregnane X Receptor (PXR)," *Proceedings of the National Academy of Sciences of the United States of America*, Vol. 99, No. 21, 2002, pp. 13801-13806. doi:10.1073/pnas.212494599

[29] S. Uno, M. Uraki, A. Ito, Y. Shinozaki, A. Yamada, A. Kawase and M. Iwaki, "Changes in mRNA Expression of ABC and SLC Transporters in Liver and Intestines of the Adjuvant-Induced Arthritis Rat," *Biopharmaceutics & Drug Disposition*, Vol. 30, No. 1, 2009, pp. 49-54. doi:10.1002/bdd.639

29

Bacterial Infection in the Limbs of Patients with Rheumatoid Arthritis during Biological Agent Therapy[*]

Hajime Yamanaka[#], Kenichiro Goto[†], Munetaka Suzuki[†]

Department of Orthopaedic Surgery, National Hospital Organization Shimoshizu Hospital, Yotsukaido City, Japan.
Email: [#]ici05323@m7.gyao.ne.jp, g10k25@yahoo.co.jp, rcjqq173@ybb.ne.jp

ABSTRACT

Biological therapies in rheumatoid arthritis (RA) are known to increase the risk of serious infections. The present study was performed to evaluate the clinical features of bacterial infections occurring in the limbs during biological therapies in patients with RA. By March 2011, 11 RA patients (14 limbs) treated with biological agents at our institution required hospitalization due to bacterial infections occurring in the limbs. These patients had an average age of 53.7 years old. Infections occurred an average of 19 months after biological treatment. Two limbs in one patient were treated with infliximab, eight limbs in six patients were treated with etanercept, one limb in one patient was treated with adalimumab, and three limbs in three patients were treated with tocilizumab. Cellulitis occurred in 7 limbs, late infections after total knee arthroplasty occurred in two limbs, early infections after orthopedic surgery occurred in three limbs, and septic arthritis occurred in two limbs. Four cases had comorbidities—liver cirrhosis and diabetes mellitus in one and three cases, respectively. All patients were treated using corticosteroid with an average dose of 4.6 mg daily. Seven limbs required surgical treatment. All patients finally recovered. Ten limbs continued treatment with biological agents. Care must be taken regarding bacterial infection in the limbs of RA patients treated by using biological agents, particularly those with comorbidities. Further studies are required to confirm means of preventing such infections in daily practice.

Keywords: Bacterial Infection; Limbs; Rheumatoid Arthritis; Biological Agents

1. Introduction

Rheumatoid arthritis (RA) is a chronic, progressive inflammatory disease that can lead to severe joint destruction and disability. Several cytokines, such as tumor necrosis factor (TNF) and interleukin-6 (IL-6), play critical roles in the pathogenesis of this disease [1]. Conventional treatment of RA involves a combination of corticosteroid and disease-modifying anti-rheumatic drugs (DMARDs), such as methotrexate. However, RA may remain active in some cases of treatment failure with traditional therapy. Drugs targeting these cytokines have been developed over the past few years to neutralize the precise pathways underlying the pathogenetic mechanisms of RA. At present, five different biological agents are available for use in RA in Japan, i.e., the TNF antagonists infliximab, etanercept, and adalimumab, the IL-6 receptor antagonist tocilizumab, and the T-cell costimulator modulator abatacept. Many studies have demonstrated improvements with regard in joint destruction and patient's daily life by using these biological agents [2-6]. In addition, these cytokines also play important roles in host defense [7-9]. Therefore, the use of biological drug therapy is accompanied by the need to study and understand the effects of modifying these key pathways on infection risk. The increased risk of bacterial and opportunistic infections in patients receiving biological drugs is well known [10]. Serious bacterial infections include not only tuberculosis respiratory infections, but also skin, urinary tract, bone, and joint infections. One of the more severe infections of bone and joints is surgical site infection of total joint arthroplasty (TJA) [11]. Although serious, TJA infection is rare in daily medical practice. There have been few comparative studies focusing on serious bacterial skin and bone and joint infections in RA patients receiving biological drugs. Such infections may be related to the effects of medications used to treat RA, particularly drugs that are potentially immunosuppressive.

The objectives of the present study were to retrospectively evaluate the clinical aspects of serious bacterial skin, bone, and joint infections requiring hospitalization in patients with RA receiving biological drugs.

All patients gave their informed consent prior to inclu-

[*]Conflict of interest statement: The authors declare that they have no competing interests.
[#]Corresponding author.
[†]Authors' contributions: K. Goto and M. Suzuki made substantial contributions to study conception and design. All authors approved the final version of this article.

sion in the study.

2. Patients and Methods

A total of 273 adult RA patients who were sequential attendees at our hospital and who had an active RA were treated with four different biological agents. During the treatment period from April 2006 to March 2011, 11 patients developed bacterial infection on 14 limbs and were hospitalized at our division (**Table 1**). All patients fulfilled the diagnostic

criteria of the American College of Rheumatology (ACR) [12]. We defined bacterial infection as septic arthritis, osteomyelitis, postoperative deep or superficial wound infection, and cellulitis, requiring hospitalization, intravenous antibiotics, or surgical therapy. Bacterial and tuberculosis pneumonia were excluded in this study. Viral infection, such as Herpes Zoster, and cases of infection after injury were also excluded. The infections were examined and diagnosed by two rheumatologists (HY, KG).

Table 1. Demographics and clinical characteristics of the patients.

No	Sex	Age	Diagnosis	Biologics	Onset period after first administered	Dose of PSL (mg/day)	Dose of MTX (mg/w)
1	F	25	Cellulitis of rt. lower leg	Infliximab	1 month	4	8
2	F	26	Cellulitis of rt. lower leg	Infliximab	16 months	4	8
3	F	58	Cellulitis of around the surgical site of rt. TKA	Etanercept	24 months	5	0
4	F	60	Late infection of rt. TKA	Etanercept	43 months	5	0
5	F	61	Late infection of rt. TKA	Etanercept	10 months	3	0
6	F	45	Cellulitis of rt. lower leg	Etanercept	40 months	5	0
7	F	47	Cellulitis of rt. lower leg with abscess	Etanercept	56 months	5	0
8	M	78	Cellulitis of rt. hand	Etanercept	3 months	3	0
9	F	59	Subcutaneous abscess after rt. TKA	Etanercept	19 months	3	0
10	F	64	Subcutaneous abscess after rt. ankle arthrodesis	Etanercept	9 months	6	0
11	F	64	Subcutaneous abscess after rt. foot arthroplasty	Adalinmab	9 months	5	0
12	F	53	Cellulitis of rt. lower leg	Tocilizumab	5 months	5	8
13	F	61	Rt. knee septic arthritis	Tocilizumab	9 months	4	8
14	M	51	Lt. knee septic arthritis	Tocilizumab	1 month	8	8

No	Past history complication	Bacteria	Therapy	Hospitalized days (days)
1	Rt. THA		Administration of antibiotics	17
2	Rt. THA		Administration of antibiotics	9
3	DM		Administration of antibiotics	9
4	DM	*Staphylococcus aureus*	Irrigation, antibiotics	40
5	None	*Staphylococcus aureus*	Irrigation, antibiotics	209
6	Bilateral-TKA PBC	*Staphylococcus aureus*	Administration of antibiotics	11
7	Bilateral-TKA PBC	*Staphylococcus aureus*	Administration of antibiotics	9
8	DM, HT	*Staphylococcus aureus*	Incision, antibiotics	35
9	HT	*Staphylococcus aureus*	Incision, antibiotics	28
10	HT	No growth	Incision, antibiotics	7
11	Angina pectoris	No growth	Incision, antibiotics	7
12	Rt. TKA breast carcinoma		Administration of antibiotics	11
13	None	*Peptostreptococcus species*	Scopic debridment	17
14	None	*Staphylococcus aureus*	Scopic debridment	33

TKA: Total Knee Arthroplasty; DM: Diabetes mellitus; THA: Total Hip Arthroplasty; PBC: Primary Biliary Cirrhosis; HT: Hypertension.

A detailed history and clinical features, including laboratory data and therapeutic method, were investigated.

3. Results

The 11 patients consisted of 2 men (2 limbs) and 9 women (12 limbs). The average age of patients was 53.7 years old (range: 25 - 78 years old), the average RA disease duration was 7.3 years (range: 1 - 18 years). The mean body mass index of the 11 patients was 25.5 (range: 20.5 - 32.3). All patients were receiving oral steroid therapy, and the average steroid dose was 4.6 mg (range: 1 - 11 mg) daily. Three of the 11 patients received methotrexate (MTX) therapy (dosage: 8 mg per week in all three patients). The mean follow-up period after discharge was 3 years 4 months (range: 3 months - 5 years 4 months).

Cellulitis occurred in 5 patients (7 limbs). Six of these were lower limbs, and cellulitis occurred after TJA in all cases. The remaining case involved the upper limb. Subcutaneous infections around the surgical site early after the operation occurred on 3 patients (3 limbs). One of the 3 surgical operations was ankle arthrodesis and the other two were foot rejection arthroplasties with swanson implant (Wright Medical Inc., Arlington, TN). Late infections after total knee arthroplasty (TKA) occurred in two patients (two limbs). Joint infections of the knee without TJA occurred in two patients (two limbs).

With regard to the biological agents, six patients (eight limbs) received etanercept (25 mg twice a week), one patient (two limbs) received infliximab (3 mg/kg, once every 8 weeks), three patients (three limbs) received tocilizumab (8 mg/kg, once every 4 weeks), and one patient (one limb) received adalimumab (40 mg once every 2 weeks).

Onset of infection occurred within one year after commencement of biological agent administration in eight limbs. However, the other cases occurred after various periods.

At the time of infection, two patients (three limbs) were also receiving treatment for diabetes mellitus and four patients (four limbs) were receiving treatment for high blood pressure. None of the patients had chronic obstructive pulmonary disorder as a comorbid condition.

Without cellulitis, we identified the bacterial species in eight limbs: *Peptostreptococcus spp.* in one case and *Staphylococcus aureus* in seven cases. However, the bacteria could not be identified in two cases, even with culture of the specimens.

About treatment, four patients (seven limbs) were cured with antibiotics only. The remaining seven patients (seven limbs) were cured by use of antibiotics and surgical treatment, such as irrigation of the wound. Finally, all patients recovered. Treatment with the same biological agent was restarted in nine patients a few months after discharge because of a worsening of RA activity due to cessation of treatment. One patient was treated with another biological agent (etanercept to tocilizumab), and one patient declined further biological agent treatment.

The average period of hospitalization was 31.6 days (range: 7 - 209 days).

Typical Case Report of Bacterial Infection on the Limb

A 47-year-old woman was diagnosed with RA and primary biliary cirrhosis (PBC) in 1999. Blood analysis indicated pancytopenia due to PBC. She underwent right TKA in 2008. As treatment with infliximab was ineffective, she was administered etanercept at a dose of 25 mg twice a week from February 2009. She developed right lower leg cellulitis suddenly in April 2010 and treatment with antibiotic (sulbactam/piperacillin; SBT/ABPC, 3 g/day) about two weeks after hospitalization, which finally healed. However, in July of the same year, she developed lower right cellulitis again with several abscesses (**Figures 1(a)** and **(b)**). Blood examination showed a C-reactive protein level of 4.9 dl/ml and white blood cell count of 1900/μl. Surgical treatment was performed with incision of the abscess and SBT/ABPC was administered at 3 g/day for 2 weeks. The patient was finally healed about 1 month after hospitalization. Pus from the abscess was cultured, and showed growth of *Staphylococcus aureus*.

4. Discussion

In this report, we presented 11 patients (14 limbs) with RA receiving biological treatment experiencing the onset of skin, bone, and joint bacterial infections. The majority were patients with infectious lesions typical of acute inflammatory

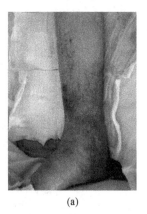 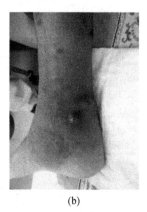

(a)   (b)

Figure 1. Clinical appearance of the right leg. (a) Anterior to the medial aspect of the right leg. Erythema with multiple, small subcutaneous hemorrhages were observed; (b) Medial aspect of the right leg. Several subcutaneous abscesses were observed.

diseases, but various clinical patterns were observed. These infections appear as rare but potentially severe complications of biological therapies.

RA patients are often treated with immunosuppressive drugs, such as glucocorticoids and MTX that contribute to the risk of infection. However, there is evidence that the underlying disease itself, the activity of the disease, and the degree of disability are independent risk factors in addition to immunosuppressive treatment. TNF and IL-6 are pleiotropic proinflammatory cytokines and play central roles in the pathogenesis of rheumatic diseases. These cytokine blockers have well-established efficacy in treatment of RA patients. However, the risk of serious infections in patients with RA treated with anti-TNF blockers was double that in patients administered placebo as controls [13]. Galloway [14] reported that anti-TNF therapy increased the risk of serious infections especially in the first 3 to 6 months of treatment.

However, less is known about the clinical features and incidence rates of bacterial infection in the limbs including postoperative infections, skin, and bone-joint infections.

Some reports [15-17] indicated a significant association between early infectious complications following orthopedic surgery and treatment with TNF inhibitors in patients with RA. Especially in TJA surgical site infection, important risk factors are primary or revision TJA within the last year, particularly when TNF blockers are not interrupted before surgery, and a daily steroid intake over 5 mg [18].

The incidence rates of bacterial infection on the limbs associated with postoperative infections, skin, and bone-joint infections in patients with RA receiving biological agents were 2.76 to 7.68 times higher than in those without biological treatment [19,20].

However, there have been no reports regarding the detailed mechanisms underlying these increased rates of infection. Several mechanisms have been postulated, including disturbance of important functions of various cells in the skin by TNF and IL-6 inhibitors [21]; increased sensitivity and reactivity of the skin to bacteria [22]; and disruption of normal wound healing reaction [23]. Moreover, complication with diabetes mellitus or respiratory disease affected patient's immune condition. Skin condition was very poor in patients using steroids. However, the details remain unclear.

Previous studies were performed to examine differences in the incidence rates of infection between biological agents, but no differences were identified [23-25]. Five different biological agents are approved for use in RA therapy in Japan. In the present study, the number of cases of infection was higher among patients treated with etanercept than in those given the other agents. However, we could not conclude that etanercept is associated with

serious infection due to the small number of patients included in this study.

Diabetes mellitus and steroid intake have previously been shown to be associated with increased risk of infection in RA [24,25]. In this study, only two patients (three limbs) were accompanied with diabetes mellitus, and although all patients had an average corticosteroid dose of 4.6 mg daily, this dose was not particularly high. We did not identify individual risk factors in this study. The small number of cases included in this study did not permit confirmation of hypotheses regarding causative relationships.

How should we guard against infectious diseases in the limbs of RA patients during biological drug use? It is unlikely that we can completely prevent infections in these cases. However, it is important to inform patients that infection on the limbs is not unusual, and to take steps to prevent such infection by skin care, avoiding excessive load on the limbs in daily living, to go immediately to hospital if signs of infection appear on the limb, etc. Medication for diabetes mellitus or respiratory disease is very important. Furthermore, it is necessary to avoid worsening the infection by consideration of surgical care immediately and patients with infectious symptoms may be hospitalized.

There were several limitations of our study. First, this was a retrospective study, and the number of patients was small. The small number of cases limited the statistical power of the study. Second, diagnosis is the most important issue. Infection was diagnosed by blood analysis, skin condition, bacteria culture analysis, etc. However, it was difficult to confirm the relation between administration of biological agents and infection. Further studies are required to clarify these points. Third, some potential risk factors (recent pulmonary infection, number of previous disease-modifying anti-rheumatic drugs (DMARDs), cumulative steroid intake, non-steroidal anti-inflammatory drugs) were not assessed because almost all patients had already been treated with RA at other hospitals before starting treatment with biological agents. Fourth, this was not a cohort and randomized control study. Our analyses were based on a limited number of episodes of limb infection. Fifth, our study did not include possible cases of mild infections that did not require hospitalization, and so may have underestimated the incidence rate.

In summary, we have demonstrated a significant complication of serious bacterial infection on the limbs of RA patients treated with biological agents. Our overall results raise concerns about how best to balance safety with effectiveness. Patients and physicians—both rheumatologists and orthopedic surgeons—must emphasize the elevated risk for awareness and vigilantly monitor for signs of infection. These findings support the need for additional investigations and development of clinical practices to prevent infection on the limbs in RA patients.

5. Conclusion

In RA patients receiving biological agents, serious bacterial infection on the limbs is rare but potentially severe complication. Physicians should exercise caution and continue to be monitored to these infections during biological agent therapy in RA patients.

REFERENCES

[1] D. L. Scott, K. A. Grindulis, G. R. Struthers, B. L. Coulton, A. L. Popert and P. A. Bacon, "Progression of Radiological Changes in Rheumatoid Arthritis," *Annals of the Rheumatic Diseases*, Vol. 43, No. 1, 1984, pp. 8-17. doi:10.1136/ard.43.1.8

[2] T. Takeuchi, H. Yamanaka, E. Inoue, H. Nagasawa, M. Nawata, K. Ikari, K. Saito, N. Sekiguchi, E. Sato, H. Kameda, S. Iwata, T. Mochizuki, K. Amano and Y. Tanaka, "Retrospective Clinical Study on the Notable Efficacy and Related Factors of Infliximab Therapy in a Rheumatoid Arthritis Management Group in Japan: One-Year Outcome of Joint Destruction (RECONFIRM-2J)," *Modern Rheumatology*, Vol. 18, No. 5, 2008, pp. 447-452. doi:10.1007/s10165-008-0077-5

[3] L. Klareskog, D. van der Heijde, J. P. de Jager, A. Gough, J. Kalden, M. Malaise, M. E. Martin, K. Pavelka, J. Sany, L. Settas, J. Wajdula, R. Pedersen, S. Fatenejad, M. Sanda, *et al.*, "Therapeutic Effect of the Combination of Etanercept and Methotrexate Compared with Each Treatment Alone in Patients with Rheumatoid Arthritis: Double-Blind Randomized Controlled Trial," *Lancet*, Vol. 363, No. 9410, 2004, pp. 675-681. doi:10.1016/S0140-6736(04)15640-7

[4] F. C. Breedveld, M. H. Weisman, A. F. Kavanaugh, S. B. Cohen, K. Pavelka and R. van Vollenhoven, "The PREMIER Study: A Multicenter, Randomized, Double-Blind Clinical Trial of Combination Therapy with Adalimumab Plus Methotrexate versus Methotrexate Alone or Adalimumab Alone in Patients with Early, Aggressive Rheumatoid Arthritis Who Had Not Had Previous Methotrexate Treatment," *Arthritis Care & Research*, Vol. 54, No. 1, 2006, pp. 26-37. doi:10.1002/art.21519

[5] N. Nishimoto and N. Takagi, "Assessment of the Validity of the 28-Joint Disease Activity Score Using Erythrocyte Sedimentation Rate (DAS28-ESR) As a Disease Activity Index of Rheumatoid Arthritis in the Efficacy Evaluation of 24-Week Treatment with Tocilizumab: Subanalysis of the SATORI Study," *Modern Rheumatology*, Vol. 20, No. 6, 2010, pp. 539-547. doi:10.1007/s10165-010-0328-0

[6] M. Schiff, "Abatacept Treatment for Rheumatoid Arthritis," *Rheumatology*, Vol. 50, No. 3, 2011, pp. 437-449. doi:10.1093/rheumatology/keq287

[7] G. Camussi, E. Albano, C. Tetta and F. Bussolio, "The Molecular Action of Tumor Necrosis Factor-Alpha," *European Journal of Biochemistry*, Vol. 202, No. 1, 1991, pp. 3-14.

[8] F. M. Brennan and I. B. McInnes, "Evidence That Cyto-kines Play a Role in Rheumatoid Arthritis," *Journal of Clinical Investigation*, Vol. 118, No. 11, 2008, pp. 3537-3545. doi:10.1172/JCI36389

[9] P. Emery, P. Durez and M. Dougados, "The Impact of T-Cell Co-Stimulation Modulation in Patients with Undifferentiated Inflammatory Arthritis or Very Early Rheumatoid Arthritis: A Clinical and Imaging Study of Abatacept," *Annals of the Rheumatic Diseases*, Vol. 69, No. 3, 2010, pp. 510-516. doi:10.1136/ard.2009.119016

[10] J. Listing, A. Strangfeld, S. Kary, R. Rau, U. von Hinueber, M. Stoyanova-Scholz, E. Gromnica-Ihle, C. Anatoni, P. Herzer, J. Kekow, M. Schneider and A. Zink, "Infections in Patients with Rheumatoid Arthritis Treated with Biologic Agents," *Arthritis Care & Research*, Vol. 52, No. 11, 2005, pp. 3403-3412. doi:10.1002/art.21386

[11] M. Gilson, L. Gossec, X. Mariette, D. Gherissi, M. H. Guyot, J. M. Berthelot, D. Wendiling, C. Michelet, P. Dellamonica, F. Tubach, M. Dougados and D. Salmon, "Risk Factors for Total Joint Arthroplasty Infection in Patients Receiving Tumor Necrosis Factor α-Blockers: A Case-Control Study," *Arthritis Research & Therapy*, Vol. 12, No. 4, 2010, p. R145. doi:10.1186/ar3087

[12] F. C. Arnett, S. M. Edworthy, D. A. Bloch, D. J. McShane, J. F. Fries, N. S. Cooper, L. A. Healey, S. R. Kaplan, M. H. Liang, H. S. Luthra, *et al.*, "The American Rheumatism Association 1987 Revised Criteria for the Classification of Rheumatoid Arthritis," *Arthritis Care & Research*, Vol. 31, No. 3, 1988, pp. 315-324. doi:10.1002/art.1780310302

[13] W. G. Dixon, K. Watson, M. Lunt, L. Hyrich, *et al.*, "Rates of Serious Infection, Including Site-Specific and Bacterial Intracellular Infection, in Rheumatoid Arthritis Patients Receiving Anti-Tumor Necrosis Factor Therapy," *Arthritis Care & Research*, Vol. 54, No. 8, 2006, pp. 2368-2376. doi:10.1002/art.21978

[14] J. B. Galloway, K. L. Hyrich, L. K. Mercer, W. G. Dixon, B. Fu, A. P. Ustianowski, K. D. Watson, M. Lunt, *et al.*, "Anti-TNF Therapy Is Associated with an Increased Risk of Serious Infections in Patients with Rheumatoid Arthritis Especially in the First 6 Months of Treatment: Updated Results from the British Society for Rheumatology Biologics Register with Special Emphasis on Risks in the Elderly," *Rheumatology*, Vol. 50, No. 1, 2011, pp. 124-131. doi:10.1093/rheumatology/keq242

[15] J. T. Giles, S. J. Bartlett, A. C. Gelber, S. Nanda, K. Fontaine, V. Ruffing and J. Bathon, "Tumor Necrosis Factor Inhibitor Therapy and Risk of Serious Postoperative Orthopedic Infection in Rheumatoid Arthritis," *Arthritis Care & Research*, Vol. 55, No. 2, 2006, pp. 333-337. doi:10.1002/art.21841

[16] C. Bibbo and J. W. Goldberg, "Infectious and Healing Complications after Elective Orthopaedic Foot and Ankle Surgery during Tumor Necrosis Factor-Alpha Inhibition Therapy," *Foot Ankle International*, Vol. 25, No. 5, 2004, pp. 331-335.

[17] A. A. Broeder, M. C. Creemers, J. Fransen, E. D. Jong, D. J. R. D. Rooij, A. Wymenga, M. D. Waal-Malefijt and F. H. J. V. D. Hoogen, "Risk Factors for Surgical Site Infections and Other Complications in Elective Surgery in Patients with Rheumatoid Arthritis with Special Attention

for Anti-Tumor Necrosis Factor: A Large Retrospective Study," *Journal of Rheumatology*, Vol. 34, No. 4, 2007, pp. 653-655.

[18] A. Strangfeld and J. Listing, "Bacterial and Opportunistic Infections during Anti-TNF Therapy," *Best Practice & Research Clinical Rheumatology*, Vol. 20, No. 6, 2006, pp. 1181-1195. doi:10.1016/j.berh.2006.08.010

[19] T. Bongarts, A. Sutton, M. Sweeting, I. Buchan, E. Matteson and V. Montori, "Anti-TNF Antibody Therapy in Rheumatoid Arthritis and the Risk of Serious Infections and Malignancies," *Journal of the American Medical Association*, Vol. 295, No. 19, 2006, pp. 2275-2285.

[20] J. D. Greenberg, G. Reed, J. M. Kremer, E. Tindall, A. Kavanaugh, C. Zheng, W. Bishai, M. C. Hochberg, *et al.*, "Association of Methotrexate and Tumor Necrosis Factor Antagonists with Risk of Infectious Outcomes Including Opportunistic Infections in the CORRONA Registry," *Annals of the Rheumatic Diseases*, Vol. 69, No. 2, 2008, pp. 380-386. doi:10.1136/ard.2008.089276

[21] H. H. Lee, I. H. Song and M. Friedrich, "Cutaneous Side-Effects in Patients with Rheumatic Diseases during Application of Tumor Necrosis Factor-α Antagonists," *British Journal of Dermatology*, Vol. 156, No. 3, 2007, pp. 486-491. doi:10.1111/j.1365-2133.2007.07682.x

[22] C. Vestergaard, C. Johansen, K. Otkjaer, M. Deleuran and L. Iversen, "Tumor Necrosis Factor-Alpha-Induced CTACK/CCL27 (Cutaneous T-Cell-Attracting Chemokine) Production in Keratinocytes Is Controlled by Nuclear Factor Kappa B," *Cytokine*, Vol. 29, No. 2, 2005, pp. 49-55. doi:10.1016/j.cyto.2004.09.008

[23] J. A. Hamilton and P. P. Tak, "The Dynamics of Macrophage Lineage Populations in Inflammatory and Autoimmune Disease," *Arthritis & Rheumatism*, Vol. 60, No. 5, 2009 1210-1221. doi:10.1002/art.24505

[24] D. M. Grennan, J. Gray, J. Loudon and S. Fear, "Methotrexate and Early Postoperative Complications in Patients with Rheumatoid Arthritis Undergoing Elective Orthopaedic Surgery," *Annals of the Rheumatic Diseases*, Vol. 60, No. 3, 2001, pp. 214-217. doi:10.1136/ard.60.3.214

[25] D. Lacaille, D. P. Guh, M. Abarahamowicz, A. H. Anis and J. M. Esdaile, "Use of Nonbiologic Disease-Modifying Anti-Rheumatic Drugs and Risk of Infection in Patients with Rheumatoid Arthritis," *Arthritis Care & Research*, Vol. 59, No. 8, 2008, pp. 1074-1081. doi:10.1002/art.23913

30

Disability Work among Argentinean Patients with Rheumatoid Arthritis

Tamborenea Maria Natalia, Silvia Moyano Caturelli, Jackeline Spengler, Grisel Olivera Roulet

Servicio Nacional de Rehabilitación (SNR), Buenos Aires, Argentina.
Email: nataliatamborenea@hotmail.com

ABSTRACT

Objective: 1) To analyze the prevalence of Work Disability (WD) in RA Argentinian patients who are attending at the National Rehabilitation Service (NRS); 2) To measure general, socioeconomics and disease characteristics in this population; 3) To characterize the associated factors of work disability in this group. **Methods:** Design cross section observational study. RA patients attending the NRS were included in consecutive form. Clinical, demographic and radiological data were collected. All patients answered about their employment status. WD was defined if the work status was unemployed due to RA, retirement prior to the normal age, or disabled pension. Comparing analysis among patients with and without paid work was done. Housewives, retired patients and students were excluded from the comparing analysis. **Results:** Three hundred and eleven patients were included (n = 311). The prevalence of WD was 44.05% (n = 137). During the study 85 (27.3%) patients were in paid employment, 48 (15.3%) were retired, 39 (12.5%) were housewives, and 2 (0.6%) patients were students. Factor associated to WD were female sex, more than 5 years of disease duration, have health insurance, education beyond high school, and greater functional limitation: HAQ > 1 and function class 3 - 4. In the multivariable logistic regression model female sex was a significant and independent predictor of WD. Having health insurance; and more than high school education were protector factors of WD in this model. **Conclusion:** WD prevalence in this sample was higher than other countries. Socioeconomics factors more than diseases factors were significant predictors of productivity loss in this sample.

Keywords: HAQ; Work Disability; Rheumatoid Arthritis

1. Introduction

Rheumatoid Arthritis is a chronic disabling condition that may affect the lives of individual patients in many ways. One of most important outcomes may be work disability [1,2].

Participation in paid employment is a major life role for most adults. People with arthritis can expect to be employed fewer years than the general population [3,4] and withdrawal from paid employment, or work disability, is a relatively common outcome of RA. It results in lost income for the patient and less productivity for society [5].

Research into WD has been reported from USA and from European countries, rates of this outcome reported range from 22% to 85% [6].

Variations in estimated rates are likely due to differences in methods, subject selection, time, available treatments and definitions of work disability.

National Rehabilitation Service (NRS) in Argentina, evaluate patients with Rheumatoid Arthritis diagnosis who request Disability Certification according to 22431

law. This law establishes the conditions for grant the disability certificate. It is a public document issued by an interdisciplinary team that performs a biopsychosocial evaluation.

The National Disability Certificate is the admission key to the health system and the principal tool for the access to complete coverage of medication and rehabilitation.

In this study we analyze the prevalence of WD in RA patients who are attending at the National Rehabilitation Service (NRS) in Argentina and determine the associated factors to this outcome in this group.

2. Patients and Methods

RA patients are attending at the NRS for tramit the National Disability Certificate. They ask for this certificate in voluntary way and the population are from Buenos Aires province and rest of the all country.

From May 2008 to August 2008 RA patients were included in consecutive form in this cross section observational study.

Clinical, demographic and radiological data were collected.

All patients answered about their employment status. The first question asked "main form of work" was unemployed, paid work, retired, housework, student or disabled.

WD was defined if the work status were unemployed due to RA, retirement prior to the normal age or disabled pension.

We analyzed the following characteristics about the disease: time of disease evolution, rheumatoid factor, functional class, radiographic erosions, HAQ-A and DAS 28 results.

For assess the association among disease characteristics and work status, were excluded for the analysis housework, students and retired patients.

3. Statistical Analysis

The sample was characterized using descriptive procedures.

To analyze categorical variables X^2 were used and Student's t-test and Mann-Whitney test for continuous variables.

The main analysis was multivariable logistic regression to assess the roles of independent variables as predictors of work disability.

The logistic regression model was constructed with the following independent variables sex, education level, health insurance, years of disease evolution, functional class, anatomic class, HAQ-A and DAS28 results. We calculated odds ratios and 95 % CIs. p values < 0.05 was considered significant.

4. Results

Three hundred and eleven patients were included (n = 311). The prevalence of WD was 44. 05% (n = 137).

Women were 87% (n = 271) of the patients, the sample was predominantly middle aged (mean age 54 years), the median time of disease evolution was 8 (4 - 15) years. Around 75.8% (n = 236) had some type of health insurance.

The 68.8% (n = 214) of the sample have education beyond high school.

The HAQ-A score was bigger than 1 in 82.2% (n = 256) of the patients and the DAS28 was more than 3.2 in the 83.3% (n = 259) of the sample. Function class was 3 or 4 in 199 patients (64.2%) and radiographies erosions were present in 234 (76%) patients. 91% (n = 285) of the population was positive for rheumatoid factor test (**Table 1**).

During the study 85 (27.3%) patients were in paid employment, 48 (15.3%) were retired, 39 (12.5%) were housewives, and 2 (0.6%) patients were students (**Table**

1).

In the comparing analysis among patients with and without paid work, were excluded housewives, retired patients and students. To avoid expected retirement-related work cessation, subjects in our analysis were lower than 65 years old, remaining 223 patients for this analysis.

There were statistical significant differences when comparing characteristics among patients with and without WD, included gender (p: 0.001), more than 5 years of disease duration (p: 0.013), have health insurance (p: 0.005), education beyond high school (p: 0.000), and greater functional limitation: HAQ-A > 1 (p: 0.017) and function class 3 - 4 (p: 0.026) (**Table 2**).

In the multivariable logistic regression model female gender was a significant and independent predictor of WD p: 0.004 OR IC 95% 3.2 (1.46 - 7.01). Having health insurance p: 0.01 OR IC 95% 0.42 (0.21 - 0.81); and more than high school education p: 0.000 IC 95% 0.25 (0.13 - 0.46) were protectors factors of WD in this model (**Table 3**).

Table 1. Sample characteristics of subjects (n = 311).

Women n (%)	271 (87)
Age, mean (range)	54 (25 - 77)
Disease duration, median (IQR)	8 (4 - 15)
Health insurance n (%)	236 (75.8)
< High school education n (%)	214 (68.8)
Paid work n (%)	85 (27.3)
Retired n (%)	48 (15.3)
Housework n (%)	39 (12.5)
Students n (%)	2 (0.6)
Unemployed due to RA n (%)	111 (35.7)
Disabled pension n (%)	26 (8.5)
Rheumatoid factor + n (%)	285 (91.6)
Function classes 3 and 4 n (%)	199 (64.2)
Radiographic erosions n (%)	234 (76)
HAQ > 1 n (%)	256 (82.3)
DAS28 > 3.2 n (%)	259 (83.3)

Table 2. Comparative analysis among patients with and without paid work (n = 223).

	WD n: 137	No WD n: 86	p	OR	95% CI
Women %	90% (124/137)	74% (64/86)	0.001	3.2	1.5 - 6.93
Disease duration > 5 years	65.6% (90/137)	48.8% (42/86)	0.013	2.	1.1 - 3.6
Health insurance	56.9% (78/137)	75.5% (65/86)	0.005	0.4	0.2 - 0.8
RF + %	92.7% (127/137)	95% (82/86)	0.42	0.61	0.1 - 2.2
High school	22.6% (31/137)	54.6% (47/86)	0.000	0.24	0.1 - 0.4
Radigraphic erosions	77% (106/137)	68.6% (59/86)	0.146	1.5	0.8 - 2.9
Function classes 3 - 4	71.5% (98/137)	56.9% (49/86)	0.026	1.89	1 - 3.4
HAQ > 1	79.5% (109/137)	65% (56/86)	0.017	2.08	1 - 4
DAS28 > 3.2	86.8% (119/137)	80% (69/86)	0.185	1.6	0.7 - 3.5

Table 3. Multivariable logistic regression model. Patients with and without paid work (n = 223).

Variable	OR 95% CI	p
Women %	3.2 (1.46 - 7.01)	0.004
Disease duration > 5 years	1.78 (0.93 - 3.4)	0.08
Health insurance	0.42 (0.21 - 0.81)	0.01
High school	0.25 (0.13 - 0.46)	0.000
HAQ > 1	1.81 (0.88 - 3.71)	0.1
Function classes 3 - 4	1.3 (0.64 - 2.68)	0.45

5. Discussion

The loss of productivity associated with RA disability places significant burden on patients, their families and society as a whole [7].

Work disability is defined in this article as work cessation due to RA, retirement prior to the normal age, or disability pension due to RA.

Rates of WD reported from USA and European countries range from 22% to 85% [6]. Recently Allaire *et al.* reported that 35.1% of RA patients in US were work disabled [8].

In this sample of RA Argentinean patients had the prevalence of WD was 44.05%, higher than the last reports from other countries. Employment status was defined for us like Allaire's study [8].

We found high prevalence of female gender, mean age of 54 years old, mean disease duration of 8 years, and high scores in DAS28 and HAQ.

Education level previous of RA diagnosis was low, and lower than others population.

Factors associated with WD in this group were female gender, absence of medical care, more than 5 years of disease duration, low education level, worse functional class and high HAQ score (**Table 2**).

Several studies agreed that medical care and education status are important socioeconomics predictors of work loss. In the same form, functional class and HAQ are predictors related to the disease [9-11].

We didn't find association between radiographic damage and disability in this group. Recent studies have demonstrated weak relationships between damage and disability in the first 10 years of disease course. It appears that inflammation contributes much more to the level of disability during the first years of disease course, whereas radiographic progression contributes more strongly after about 10 years of disease duration [12]. In our study patients had 8 years of disease duration approximately and high score of DAS28.

In the multivariable analysis were significant and independent predictors of WD female gender, absence of medical plan and education below high school.

Female gender has been reported to be an independent risk factor for WD in RA in several studies. RA more frequently starts early in females indicating that females are exposed to the inflammation longer than males [13].

M. Wallenius *et al.* [14] found fourfold increased risk in females, and reported differences in pain perceptions and worse mental health among genders could contribute to this point.

Health insurance absence in our country is associated

to difficulties in access to the medical system, delay to start specific treatment and less possibilities to obtain the new available drugs. It results in worse disease evolution and disability increase.

Fewer years of schooling often result in a physically demanding occupation with fewer possibilities for vocational rehabilitation [15].

The HAQ disability has been a correlate of permanent work disability in almost all studies [16-18]. In this sample HAQ wasn't a significant independent predictor of WD. However, this is a cross section study and HAQ score was measured at the moment of processing disability certificate, and not in the moment that the patient developed work loss.

There are several limitations in our study. Patients who ask for disability certificate have probably more severs forms of the disease, and in this point our results can be overestimated. Sample size of 311 patients does not allow extrapolating the results to all patients with Rheumatoid Arthritis in our country. In this study was not recorded the type of patient's work. Due to the study design, we can not establish a temporal relationship between disability and work loss.

In conclusion, our data suggest that work disability among persons with RA in Argentina is still a substantial problem. We need design prospective cohort studies to estimate the prevalence of WD in this country and identify the real impact of RA on paid work.

REFERENCES

[1] D. L. Scott and S. Steer, "The Course of Established Rheumatoid Arthritis," *Best Practice & Research Clinical Rheumatology*, Vol. 21, No. 5, 2007, pp. 943-967. doi:10.1016/j.berh.2007.05.006

[2] Saralynn and H. A. ScD, "Update on Work Disability in Rheumatic Diseases," *Current Opinion in Rheumatology*, Vol. 13, No. 2, 2001, pp. 93-98. doi:10.1097/00002281-200103000-00001

[3] K. Puolakka, H. Kautiainen, *et al.*, "Monetary Value of Lost Productivity over a Five-Year Follow Up in Early Rheumatoid Arthritis Estimated on the Basis of Official Register Data on Patients' Sickness Absence and Gross Income: Experience from the FIN-RACo Trial," *Annals of the Rheumatic Diseases*, Vol. 65, No. 7, 2006, pp. 899-904. doi:10.1136/ard.2005.045807

[4] A. Joung, J. Dixey, *et al.*, "How Does Functional Disability in Early Rheumatoid Arthritis Affect Patients and Their Lives? Results from 5 Years of Follow-Up in 732 Patients from the Early RA Study," *Rheumatology*, Vol. 39, No. 6, 2000, pp. 603-611. doi:10.1093/rheumatology/39.6.603

[5] A.-C. Rat and M.-C. Boissier, "Rheumatoid Arthritis: Direct and Indirect Costs," *Joint Bone Spine*, Vol. 71, No. 6, 2004, pp. 518-524. doi:10.1016/j.jbspin.2004.01.003

[6] E. M. Barret, D. G. Scott, *et al.*, "The Impact of Rheumatoid Arthritis on Employment Status in the Early Years of Desease: A UK Community Based Study," *Rheumatology*, Vol. 39, No. 12, 2000, pp. 1403-1409. doi:10.1093/rheumatology/39.12.1403

[7] A. A. Kalla and M. Tikly, "Rheumatoid Arthritis in the Developing World," *Best Practice & Research Clinical Rheumatology*, Vol. 17, No. 5, 2003, pp. 863-875. doi:10.1016/S1521-6942(03)00047-0

[8] S. Allaire, F. Wolfe, *et al.*, "Contemporany Prevalence and Incidence of Work Disability Associated with Rheumatoid Arthritis in US," *Arthritis Care & Research*, Vol. 59, No. 4, 2008, pp. 474-480. doi:10.1002/art.23538

[9] A. Young, J. Dixey, *et al.*, "Which Patients Stop Working Because of Rheumatoid Arthritis? Results of Five Years' Follow Up in 732 Patients from the Early RA Study (ERAS)," *Annals of the Rheumatic Diseases*, Vol. 61, No. 4, 2002, pp. 335-340. doi:10.1136/ard.61.4.335

[10] M. J. Plant and M. M. O'Sullivan, "What Factors Influence Functional Ability in Patients with Rheumatoid Arthritis. Do They Alter over Time?" *Rheumatology*, Vol. 44, No. 9, 2005, pp. 1181-1185. doi:10.1093/rheumatology/keh707

[11] K. Puolakka, H. Kautiainen, T. Möttönen, *et al.*, "Predictors of Productivity Loss in Early Rheumatoid Arthritis: A 5-Year-Follow-Up Study," *Annals of the Rheumatic Diseases*, Vol. 64, No. 1, 2005, pp. 130-133. doi:10.1136/ard.2003.019034

[12] T. K. Kvein, "Epidemiology of Disability in Rheumatoid Arthritis," *Rheumatology*, Vol. 41, No. 2, 2002, pp. 121-123. doi:10.1093/rheumatology/41.2.121

[13] T. K. Kvien, T. Uhlig, *et al.*, "Epidemiological Aspects of Rheumatoid Arthritis: The Sex Ratio," *Annals of the New York Academy of Sciences*, Vol. 1069, 2006, pp. 212-222. doi:10.1196/annals.1351.019

[14] M. Wallenius, J. F. Skomsvoll, *et al.*, "Comparison of Work Disability and Health-Related Quality of Life between Males and Females with Rheumatoid Arthritis below the Age of 45 Years," *Scandinavian Journal of Rheumatology*, Vol. 38, No, 3, 2008, pp. 178-183. doi:10.1080/03009740802400594

[15] A. Macedo, S. Oakley, *et al.*, "An Examination of Work Instability, Functional Impairment, Ant Disease Activity in Employed Patients with Rheumatoid Arthritis," *The Journal of Rheumatology*, Vol. 36, No. 2, 2009, pp. 1-6. doi:10.3899/jrheum.071001

[16] C. Han, J. Smolen, *et al.*, "Comparision of Employability Outcomes among Patients with Early or Long-Standing Rheumatoid Arthritis," *Arthritis Care & Research*, Vol. 59, No. 4, 2008, pp. 510-514. doi:10.1002/art.23541

[17] S. Lillegraven and T. K. Kvien, "Measuring Disability and Quality of Life in Established Rheumatoid Arthritis," *Best Practice & Research Clinical Rheumatology*, Vol. 21, No. 5, 2007, pp. 827-840. doi:10.1016/j.berh.2007.05.004

[18] P. Katz and A. Morris, "Subclinical Disability in Valued Life Activities among Individuals with Rheumatoid Arthritis," *Arthritis Care & Research*, Vol. 59, No. 10, 2008, pp. 1416-1423. doi:10.1002/art.24110

31

Is Chemokine Receptor CCR9 Required for Synovitis in Rheumatoid Arthritis? Deficiency of CCR9 in a Murine Model of Antigen-Induced Arthritis

Alison Cartwright[1], Sophie King[2], Jim Middleton[1,2], Oksana Kehoe[1]

[1]Keele University at Robert Jones and Agnes Hunt Orthopaedic Hospital, Oswestry, UK; [2]Faculty of Medicine and Dentistry, School of Oral and Dental Sciences, University of Bristol, Bristol, UK.
Email: Alison.Cartwright@rjah.nhs.uk

ABSTRACT

Objectives: Monocytes/macrophages accumulate in the synovial membrane in rheumatoid arthritis and play a key role in disease pathogenesis, contributing to inflammation, cartilage destruction and bone erosion. Identification of molecules involved in monocyte/macrophage recruitment in inflammation is crucial for development of therapeutic interventions. Chemokine receptor CCR9 is up-regulated on these cells in peripheral blood and synovium of rheumatoid patients. This study investigated the course of antigen-induced arthritis in CCR9 deficient C57BL/6 mice in comparison to wild type animals to determine whether CCR9 is critical for disease severity and progression. **Methods:** Methylated bovine serum albumin was used for induction of uni-lateral arthritis by direct injection into the knee joints of preimmunized animals. Arthritis is confined to the injected joint allowing comparison with the normal opposing joint. Clinical severity of arthritis was assessed by measuring swelling in the arthritic joint in comparison to the normal joint. Histological analysis was performed to assess the extent of leukocyte infiltration and cartilage depletion. **Results:** Levels of swelling were not significantly different between wild type and CCR9 deficient mice. Similarly there was no significant difference in histological severity of arthritis when comparing CCR9-deficient mice to wild type mice. **Conclusions:** CCR9 was not required for development of synovial inflammation and cartilage destruction in the antigen-induced model of arthritis in C57BL/6 mice in this study. This may reflect a true lack of a pathogenic role of CCR9 on monocyte/macrophage function *in vivo* or it may reflect differences in the current antigen-induced arthritis model when compared to human RA.

Keywords: Chemokine Receptor CCR9; Rheumatoid Arthritis; Inflammation; Antigen-Induced Arthritis; Mouse Model; Monocytes/Macrophages

1. Introduction

Rheumatoid Arthritis (RA) is a chronic inflammatory disease characterized by the accumulation of leukocytes in the synovial membrane and fluid of affected joints. Chemokine receptors on leukocytes mediate the persistent recruitment of these cells and identification of involved receptors offers potential for development of therapeutic interventions. Monocytes/macrophages play a key role in RA, contributing to inflammation, cartilage destruction and bone erosion. Monocytes migrate from the blood across the vascular endothelium into the synovium where they differentiate into macrophages. Activated macrophages produce large quantities of pro-inflammatory cytokines and chemokines including interleukin-1beta (IL-1β), tumour necrosis factor alpha (TNFα), IL-6, chemokine ligands CXCL8, CCL2 and CCL3, and also proteases such as matrix metalloproteinase MMP-9 and MMP-12

[1,2]. The degree of macrophage infiltration correlates to the radiological progression of joint destruction [3].

Chemokine receptor CCR9 is constitutively expressed on T lymphocytes in the small intestine, thymus, lymph node and spleen [4,5] with involvement in T cell recruitment to the small intestine and T cell development and migration within the thymus.

CCR9 mediates migration of malignant cluster of differentiation 4+ (CD4+) T lymphocytes into various organs such as the lymph nodes, liver, spleen, lungs and intestinal tract in T-cell lineage acute lymphocytic leukaemia (T-ALL) [6]. CCR9 and its ligand CCL25 were found to be highly over-expressed on T-ALL CD4+ T cells when compared to normal CD4+ T cells. Human cutaneous melanoma cells are suggested to metastasize to the small intestine via action of CCR9 [7]. CCR9 also has roles in the metastatic spread of tumour cells in prostate cancer [8] and ovarian cancer [9] and the CCR9/ CCL25 axis is also involved in breast cancer cell migration and invasion [10].

CCR9 is expressed in inflammation with involvement in T cell recruitment in inflammatory bowel disease. A potent human CCR9 small molecule antagonist: GSK-1605786 (CCX-282; Traficet-EN) is being developed by GlaxoSmithKline plc under licence from ChemoCentryx Inc., for potential treatment of inflammatory bowel disease including Crohn's disease [11,12]. It is currently being used to conduct clinical trials with the aim that it will inhibit lymphocyte migration to the small intestine and ameliorate inflammation occurring in Crohn's disease.

CCR9 expression has been observed on monocytes/ macrophages but not on T or B cells in the synovium, with expression increasing in inflamed synovium in RA [13]. The number of $CCR9^+$ $CD14^+$ monocytes/ macrophages increases significantly in RA synovium compared to non-RA tissue. The differentiation of monocytes into macrophages within this tissue is suggested to involve CCR9 and its sole ligand CCL25, particularly under inflammatory conditions [13]. Expression of CCR9 also increases significantly on Peripheral Blood (PB) monocytes in RA suggesting a role for CCR9 and CCL25 in the pathogenesis of this disease.

This study investigated whether CCR9/CCL25 interactions are critical for the development of inflammation in a murine model of Antigen-Induced Arthritis (AIA). AIA is a mono-articular disease model caused by the direct injection of antigen into the knee joint of a pre-immunized animal. Arthritis is confined to the injected joint allowing comparison with the normal opposing joint. The model was used to compare hyperplasia, leukocyte infiltration, and cartilage erosion in the synovial joint of CCR9-deficient ($CCR9^{-/-}$) and wild-type (WT, $CCR9^{+/+}$) mice, with the aim of investigating the role played by CCR9 in this experimental model which forms a close experimental analogue of human RA [14,15]. The CCR9 deficient mice used in this study were C57BL/6 strain in which the model of methylated bovine serum albumin (mBSA) AIA shows good severity and chronicity [15]. The AIA model has the following characteristics:

1) preimmunisation induces humoral and cell-mediated immunity;

2) leukocytes: lymphocytes, plasma cells, macrophages and neutrophils, migrate into the injected joint;

3) uni-lateral arthritis with controlled onset;

4) pannus formation resulting in erosion of cartilage and bone;

5) antigen-specific local hyper-reactivity and antigen retention in cartilage;

6) chronicity by repeated flares.

2. Methods

2.1. Animals

Experiments were conducted in 7 to 8 week old inbred, male C57BL/6 wild-type ($CCR9^{+/+}$) mice (Charles River UK, Margate, UK) and CCR9-deficient ($CCR9^{-/-}$) C-57BL/6 mice bred in-house from breeding pairs (MRC Harwell, Oxfordshire, UK). Animals were maintained under "conventional regime" and according to the institutional and national guide for care and use of laboratory animals. Procedures were conducted in accordance with Home Office Project License PPL-40/3047.

2.2. Induction of Antigen-Induced Arthritis (AIA)

Mice were immunized subcutaneously with 100 µl of an emulsion of 1 mg/ml·mBSA in Phosphate Buffered Saline (PBS) mixed with an equal volume of complete Freund's adjuvant [16]. At the same time they were injected intraperitoneally with 160 ng heat-inactivated *Bordetella pertussis* toxin in 100 µl PBS (all reagents were from Sigma, Gillingham, UK). At one week the immune response was boosted by subcutaneous injection again with 100 µl of 1mg/ml mBSA in PBS mixed with an equal volume of complete Freund's adjuvant. At three weeks AIA was induced by injecting 10 µl·10 mg/ml mBSA in PBS intraarticularly into the right hind knee joint and 10 µl PBS into the left knee joint to act as control (day 0).

2.3. Clinical Assessment of Arthritis

Severity of arthritis was assessed by comparing the right hind limb joint in which AIA had been induced, with the left hind limb joint which acted as control. Both knee joint diameters were measured before and at 1, 2, 3, 5, 7, 14 and 21 days after arthritis induction using a digital micrometer (Kroeplin GmbH, Schlüchtern, Germany) to monitor swelling.

2.4. Histological Assessment of Arthritis

Animals were killed at day 3, 14 and 21 after induction of arthritis, with a minimum of 5 animals at each time point. For AIA in CCR9-deficient mice 18 animals were used over two experiments. 7 animals were sacrificed at day 3, 6 animals at day 14 and 5 animals at day 21. For AIA in WT mice 66 animals were used over 8 experiments. 20 animals were sacrificed at day 3, 23 animals at day 14, and 23 animals at day 21.

Knee joints were removed and fixed in neutral buffered formal saline. Decalcification in formic acid, embedding in paraffin and sectioning (of 4 µm thickness) was carried out by the histology department, RJAH Orthopaedic Hospital.

Serial sections were stained with Haematoxylin and Eosin (H & E) and safranin O-fast green. Sections were examined at ×100 and ×200 magnifications. Scoring of sections was carried out blind [16]. H&E sections were used to score synovial hyperplasia from 0 (normal: lining 1 cell thick) to 3 (severe: lining 4 or more cells thick); cellular exudate from 0 (no cells present in joint cavity) to 3 (20 or more cells present in joint cavity), and synovial leukocyte infiltration, from 0 (no infiltration) to 5 (extensive infiltration). Safranin O stains proteoglycans in cartilage orange/red in colour and stained sections were used to score cartilage depletion based on loss of red staining on femoral and tibial condyles, from 0 (no apparent loss of colour intensity) to 3 (extensive loss of cartilage staining). Parameters were then summed to give an arthritis index.

2.5. Immunohistology

Sections were deparaffinized, rehydrated and antigen retrieval carried out overnight at 50°C in 100 mM Tris/HCl, pH 9.0. Slides were rinsed in PBS and incubated with goat anti-mouse CCR9 (4 µg/ml; Genetex, Source BioScience, Nottingham, UK) and goat IgG control (R & D Systems, Abingdon, UK) for 60 minutes. The sections were rinsed in PBS and then further incubated with donkey anti-goat Alexa 594 (1:100; Molecular Probes, Invitrogen, Paisley, UK) in 10% mouse serum for 30 minutes. Sections were rinsed in PBS and nuclear staining was performed with 4',6-diamidino-2-phenyl indole dihydrochloride (DAPI; 2 µg/ml in PBS; Sigma) for 3 minutes before rinsing and mounting.

2.6. Statistical Analysis

GraphPad Prism Version 5.01 was used for all statistical analysis. Joint swelling was compared between CCR9 deficient and WT mice by 2-way analysis of variance (ANOVA) followed by Bonferroni post tests to compare swelling at each time point. Comparisons were made between the arthritis index for CCR9 deficient and WT mice at days 3, 14 and 21 by Kruskal-Wallis test followed by Dunn's post test. Individual parameters comprising the arthritis index were also compared by Kruskal-Wallis test followed by Dunn's post test. Values of $p < 0.05$ were considered statistically significant.

3. Results

3.1. Clinical Assessment of Knee Joints

Joint swelling was measured following intra-articular injection with mBSA or PBS at day 0. The difference in knee joint diameter between the right limb in which arthritis had been induced, and the left limb (PBS injected)

which acted as control, was recorded for each animal over a 21 day period (**Figure 1**). Animals were sacrificed at days 3, 14 and 21 for assessment of inflammatory parameters by histology. Joints were measured for remaining animals in each experiment. Both WT and CCR9 deficient mice demonstrated significant joint swelling (**Figure 1**; $p < 0.0001$) following injection of mBSA to induce arthritis, and swelling was most severe at 1 day post injection. Swelling then reduced by approaching 50% at day 2 in both strains of mice, and subsequently returned to approximately normal by day 21. However levels of swelling were not significantly different between WT and CCR9 deficient mice when analyzed by 2-way ANOVA with Bonferroni post tests to analyse the difference in swelling between strains at each time point ($p > 0.05$).

3.2. Histopathological Assessment of Knee Joints

Figures 2 and **3** show representative micrographs from CCR9$^{+/+}$ and CCR9$^{-/-}$ mice. A pronounced arthritis was induced by intra-articular injection of mBSA which was not observed in contra-lateral control joints from the same animals. In both CCR9$^{-/-}$ (**Figure 2(a)**) and WT mice (**Figure 2(c)**) arthritis was characterized by the hyperplasia (thickening) of the synovial lining layer and infiltration of leukocytes in the sub-lining of the joint. Contra-lateral control joints from the same animals showed that they did not become inflamed (**Figures 2(b)** and **(d)**). Synovial exudate was present in the joints with AIA and consisted of neutrophils within the joint space.

The AIA model is characterized by cartilage depletion

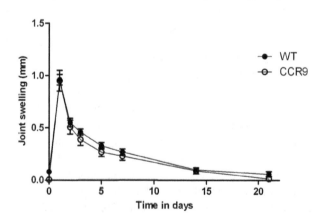

Figure 1. Joint swelling following antigen-induced arthritis in wild type (CCR9$^{+/+}$) and CCR9 deficient (CCR9$^{-/-}$) mice. AIA was induced in preimmunized CCR9$^{-/-}$ and CCR9$^{+/+}$ mice by intraarticular injection of mBSA in PBS. Data represent mean ± standard error for swelling measurements for all mice remaining in the experiment before sacrifice for histology. For measurements on CCR9 deficient animals at days 0 - 3: n = 18; days 5 - 14: n = 13, and day 21, n = 7. For WT animals n = 66 at days 0 - 3; n = 47 at days 5 - 14 and n = 27 at day 21.

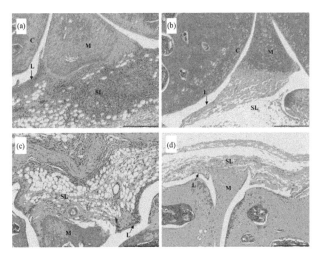

Figure 2. Antigen-induced arthritis in CCR9-deficient (CCR9$^{-/-}$) and wild type (CCR9$^{+/+}$) mice. Representative haematoxylin and eosin stained sections are shown for CCR9$^{-/-}$ (a) and (b) and CCR9$^{+/+}$ (c) and (d) mice sacrificed on day 3, showing antigen-induced arthritis (a) and (c) and contra-lateral controls (b) and (d). (c), cartilage; L, synovial lining; SL, synovial sub-lining; M, meniscus; scale bar represents 200 μm.

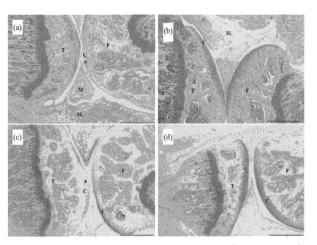

Figure 3. Antigen-induced arthritis in CCR9$^{-/-}$ and CCR9$^{+/+}$ mice. Representative haematoxylin and safranin O-fast green stained sections are shown for CCR9$^{-/-}$ (a) and (b) and CCR9$^{+/+}$ (c) and (d) mice sacrificed on day 3, showing antigen-induced arthritis (a) and (c) and contra-lateral controls (b) and (d). (c), cartilage; SL, sub-lining: M, meniscus; T, tibia; F, femur; (*) = region of proteoglycan depletion; scale bar represents 500 μm.

which occurs due to proteoglycan loss, and this was visualized as loss of red staining (**Figure 3(a)** and **(c)**) when stained with Safranin O-fast green. Depletion of cartilage can be seen on the femoral condyle (**Figure 3(a)**) of a CCR9$^{-/-}$ mouse at day 3 of AIA. The marked area (*) shows a region of proteoglycan depletion. Likewise, cartilage depletion marked by (*) can be observed on the tibial condyle in a wild type mouse at day 3 (**Figure 3(c)**) of AIA. The contra-lateral controls for the same animals show that the cartilage did not become depleted (**Figures 3(b)** and **(d)**).

The severity of arthritis was quantified by histopathological assessment of joint sections from CCR9$^{+/+}$ and

CCR9$^{-/-}$ mice sacrificed at 3, 14 and 21 days following induction of arthritis. 4 parameters were scored: synovial hyperplasia (thickening of the lining layer), cellular exudate, cartilage depletion/bone erosion and synovial infiltration and scores were summed to give an arthritis index (**Table 1**) [16]. Although arthritis developed following intraarticular injection of mBSA, joints from CCR9 deficient mice showed limited pathological changes.

Hyperplasia did not alter significantly with time in either the wild type or knockout mice or indeed between the 2 strains (p > 0.05). Infiltration of leukocytes in the sub-lining was highest at day 3 in both mouse strains and declined over the course of the model as did synovial exudate, with no significant difference observed between

Table 1. Joint inflammation and cartilage damage on day 3, 14 and 21 of antigen-induced arthritis.

Day	Strain	Hyperplasia (0 - 3)	Synovial infiltrate (0 - 5)	Synovial exudate (0 - 3)	Cartilage depletion (0 - 3)	Arthritis index
3	CCR9$^{-/-}$	1.64 ± 0.28	3.07 ± 0.33	1.71 ± 0.29	1.36 ± 0.28	7.93 ± 0.70
	CCR9$^{+/+}$	2.17 ± 0.25	2.57 ± 0.25	1.10 ± 0.25	1.10 ± 0.21	6.93 ± 0.71
14	CCR9$^{-/-}$	1.42 ± 0.20	1.33 ± 0.48	1.00 ± 0.26	0.75 ± 0.25	4.50 ± 0.90
	CCR9$^{+/+}$	2.05 ± 0.27	2.09 ± 0.40	1.00 ± 0.40	1.23 ± 0.22	6.36 ± 1.09
21	CCR9$^{-/-}$	1.90 ± 0.40	1.00 ± 0.47	1.00 ± 0.55	0.80 ± 0.58	4.70 ± 1.63
	CCR9$^{+/+}$	1.44 ± 0.21	1.38 ± 0.20	0.85 ± 0.22	1.21 ± 0.27	4.88 ± 0.71

Histopathological analysis of sections from CCR9$^{-/-}$ and CCR9$^{+/+}$ mice sacrificed at day 3, 14 and 21 of AIA. Hyperplasia and cellular infiltration of the synovial membrane and cellular exudate into the synovial cavity were observed in haematoxylin and eosin-stained sections. Cartilage depletion was observed in haematoxylin and safranin O-fast green-stained sections. Histological scoring was carried out blind at ×100 and ×200 magnification. Data are mean values ± standard error. For CCR9$^{-/-}$ animals, day 3 n = 7, day 14 n = 6, day 21 n = 5; for CCR9$^{+/+}$ animals, day 3 n = 20, day 14 n = 23, day 21 n = 23.

strains (p > 0.05). Cartilage depletion was greatest at day 3 in CCR9 deficient mice, and declined by day 14, whereas it did not change much in the wild type animals. The overall arthritis index was greatest at day 3 with a higher score in CCR9 deficient mice. It declined by day 14 in both mouse strains, although the reduction was greater in the knockout mice. By day 21 it was the same for both strains. Kruskal-Wallis tests with Dunn's post tests were carried out to compare the arthritis index and each individual parameter and showed that there was no significant difference between the CCR9-deficient and wild type mice.

3.3. CCR9 Expression in Synovium

CCR9 expression was examined by immunohistochemistry on paraffin embedded synovial sections obtained from WT mice sacrificed at day 3 of AIA. The receptor was detected in all animals observed on infiltrated leukocytes in the synovium (**Figure 4**). Investigation of CCR9 expression on CCR9$^{-/-}$ mice sacrificed at day 3 of AIA showed that infiltrated leukocytes and also stromal cells were CCR9 negative (data not shown).

4. Discussion

To investigate the requirement for chemokine receptor CCR9 in synovitis in RA, a mouse AIA model was used

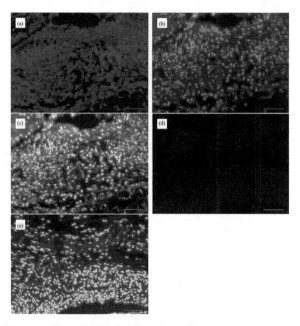

Figure 4. Expression of CCR9 by infiltrating leukocytes in CCR9$^{+/+}$ mice sacrificed on day 3 of antigen-induced arthritis. Sections were stained with antibody to CCR9 (a) and DAPI nuclear stain (b). (c) represents a merge of images (a) and (b). (d) is the isotype control for CCR9 and (e) is the same field of view stained with DAPI. The scale bar represents 100 μm.

which forms a close experimental analogue of human RA [14]. AIA was induced in WT and CCR9$^{-/-}$ mice. The severity of the inflammatory response was determined firstly by monitoring joint swelling over the 21 day time course of the arthritis model which showed that there was no significant difference in joint swelling between the two mouse strains. Secondly, histological assessment of joint sections from mice sacrificed at days 3, 14 and 21 showed that again, there was no significant difference in severity of arthritis when comparing CCR9-deficient mice to WT mice.

We then examined expression of CCR9 in WT arthritic joints at the peak of synovitis (day 3) observing strong expression of CCR9 on infiltrating leukocytes in the synovium. This observation agrees with our finding that CCR9 is expressed intensely on a subset of infiltrating leukocytes in human rheumatoid synovium [13]. The examination of corresponding sections from CCR9$^{-/-}$ mice showed joints were indeed CCR9 negative although synovia were equally infiltrated by leukocytes. Therefore although leukocytes recruited to the inflamed synovium in WT animals were populations positive for CCR9, expression of this receptor does not appear critical for leukocyte recruitment and development of arthritis in the AIA model in C57BL/6 mice.

The AIA model includes the initial adaptive immune response during which mBSA presentation to T cells stimulates T cell proliferation and down stream activation of B cells and production of antibodies to mBSA. This model also includes the inflammatory effector phase of disease in which neutrophils and mononuclear cells migrate into the joint producing swelling, cartilage depletion and bone erosions. Disease severity may be reduced in CCR9 deficient mice if the receptor is critical to either stage. In humans expression of CCR9 increased on rheumatoid monocytes/macrophages in blood and synovium but the receptor was not detected on synovial lymphocytes [13]. Furthermore, CCR9 expression was low on neutrophils (personal communication from Dr Caroline Schmutz) so CCR9 absence may not directly affect lymphocyte or neutrophil recruitment.

CCR9 is suggested to be involved in the differentiation of monocytes into macrophages once they have been recruited to the synovium [13] so CCR9 deficiency may impede the effector phase of the disease, inhibiting differentiation and activation of monocytes/macrophages so restricting production of proinflammatory cytokines such as TNFα and IL-6. It is possible however, that in the current study CCR9 may not be involved in differentiation of monocytes to macrophages. There may be differences between human RA and the AIA mouse model, or CCR9 may be expressed on a non-pathogenic phenotypic subset of monocytes/macrophages in the mouse [17].

K/BxN mice spontaneously develop an arthritis that is similar to human RA [18]. K/BxN mice produce arthritogenic autoantibodies which induce arthritis when transferred to recipient mouse strains. Jacobs *et al.*, (2010) used the K/BxN serum-transfer model to investigate involvement of various chemokine receptors in the effector phase of autoantibody-mediated arthritis. K/BxN serum was transferred into CCR9$^{-/-}$ mice but ensuing arthritis assessed over a 20 day period was not assessed as significantly different from heterozygote controls demonstrating that CCR9 was not critical for development of synovitis in this model. CXCR2 was found to be necessary for development of arthritis and recruitment of neutrophils to the joints [19]. However, other receptors such as CCR1-7, CXCR3 and CXCR5 were not required in the model although some have been shown to function in arthritis using adaptive immune response models. It would therefore be interesting to examine function of CCR9 in other murine arthritis models.

CCR9 involvement in inflammation has been demonstrated in mouse models of hepatitis where CCR9^{+} macrophages were required for the induction of acute liver inflammation [20]. CCR9^{+} macrophages produced TNFα, stimulating naïve CD4^{+} T cells to become Th1 cells producing interferon-gamma. Additionally, PB from acute hepatitis patients had increased numbers of CCR9^{+} monocytes compared to controls. Therefore the importance of macrophage CCR9 may vary between different inflammatory diseases

CCR9 and its ligand CCL25 mediate T cell migration to the small intestine under both homeostatic [4,21] and inflammatory conditions [22,23]. CCR9 is implicated in pathogenesis of small intestinal Crohn's disease, a chronic inflammatory bowel disease characterised by an influx of T cells. CCR9^{+} T cells are elevated in the blood and CCL25 is increased in the intestine in areas close to lymphocytic infiltrates [22]. A mouse model of Crohn's disease is provided by TNF-ΔARE mice which have raised levels of TNFα leading to spontaneous development of severe small intestinal inflammation with similarities to Crohn's disease [12]. The CCR9 small molecule antagonist CCX-282-B, which has been developed for potential treatment of inflammatory bowel disease including Crohn's disease [11,12], provided complete protection from severe intestinal inflammation in this mouse model. In contrast, Apostolaki *et al.* (2008) determined that development of inflammation in TNF-ΔARE mice occurred in the genetic absence of CCR9 and also CCL25 demonstrating a difference between pharmacological inhibition and genetic manipulation of CCR9 [24]. This suggests that gene deficient mice may use alternate genes to compensate for the function of the missing gene. It would therefore be interesting to use the CCR9 antagonist

CCX-282-B in our AIA model in WT mice to investigate whether synovial inflammation could be similarly prevented.

CCR9 is not indispensable for lymphocyte recruitment into the small intestine or for T cell development in the thymus. Wurbel *et al.* (2001) generated a CCR9$^{-/-}$ mouse strain in which the absence of CCR9 had no major effect on thymocyte development as a time lag of only one day was observed in the appearance of CD4^{+}CD8^{+} cells [25]. When they looked at the ratio of intraepithelial lymphocytes (IELs) to epithelial cells in small intestine it was decreased 2-fold in the CCR9 knockout compared to wild type mouse. Further analysis of the isolated IEL subsets showed that the reduction was due to low numbers of the TCR$\gamma\delta$ subset. This subset had actually decreased 5-fold in CCR9 knockout compared to wild type mice. Although the absence of CCR9 was obviously effecting IEL populations, the overall effect was not greater probably as a result of the action of other chemokine receptors expressed on intestinal lymphocytes. Receptors such as CXCR4, CCR6, CXCR3 and CCR5 may be able to recruit and retain lymphocytes so compensating for absence of CCR9.

5. Conclusion

CCR9 deficient mice developed arthritis not significantly different in severity to wild type animals. The data from the AIA model demonstrate that recruitment of inflammatory leukocytes into the arthritic joint does not critically require the function of CCR9 in C57BL/6 mice in this arthritis model.

6. Acknowledgements

We thank Pat Evans, Martin Pritchard and Nigel Harness for their histological expertise, staff at the Life Science Support Unit of Liverpool John Moores University for breeding and keeping of the mice, and Anwen Williams for help in setting up the animal model.

This work was supported by Keele University and the Medical Research Council (grant number G0401634). Disclosure statement: The authors have declared no conflicts of interest.

REFERENCES

[1]   Y. Ma and R. M. Pope, "The Role of Macrophages in Rheumatoid Arthritis," *Current Pharmaceutical Design*, Vol. 11, No. 5, 2005, pp. 569-580. doi:10.2174/1381612053381927

[2]   R. W. Kinne, B. Stuhlmüller and G. R. Burmester, "Cells of the Synovium in Rheumatoid Arthritis: Macrophages," *Arthritis Research and Therapy*, Vol. 9, 2007, p. 224. doi:10.1186/ar2333

[3]   D. Mulherin, O. Fitzgerald and B. Bresnihan, "Synovial Tissue Macrophage Populations and Articular Damage in Rheumatoid Arthritis," *Arthritis and Rheumatism*, Vol. 39, No. 1, 1996, pp. 115-124. doi:10.1002/art.1780390116

[4]   B. A. Zabel, W. W. Agace, J. J. Campbell, H. M. Heath, D. Parent, A. I. Roberts, E. C. Ebert, N. Kassam, S. Qin, M. Zovko, G. J. LaRosa, L. L. Yang, D. Soler, E. C. Butcher, P. D. Ponath, C. M. Parker and D. P. Andrew, "Human G Protein-Coupled Receptor GPR-9-6/CC Chemokine Receptor 9 Is Selectively Expressed on Intestinal homing T Lymphocytes, Mucosal Lymphocytes, and Thymocytes and Is Required for Thymus-Expressed Chemokine-Mediated Chemotaxis," *Journal of Experimental Medicine*, Vol. 190, No. 9, 1999, pp. 1241-1256. doi:10.1084/jem.190.9.1241

[5]   E. J. Kunkel, J. J. Campbell, G. Haraldsen, J. Pan, J. Boisvert, A. I. Roberts, E. C. Ebert, M. A. Vierra, S. B. Goodman, M. C. Genovese, A. J. Wardlaw, H. B. Greenberg, C. M. Parker, E. C. Butcher, D. P. Andrew and W. W. Agace, "Lymphocyte CC Chemokine Receptor 9 and Epithelial Thymus-Expressed Chemokine (TECK) expression Distinguish the Small Intestinal Immune Compartment: Epithelial Expression of Tissue-Specific Chemokines as an Organizing Principle in Regional Immunity," *Journal of Experimental Medicine*, Vol. 192, No. 5, 2000, pp. 761-768. doi:10.1084/jem.192.5.761

[6]   Q. P. Zhang, Q. Li, C. S. Hu, X. L. Zhang, B. J. Huang, M. Z. Huang, C. M. Lao, J. S. He, Q. P. Gao, K. J. Zhang, Z. M. Sun, X. J. Zhang, J. Y. Liu and J. Q. Tan, "Selectively Increased Expression and Functions of Chemokine Receptor CCR9 on CD4$^+$ T cells from Patients with T-Cell Lineage Acute Lymphocytic Leukaemia," *Cancer Research*, Vol. 63, No. 19, 2003, pp. 6469-6477.

[7]   F. F. Amersi, A. M. Terando, Y. Goto, R. A. Scolyer, J. F. Thompson, A. N. Tran, M. B. Faries, D. L. Morton and D. S. Hoon, "Activation of CCR9/CCL25 in Cutaneous Melanoma Mediates Preferential Metastasis to the Small Intestine," *Clinical Cancer Research*, Vol. 14, 2008, pp. 638-645. doi:10.1158/1078-0432.CCR-07-2025

[8]   S. Singh, U. P. Singh, J. K. Stiles, W. E. Grizzle and J. W. Lillard Jr., "Expression and Functional Role of CCR9 in Prostate Cancer Cell Migration and Invasion," *Clinical Cancer Research*, Vol. 18, No. 21, 2004, pp. 8743-8750. doi:10.1158/1078-0432.CCR-04-0266

[9]   E. L. Johnson, R. Singh, S. Singh, C. M. Johnson-Holiday, W. E. Grizzle, E. E. Partridge and J. W. Lillard Jr., "CCL25-CCR9 Interaction Modulates Ovarian Cancer Cell Migration, Metalloproteinase Expression, and Invasion," *World Journal of Surgical Oncology*, Vol. 8, 2010, p. 62. doi:10.1186/1477-7819-8-62

[10]   C. Johnson-Holiday, R. Singh, E. Johnson, S. Singh, C. R. Stockard, W. E. Grizzle and J. W. Lillard Jr., "CCL25 Mediates Migration, Invasion and Matrix Metalloproteinase Expression by Breast Cancer Cells in a CCR9-Dependent Fashion," *International Journal of Oncology*, Vol. 38, No. 5, 2011, pp. 1279-1285.

[11]   B. Eksteen and D. H. Adams, "GSK-1605786, a Selective Small-Molecule Antagonist of the CCR9 Chemokine Receptor for the Treatment of Crohn's Disease," *Drugs*, Vol. 13, No. 7, 2010, pp.472-781.

[12]   M. J. Walters, Y. Wang, N. Lai, T. Baumgart, B. N. Zhao, D. J. Dairaghi, P. Bekker, L. S. Ertl, M. E. Penfold, J. C. Jaen, S. Keshav, E. Wendt, A. Pennell, S. Ungashe, Z. Wei, J. J. Wright and T. J. Schall, "Characterization of CCX282-B, an Orally Bioavailable Antagonist of the CCR9 Chemokine Receptor, for Treatment of Inflammatory Bowel Disease," *Journal of Pharmacology and Experimental Therapeutics*, Vol. 335, No. 1, 2010, pp. 61-69. doi:10.1124/jpet.110.169714

[13]   C. Schmutz, A. Cartwright, H. Williams, O. Haworth, J. H. Williams, A. Filer, M. Salmon, C. D. Buckley and J. Middleton, "Monocytes/Macrophages Express CCR9 in Rheumatoid Arthritis and CCL25 Stimulates Their Differentiation," *Arthritis Research and Therapy*, Vol. 12, No. 4, 2010, p. R161. doi:10.1186/ar3120

[14]   D. Brackertz, G. F. Mitchell and I. R. Mackay, "Antigen-Induced Arthritis in Mice," *Arthritis and Rheumatism*, Vol. 20, No. 3, 1977, pp. 841-850. doi:10.1002/art.1780200314

[15]   W. B. van den Berg, L. A. Joosten and P. L. van Lent, "Murine Antigen-Induced Arthritis," *Methods in Molecular Medicine*, Vol. 136, No. 2, 2007, pp. 243-253. doi:10.1007/978-1-59745-402-5_18

[16]   M. A. Nowell, P. J. Richards, S. Horiuchi, N. Yamamoto, S. Rose-John, N. Topley, A. S. Williams and S. A. Jones, "Soluble IL-6 Receptor Governs IL-6 Activity in Experimental Arthritis: Blockade of Arthritis Severity by Soluble Glycoprotein," *Journal of Immunology*, Vol. 171, 2003, pp. 3202-3209.

[17]   A. Mantovani, A. Sica and M. Locati, "New Vistas on Macrophage Differentiation and Activation," *European Journal of Immunology*, Vol. 37, No. 1, 2007, pp. 14-16. doi:10.1002/eji.200636910

[18]   M. Corr and B. Crain, "The Role of FcgammaR Signaling in the K/B × N Serum Transfer Model of Arthritis," *Journal of Immunology*, Vol. 169, No. 11, 2002, pp. 6604-6609.

[19]   J. P. Jacobs, A. Ortiz-Lopez, J. J. Campbell, C. J. Gerard, D. Mathis and C. Benoist, "Deficiency of CXCR2, but Not Other Chemokine Receptors, Attenuates a Murine Model of Autoantibody-Mediated Arthritis," *Arthritis and Rheumatism*, Vol. 62, No. 7, 2010, pp. 1921-1932.

[20]   N. Nakamoto, H. Ebinum, T. Kanai, P. S. Chu, Y. Ono, Y. Mikami, K. Ojiro, M. Lipp, P. E. Love, H. Saito and T. Hibi, "CCR9($^+$) Macrophages Are Required for Acute Liver Inflammation in Mouse Models of Hepatitis," *Gastroenterology*, Vol. 142, No. 2, 2012, pp. 366-376. doi:10.1053/j.gastro.2011.10.039

[21]   B. Johansson-Lindbom and W. W. Agace, "Generation of Gut-Homing T Cells and Their Localization to the Small Intestinal Mucosa," *Immunological Reviews*, Vol. 215, 2007, pp. 226-242. doi:10.1111/j.1600-065X.2006.00482.x

[22]   K. A. Papadakis, J. Prehn, S. T. Moreno, L. Cheng, E. A. Kouroumalis, R. Deem, T. Breaverman, P. D. Ponath, D. P. Andrew, P. H. Green, M. R. Hodge, S. W. Binder and S. R. Targan, "CCR9-Positive Lymphocytes and Thymus-

Expressed Chemokine Distinguish Small Bowel from Colonic Crohn's Disease," *Gastroenterology*, Vol. 121, No. 2, 2001, pp. 246-254. doi:10.1053/gast.2001.27154

[23] C. Koenecke and R. Förster, "CCR9 and Inflammatory Bowel Disease," *Expert Opinion on Therapeutic Targets*, Vol. 13, No. 3, 2009, pp.297-306. doi:10.1517/14728220902762928

[24] M. Apostolaki, M. Manoloukos, M. Roulis, M. A. Wurbel, and W. Müller, "Role of $\beta7$ Integrin and the Chemokine/Chemokine Receptor Pair CCL25/CCR9 in Modelled TNF-Dependent Crohn's Disease," *Gastroentero-logy*, Vol. 134, No. 7, 2008, pp. 2025-2035. doi:10.1053/j.gastro.2008.02.085

[25] M. A. Wurbel, M. Malissen, D. Guy-Grand, E. Meffre, M. C. Nussenzweig, M. Richelme, A. Carrier and B. Malissen, "Mice Lacking the CCR9 CC-Chemokine Receptor Show a Mild Impairment of Early T- and B-Cell Development and a Reduction in T-Cell Receptor Gamma-delta($^+$) Gut Intraepithelial Lymphocytes," *Blood*, Vol. 98, No. 9, 2001, pp. 2626-2632. doi:10.1182/blood.V98.9.2626

32

The Relationship between Bone Mineral Density and Dietary Intake in Moroccan Children with Juvenile Idiopathic Arthritis

A. Hassani[1], S. Rostom[1], D. El Badri[1], I. Bouaadi[1], A. Barakat[2], B. Chkirat[2], K. Elkari[3], R. Bahiri[1], B. Amine[1], N. Hajjaj-Hassouni[1]

[1]Department of Rheumatology, El Eyachi Hospital, University Hospital of Rabat-Sale, Sale, Morocco; [2]Department of Pediatrics, Hospital of Children, University Hospital of Rabat-Sale, Rabat, Morocco; [3]Department of Nutrition, Faculty of Science of Kenitra, University Ibn Tofaïl, Kenitra, Morocco.
Email: hassaniasmae5@gmail.com

ABSTRACT

Background and Objective: The aim of this study was to evaluate the association between dietary intake and bone mineral density in children with juvenile idiopathic arthritis (JIA). **Methods:** A cross-sectional study carried out in Morocco between May 2010 and June 2011, covering out patients with JIA. The characteristics of patients were collected. The nutritional status was assessed by a food questionnaire including data of food intake during 7 consecutive days using 24-hour dietary recall. Food intake was quantified using the software Bilnut (Bilnut version 2.01, 1991). Bone mineral density (BMD in g/cm^2) was measured by DXA method (X-ray absorptiometry) on a Lunar Prodigy. **Results:** The study consisted of 33 patients with JIA (4 - 16 years old). The median age of patients was 10.4 ± 4.3 years. Median disease duration was 2 (1 - 4.5) years. The group of patients with low dietary intake of proteins was associated with low BMD (p = 0.03). Low BMD was related with low intake of magnesium (p = 0.007) and vitamin C (p = 0.04) in children aged between 4 and 9 years. Low intake of vitamin E and folate was associated with high BMD in the other range of children (p < 0.001). **Conclusion:** This study suggests that low intake of protein and of some micronutrients (magnesium, vitamin C, vitamin E and folate) influence bone mass in children with JIA. Prospective studies with a larger number of patients seem to be necessary in order to confirm our findings.

Keywords: Juvenile Idiopathic Arthritis; Macronutrients; Vitamins; Trace Elements; Bone Mineral Density

1. Background

Osteoporosis is currently estimated to be a major health threat [1]. It's defined by a disease characterized by loss of bone masse, accompanied by microarchitectural deterioration of bone tissue, which leads to an unacceptable increase in the risk of fracture [2]. About 90% of total adult mass is accrued by age 20, and a signification proportion of this is archived during puberty alone [3].

Juvenile idiopathic arthritis (AJI) is one of the commonest rheumatic diseases of children [4]. In one hand, several studies demonstrate reduced bone mineral density (BMD) in children with JIA [5,6]. In the other hand, JIA is often associated with poor nutritional status [7]. Nutrition is a key factor, not only for bone growth, but also for its mineralization [5]. The acquisition of adequate mineralization during childhood has proven to be a key event in the prevention of osteoporosis in adults [8]. Recent studies on various dietary components have shown that there is some correlation between their daily food intake and the genesis of osteoporosis and its fracture complications [9]. An inadequate nutrition (especially intake of macronutrients, trace elements and vitamins), can be associated with an increase in bone remodeling leading to significant loss of bone and an increase fracture risk [10]. There are few studies available in the literature assessing the relation sheep between dietary intake and bone mineral density in children. In addition, there are no studies in a Moroccan population that evaluate the same subject. The aim of this study was to assess the relationship between the dietary intake and bone mineral density in Moroccan children and adolescents with JIA.

2. Materials and Methods

2.1. Data Collection

It was a cross sectional study of children with JIA over a

---

*The authors declare that they have no conflicts of interest concerning this article.

period of 13 months (between May 2010 and June 2011) at the department of rheumatology of El Eyachi University hospital and department of pediatrics of university hospital of children of Rabat-Sale. Informed consent was obtained by parents from all subjects and the study was approved by ethics committee of our university hospital.

The diagnosis of JIA was based on the criteria of the International League of Association for Rheumatology (ILAR) [11]. Patients were recruited in consultation or during hospitalization. We excluded patients with any other chronic disease (endocrinal, neurological, cardiac, and renal) that affect bone metabolism. The disease and patients characteristics considered as explanatory measures were: age (year), gender, diagnosis (JIA subtype), disease duration (years), disease activity was assessed using a visual analogical scale (VAS), functional disability was determined by using the Moroccan version of Childhood Health Assessment Questionnaire (CHAQ) [12], number of tender joints, number of swollen joints and the erythrocyte sedimentation rate (ESR). Treatment with NSAIDs, corticosteroid and disease modifying antirheumatic drugs (DMARDs) was determined.

2.2. BMD Assessment

All BMD measurements were obtained with the same DXA instrument (Lunar Prodigy; GE Lunar, Madison, WI). BMD (g/cm²) was measured in the lumbar spine (L1-L4) and total body. The lumbar spine and the total body BMD values were transformed into Z scores by comparing them with age- and sex-specific reference values for this equipment [13,14]. According to the International Society for Clinical Densitometry recommendations osteoporosis was defined as a Z-score less than 2 with a fracture history. Low BMD was defined as a Z-score less than 2 without a significant fracture history [15].

2.3. Dietary Evaluation

Nutrient intake was determined using the 24 hour diet recall during 7 consecutive days [16]. The food questionnaire had two parts; the first identified all foods consumed during the day previous to the interview; the second part; specified food frequency to appreciate food eating habits. Two nutritionists analyzed the food dietary to quantify the food consumed from the recorded information. Nutrient intake was analyzed by software bilnut (Bilnut version 2.01, 1991), validated and standardized. The dietary intake of macro and micronutrients were assessed against the recommended dietary allowances (RDA) [17]. The analysis of micronutrients was made according to the age (group between 4 years and 9 years and group between 10 years to 16 years). We considered

that 50% to 60% as the appropriate percentage of calories from carbohydrates, between 10% and 15% the percentage related to proteins and between 25% to 30% the percentage of lipids [7].

2.4. Anthropometric Measures

Weight (kg) and height (m) were measured according to the recommendation of the World Health Organization (WHO). The results of the BMI (Kg/m²) were compared with reference values of Hammer et al. [18,19].

2.5. Statistics

Analysis was carried out using the statistical package for the social sciences (SPSS) version 16.0. Data for patients were presented as mean ± standard deviation or median (IQ) for continuous variables and as frequencies and percentage for categorical variables. For dietary intake of macronutrients, we are divided patients on 3 groups, low, normal and high dietary intake, and we used one way Anova test to compare values of BMD (g/cm²) between the 3 groups. As regards micronutrient intake, Student's t-test for independent samples was used to compare values of BMD (g/cm²) between two groups: with low and with normal dietary intake of micronutrients. Significance level was p value less than 0.05.

3. Results

Thirty three patients where included in this study. The mean age of our patients was 10.4 ± 4.35. 54.5% of our patients were males. The median disease duration was equal to 2 (1 - 4.5) years. Eleven patients (33.3%) had a low BMD in lumbar spine, and nine (27%) in total body, and no patient had an osteoporosis. Demographic and clinical characteristics of patients are described in **Table 1**.

We found that patients with JIA had an excessive intake of proteins, carbohydrates and lipids in 30.3%, 63.6% and 54.5% of the cases respectively. Moreover all patients had a low consumption of micronutrients.

Low intake of proteins was associated with a low BMD (p = 0.03) (**Table 2**). No difference was observed between dietary intake of glucids and lipids, and BMD (**Table 2**).

Daily mean intake of micronutrients show that low dietary intake of vitamin C was associated with an increase on BMD (p = 0.04) and low dietary intake of magnesium was associated with decreased BMD (p < 0.0001) in children aged between 4 and 9 years (**Table 3**). Low intake of vitamin E and folate was associated with increased BMD in children between 10 and 16 years (p < 0.001) (**Table 4**).

4. Discussion

In our study, we show that low dietary intake of proteins was associated to reduce bone density. It has been suggested that dietary protein intake may be a risk factor for

Table 1. Clinical characteristics of patients.

Characteristics AJI	(n = 33)
Age (year)[1]	10.45 ± 4.35
Sex males[2]	18 (54.5)
DAS28 ESR[1]	5.30 ± 1.10
Disease duration (year)[3]	2 [1 - 4.5]
Visual analogical scale (0 - 10)[3]	20 [10 - 50]
CHAQ score (0 - 3)[3]	0.5 [0 - 1.6]
JIA clinical subtypes[2]	
Oligoarticular	9 [27 - 3]
Polyarticular	16 [48 - 5]
Systemic	8 [24 - 2]
Nutritional status[2]	
Underweight	9 (27.3)
Normal	16 (48.5)
Obesity	8 (24.2)
BMD lumber spine (g/cm²)[3]	0.6 [0.1 - 1]
BMD total body (g/cm²)[3]	0.7 [0.3 - 1.1]
Z score lumber spine < –2[2]	11 (33.3)
Z score total body < –2[2]	9 (27.3)
NSAID[2] (yes)	26 (78.7)
DMARDs[2] (yes)	17 (51.6)
Oral corticosteroid[2] (yes)	14 (42.4)

DAS28 = disease activity score; CHAQ = Childhood Health Assessment Questionnaire; JIA = juvenile idiopathic arthritis; BMD = bone mineral density; NSAID = non-steroidal inflammatory drugs; DMARDs: Disease-Modifying Anti-Rheumatic Drugs. [1]Mean ± S.D.; [2]Number and percentage; [3]Median and IQR.

osteoporosis, especially in childhood, and high-protein diets are associated with increased bone loss [5]. Two mechanisms are discussed. The protein metabolism is accompanied by a significant production of amino acids that can promote osteoclast function and bone resumption. Also, protein intake may be involved indirectly in the genesis of osteoporosis by altering the metabolism of insulin like growth factor (IGF)-I [20,21].

Zhang Q. *et al.*, found that higher protein intake, especially from animal foods, appeared to have a negative effect on bone mass accrual in pubertal girls, which is different with our data [22]. In the study of Vatanparast H, they found that protein intake has a beneficial effect on bone mass of young adult females when calcium intake is adequate; protein, in the absence of sufficient calcium, does not confer as much benefit to bone [23]. In the longitudinal study including 560 women aged between 14 and 40 years, they suggest that a higher protein intake does not have an adverse effect on bone, and low intake on vegetal protein is associated with a less bone mass, [24].

Moreover, many scientists have examined the relationship between types of protein and urinary calcium excretion, and found that animal protein was associated with increased urinary calcium excretion, soy protein was not. There is sufficient evidence suggesting soy isoflavones may have potential benefits for bone, but a relationship has not been established between the consumption of ipriflavone and maintenance of bone mineral density [25].

These studies were conducted in healthy subjects, while our population is made of children with chronic inflammatory arthritis and who take corticosteroids which could lower their bone mineral density and subsequent can may explain our results.

In our study, we found that dietary intake of glucids and lipids were not associated with bone mass. Epidemi-

Table 2. Association between daily macronutrients intake and BMD in children with JIA.

BMD (g/cm²)		Lumber spine	p	Total body	p
Proteins (% of energy)	Low	0.510 ± 0.155		0.735 ± 0.049	
	Normal	0.833 ± 0.192	**0.03**	0.840 ± 0.134	0.2
	High	0.627 ± 0.230		0.246 ± 0.205	
Glucids (% of energy)	Low	0.619 ± 0.260		0.726 ± 0.179	
	Normal	0.714 ± 0.242	0.4	0.785 ± 0.239	0.4
	High	0.733 ± 0.193		0.826 ± 0.112	
Lipids (% of energy)	Low	0.723 ± 0.180		0.752 ± 0.179	
	Normal	0.710 ± 0.323	0.7	0.908 ± 0.202	0.2
	High	0.652 ± 0.245		0.749± 0.147	

BMD: bone mineral density; JIA: juvenile idiopathic arthritis. Values are the mean ± SD; p, descriptive level of one way Anova. Low dietary intake of proteins was associated with low BMD in lumber spine.

Table 3. Association between daily micronutrients intake and BMD in children with JIA aged between 4 and 9 years.

BMD (g/cm²)	Lumber spine	p	Total body	p
Calcium (mg)				
Low	0.552 ± 0.209	0.7	0.720 ± 0.068	0.2
Normal	0.600 ± 0.001		0.650 ± 0.070	
Phosphorus (mg)				
Low	0.574 ± 0.223	0.6	0.713 ± 0.085	0.8
Normal	0.522 ± 0.093		0.705 ± 0.010	
Magnesium (mg)				
Low	0.100 ± 0.000	**0.007**	0.700 ± 0.000	0.8
Normal	0.594 ± 0.146		0.711 ± 0.073	
Fer (mg)				
Low	0.563 ± 0.234	0.9	0.725 ± 0.079	0.3
Normal	0.552 ± 0.104		0.684 ± 0.047	
Zinc (mg)				
Low	0.587 ± 0.261	0.6	0.727 ± 0.091	0.4
Normal	0.531 ± 0.103		0.694 ± 0.044	
Vitamin B1 (mg)				
Low	0.574 ± 0.223	0.6	0.723 ± 0.075	0.3
Normal	0.522 ± 0.093		0.680 ± 0.054	
Vitamin C (mg)				
Low	0.562 ± 0.234	0.9	0.738 ± 0.064	**0.04**
Normal	0.530 ± 0.100		0.634 ± 0.052	
Vitamin E (mg)				
Low	0.563 ± 0.200	0.7	0.711 ± 0.073	0.8
Normal	0.500 ± 0.001		0.700 ± 0.001	
Folate (µg)				
Low	0.560 ± 0.208	0.9	0.720 ± 0.068	0.2
Normal	0.550 ± 0.070		0.650 ± 0.070	

BMD: bone mineral density; JIA: juvenile idiopathic arthritis. Values are the mean ± SD; p, descriptive level of Student's t-test. Low intake of magnesium and vitamin C was associated with decreased BMD in lumber spine, and increased BMD in total body respectively.

Table 4. Association between daily micronutrients intake and BMD in children with JIA aged between 10 and 16 years.

BMD (g/cm²)	Lumber spine	p	Total body	p
Calcium (mg)				
Low	0.805 ± 0.250	0.9	0.761 ± 0.229	0.5
Normal	0.800 ± 0.001		0.900 ± 0.001	
Phosphorus (mg)				
Low	0.805 ± 0.250	0.9	0.761 ± 0.229	0.5
Normal	0.800 ± 0.001		0.900 ± 0.001	
Magnesium (mg)				
Low	0.773 ± 0.245	0.2	0.753 ± 0.241	0.4
Normal	0.973 ± 0.180		0.876 ± 0.040	
Fer (mg)				
Low	0.784 ± 0.241	0.3	0.758 ± 0.234	0.4
Normal	0.980 ± 0.254		0.900 ± 0.001	
Zinc (mg)				
Low	0.773 ± 0.245	0.2	0.753 ± 0.241	0.4
Normal	0.973±0.180		0.876 ± 0.040	
Vitamin B1 (mg)				
Low	0.805 ± 0.250	0.6	0.766 ± 0.229	0.8
Normal	0.800 ± 0.001		0.900 ± 0.001	
Vitamin C (mg)				
Low	0.829 ± 0.222	0.2	0.789 ± 0.228	0.3
Normal	0.600 ± 0.424		0.630 ± 0.190	
Vitamin E (mg)				
Low	0.805 ± 0.243	**<0.001**	0.761 ± 0.229	**<0.001**
Normal	0.500 ± 0.001		0.600 ± 0.001	
Folate (µg)				
Low	0.805 ± 0.243	**<0.001**	0.789 ± 0.228	**<0.001**
Normal	0.500 ± 0.001		0.600 ± 0.001	

BMD: bone mineral density; JIA: juvenile idiopathic arthritis. Values are the mean ± SD; p, descriptive level of Student's t-test. Low dietary intake of vitamin E and folats was associated with high BMD in both lumber spine and total body.

ological data indicate that high-fat diets, especially those rich in saturated fatty acids, may contribute to reduced bone density and increased fracture risk, in older as well as younger people [26]. One other study that assessed the relation of dietary fat to hip bone mineral density (BMD) in men and women indicated that BMD is negatively associated with saturated fat intake [27]. Several studies have shown the importance of individual fatty acids in enterocyte membrane dynamics, Vitamin D3 activity, and prostaglandin formation, which can have important effects on intestinal calcium absorption as well as urinary calcium excretion [28]. Also, dietary lipids can influence GH and osteoblast formation [21].

In their study, Rubinacci A. *et al.*, show the presence of positive relationships between bone mineral content (BMC) and lipid intakes in the population of women in early menopause, but they have no association between glucids intakes and BMC [29]. In animal study, it has been demonstrated in a group of rats with a diet rich on fructo-oligosaccharides decreased content bone on calcium and phosphorus and resistance bone, compared to a control group [30]. But these results are contradictory with data of other studies.

Regarding the dietary intake of micronutrients, our results show that low intake of magnesium is related with a low bone mineral density. Rude *et al.* tested the effects of deficient diets on bone tissue in rats [31]. The results showed the histology decreased trabecular bone volume, increased osteoclast activity without activation of osteoblasts and biologically hypercalcemia, a decrease in serum parathyroid hormone (PTH) and 1, 25 (OH) vitamin D. Thus, the Mg depletion would lead to bone resorption uncoupled could exert inhibitory effect on PTH. In the data of the literature, small epidemiologic studies suggest that an excessive magnesium intake was associated with higher BMD in elderly men and women [32,33]. In clinical trials of magnesium supplementation, there is a little evidence that magnesium is essential to prevent osteoporosis in the general population [34,35]. Also, one recent study from the WHI suggested that higher intakes of magnesium were associated with a risk of wrist fracture [36].

Vitamin C is an essential cofactor for collagen formation and synthesis of hydroxyproline and hydroxylysine. A several studies show a positive association between vitamin C and bone mass. Low intakes of vitamin C are associated with loss of BMD [37,38]. Celia J. Prynne *et al.*, explored the association between bone mineral status and fruit and vegetable intakes in adolescent boys and girls (aged 16 - 18 y), young women (aged 23 - 37 y), and older men and women (aged 60 - 83 y). In boys, significant positive associations were found between dietary vitamin C and BMC and BMD. No significant univariate

association was found in the girls, and a significant negative association with BMD was found in the older women [39]. One study found that higher intake on vitamin C was associated with fewer fractures; however, there are no randomized clinical trials, [40]. In our study, we found a significant association between low intake of vitamin C and increased bone mineral density, which is contradictory with the literature data.

In our data, we showed a negative association between intake of vitamin E and BMD. In a Japanese study including 441 women aged 20 to 35 years, they found that increased vitamin E intake was associated with greater total spine BMD [41]. Farrell V. A. *et al.* showed that dietary vitamin E intake did not have any similar BMD association [42].

Folate, vitamin B2 (riboflavin), and vitamin B12 may affect bone directly or through an effect on plasma homocysteine levels [43]. In the current study, decreased intake of folate was associated with high BMD. In a study of Rejnmark L. *et al.*, they found that high dietary intake of folate exerts positive effects on BMD [31]. Also, Rivas A. *et al.* showed that the BMD was signifycantly associated with the intake of folate [44].

There was no association between BMD and the other micronutrients.

Our study is limited by its cross-sectional design, sample size and non-controlled design, but identification of relationship between nutrition and bone status it so important and especially in children with rheumatoid arthritis like juvenile idiopathic arthritis. Thus, more research on the role of diet on bone health is required. In addition, more emphasis should be placed on understanding the role of diet and nutrition on bone health during childhood and adolescence.

5. Conclusion

This study showed that in children with JIA, adequate dietary intake of proteins and magnesium can have a beneficial effect on the bone mass; low dietary intake of vitamin C, vitamin E and folate exerts positive effects on BMD; but further studies are needed to confirm this association.

REFERENCES

[1] America's Bone Health, "The State of Osteoporosis and Low Bone Mass in Our Nation," *A Report of the National Osteoporosis Foundation*, 2002.

[2] J. E. McDonagh, "Osteoporosis in Juvenile Idiopathic Arthritis," *Current Opinion in Rheumatology*, Vol. 13, No. 5, 2001, pp. 399-404. doi:10.1097/00002281-200109000-00010

[3] K. D. Cashman, "Calcium Intake, Calcium Bioavailability

and Bone Health," *British Journal of Nutrition*, Vol. 87, No. S2, 2002, pp. S169-S177.
doi:10.1079/BJN/2002534

[4]   J. T. Cassidy and R. E. Petty, "Chronic Arthritis in Childhood," In: J. T. Cassidy and R. E. Petty, Eds., *Textbook of Pediatric Rheumatology*, 5th Edition, Elsevier Saunders, Philadelphia, 2005, pp. 206-260.
doi:10.1016/B978-1-4160-0246-8.50015-2

[5]   M. A. Franch, M. P. Redondo Del Rıo, L. S. Cortina, "Nutricion Infantily Saludosea," *Anales de Pediatría*, Vol. 72, No. 1, 2010, pp. 80.e1-80.e11.

[6]   C. E. Rabinovich, "Bone Mineral Status in Juvenile Rheumatoid Arthritis," *Journal of Rheumatology*, Vol. 27, No. Suppl 58, 2000, pp. 34-38.

[7]   M. C. Caetano, T. T. Ortiz, M. T. Terreri, *et al.*, "Inadequate Dietary Intake of Children and Adolescents with Juvenile Idiopathic Arthritis and Systemic Lupus Erythematosus," *Journal of Pediatrics*, Vol. 85, No. 6, 2009, pp. 509-515. doi:10.1590/S0021-75572009000600007

[8]   M. Romera and L. Serra, "Nutricion y Osteoporosis," In: L. L. Serra, *et al.*, Eds., Nutricion y Salud Publica, Masson, 1995, pp. 269-275.

[9]   K. Michaelsson, L. Holmberg, H. Mallmin, *et al.*, "Diet and Hip Fracture Risk: A Case-Control Study. Study Group of the Multiple Risk Survey on Swedish Women for Eating Assessment," *International Journal of Epidemiology*, Vol. 24, No. 4, 1995, pp. 771-782.

[10] J. W. Nieves, "Nutrition and Osteoporosis," In: S. Cummings, F. Cosman and S. Jamal, Eds., *Osteoporosis: An Evidence Based Approach to the Prevention and Management*, American College of Physicians, Philadelphia, 2002.

[11] R. E. Petty, *et al.*, "International League of Associations for Rheumatology Classification of Juvenile Idiopathic Arthritis," *Journal of Rheumatology*, Vol. 31, No. 2, 2004, pp. 390-392.

[12] S. Rostom, B. Amine, R. Bensabbah, *et al.*, "Psychometric Properties Evaluation of the Childhood Health Assessment Questionnaire (CHAQ) in Moroccan Juvenile Idiopathic Arthritis," *Rheumatology International*, Vol. 30, No. 7, 2010, pp. 879-885.
doi:10.1007/s00296-009-1069-2

[13] W. Wacker and H. S. Barden, "Pediatric Reference Data for Male and Female Total Body and Spine BMD and BMC," *Meeting of the International Society of Clinical Densitometry*, Denver, 20-22 July 2001.

[14] G. S. Bhudhikanok, M. C. Wang, K. Eckert, *et al.*, "Differences in Bone Mineral in Young Asian and Caucasian Americans May Reflect Differences in Bone Size," *Journal of Bone and Mineral Research*, Vol. 11, No. 10, 1996, pp. 1545-1556.
doi:10.1002/jbmr.5650111023

[15] E. M. Lewiecki, C. M. Gordon, S. Baim, *et al.*, "International Society for Clinical Densitometry 2007 Adult and Pediatric Official Positions," *Bone*, Vol. 43, No. 6, 2008, pp. 1115-1121. doi:10.1016/j.bone.2008.08.106

[16] K. El Kari, L. Borghos, N. Benajiba, *et al.*, "Daily Vitamin A Intake and Nutritional Disorders in Preschool Children: Case of the Northwest Area of Morocco," *Report of the 22nd International Vitamin A Consultative Group Meeting*, Vol. T38, 2004, p. 54

[17] G. Nantel and K. Tontisirin, "Human Vitamin and Mineral Requirements. Report of a Joint FAO/WHO Expert Consultation Food and Nutrition Division 2001," 2011. http://www.fao.org/es/esn/vitrni/vitrni.html.FAO/WHO

[18] D. L. Hammer, H. C. Kraemer, D. M. Wilson, *et al.*, "Standardized Percentile Curves of Body-Mass-Index for Children and Adolescents," *American Journal of Clinical Nutrition*, Vol. 145, 1991, pp. 259-263.

[19] D. M. A. Chaud, M. O. E. Hilário, G. Yanaguibashi and O. M. S. Amancio, "Avaliações Dietética e Antropométrica em Pacientes com Artrite Reumatóide Juvenil," *Revista da Associação Médica Brasileira*, Vol. 49, No. 2, 2003.

[20] G. Geinoz, C. H. Rapin, R. Rizzoli, *et al.*, "Relationship between Bone Mineral Density and Dietary Intakes in the Elderly," *Osteoporosis International*, Vol. 3, No. 5, 1993, pp. 242-248. doi:10.1007/BF01623827

[21] M. Sarazin1, C. Alexandre and T. Thomas, "Influence on Bone Metabolism of Dietary Trace Elements, Protein, Fat, Carbohydrates, and Vitamins," *Joint Bone Spine*, Vol. 67, No. 5, 2000, pp. 408-418.

[22] Q. Zhang, G. Ma, H. Greenfield, *et al.*, "The Association between Dietary Protein Intake and Bone Mass Accretion in Pubertal Girls with Low Calcium Intakes," *British Journal of Nutrition*, Vol. 103, No. 5, 2010, pp. 714-723.
doi:10.1017/S0007114509992303

[23] H. Vatanparast, D. A. Bailey, A. D. Baxter-Jones, *et al.*, "The Effects of Dietary Protein on Bone Mineral Mass in Young Adults May Be Modulated by Adolescent Calcium Intake," *Journal of Nutrition*, Vol. 137, No. 12, 2007, pp. 2674-2679.

[24] J. M. Beasley, L. E. Ichikawa, B. A. Ange, *et al.*, "Is protein Intake Associated with Bone Mineral Density in Young Women? Scholes," *American Journal of Clinical Nutrition*, Vol. 91, No. 5, 2010, pp. 1311-1316.
doi:10.3945/ajcn.2009.28728

[25] S. Bawa, "The Significance of Soy Protein and Soy Bioactive Compounds in the Prophylaxis and Treatment of Osteoporosis," *Journal of Osteoporosis*, 2010, Article ID 891058. doi:10.4061/2010/891058

[26] R. L. Corwin, "Effects of Dietary Fats on Bone Health in Advanced Age," *Prostaglandins, Leukotrienes and Essential Fatty Acids*, Vol. 68, No. 6, 2003, pp. 379-386.
doi:10.1016/S0952-3278(03)00062-0

[27] R. L. Corwin, T. J. Hartman, S. A. Maczuga, *et al.*, "Dietary Saturated Fat Intake Is Inversely Associated with Bone Density in Humans: Analysis of NHANES III," *Journal of Nutrition*, Vol. 136, No. 1, 2006, pp. 159-165.

[28] M. C. Kruger and D. F. Horrobin, "Calcium Metabolism, Osteoporosis and Essential Fatty Acids: A Review," *Progress in Lipid Research*, Vol. 36, 1997, pp. 131-151.
doi:10.1016/S0163-7827(97)00007-6

[29] A. Rubinacci, M. Porrini, P. Sirtori, *et al.*, "Nutrients,

Anthropometric Characteristics and Osteoporosis in Women in the Recent and Late Postmenopausal Period," *Minerva Medica*, Vol. 83, No. 9, 1992, pp. 497-506

[30] L. Tjäderhane and M. Larmas, "A High Sucrose Diet Decreases the Mechanical Strength of Bones in Growing Rats," *Journal of Nutrition*, Vol. 128, No. 10, 1998, pp. 1807-1810.

[31] R. K. Rude, M. E. Kirchen, H. E. Gruber, *et al.*, "Magnesium Deficiency Induces Bone Loss in the Rat," *Mineral and Electrolyte Metabolism*, Vol. 24, No. 5, 1998, pp. 314-320. doi:10.1159/000057389

[32] J. W. Nieves, "Osteoporosis: The Role of Micronutrients 1-4," *American Journal of Clinical Nutrition*, Vol. 81, 2005, pp. 1232S-1239S

[33] K. L. Tucker, M. T. Hannan, H. Chen, *et al.*, "Potassium, Magnesium, and Fruit and Vegetable Intakes Are Associated with Greater Bone Mineral Density in Elderly Men and Women," *American Journal of Clinical Nutrition*, Vol. 69, No. 4, 1999, pp. 727-736.

[34] F. H. Nielsen, "Studies on the Relationship between Boron and Magnesium Which Possibly Affects the Formation and Maintenance of Bones," *MagTr Elementary*, Vol. 9, 1990, pp. 61-69.

[35] G. Stendig-Lindberg, R. Tepper and I. Leichter, "Trabecular Bone Density in a Two Year Controlled Trial of Peroral Magnesium in Osteoporosis," *Magnesium Research*, Vol. 6, 1993, pp. 155-163.

[36] R. D. Jackson, T. Bassford, J. Cauley, *et al.*, "The Impact of Magnesium Intake on Fractures: Results from the Women's Health Initiative Observational Study (WHI-OS)," ASBMR, 2003.

[37] L. M. Odaland, R. L. Mason and A. I. Alexeff, "Bone Density and Dietary Findings of 409 Tennessee Subject. I. Bone Density Considerations," *American Journal of Clinical Nutrition*, Vol. 25, 1972, pp. 905-907.

[38] S. G. Leveille, A. Z. LaCroix, T. D. Koepsell, *et al.*, "Dietary Vitamin C and Bone Mineral Density in Postmenopausal Women in Washington State, USA," *Journal of Epidemiology & Community Health*, Vol. 51, No. 5, 1997, pp. 479-485. doi:10.1136/jech.51.5.479

[39] C. J. Prynne, G. D. Mishra, M. A. O'Connell, *et al.*, "Fruit and Vegetable Intakes and Bone Mineral Status: A Cross-Sectional Study in 5 Age and Sex Cohorts," *Journal of Clinical Nutrition*, Vol. 83, 2006, pp. 1420-1428

[40] S. Kaptoge, A. Welch, A. McTaggart, *et al.*, "Effects of Dietary Nutrients and Food Groups on Bone Loss from the Proximal Femur in Men and Women in the 7th and 8th Decades of Age," *Osteoporosis International*, Vol. 14, No. 5, 2003, pp. 418-428. doi:10.1007/s00198-003-1391-6

[41] R. Chan, J. Woo, W. Lau, J. Leung, *et al.*, "Effects of Lifestyle and Diet on Bone Health in Young Adult Chinese Women Living in Hong Kong and Beijing," *Food and Nutrition Bulletin*, Vol. 30, No. 4, 2009, pp. 370-378.

[42] V. A. Farrell, M. Harris and T. G. Lohman, *et al.*, "Comparison between Dietary Assessment Methods for Determining Associations between Nutrient Intakes and Bone Mineral Density in Postmenopausal Women," *Journal of the American Dietetic Association*, Vol. 109, No. 5, 2009, pp. 899-904. doi:10.1016/j.jada.2009.02.008

[43] L. Rejnmark, P. Vestergaard, A. P. Hermann, *et al.*, "Dietary Intake of Folate, but Not Vitamin B2 or B12, Is Associated with Increased Bone Mineral Density 5 Years after the Menopause: Results from a 10-Year Follow-Up Study in Early Postmenopausal Women," *Calcified Tissue International*, Vol. 82, No. 1, 2008, pp. 1-11. doi:10.1007/s00223-007-9087-0

[44] A. Rivas1, A. Romero, M. Mariscal, *et al.*, "Validation of Questionnaires for the Study of Food Habits and Bone Mass," *Nutricion Hospitalaria*, Vol. 24, No. 5 2009, pp. 521-528.

Permissions

List of Contributors

Ramanjaneya V. R. Mula and Rangaiah Shashidharamurthy
Department of Pharmaceutical Sciences, Philadelphia College of Osteopathic Medicine, School of Pharmacy, Suwanee, USA

Ethelina Cargnelutti and María Silvia Di Genaro
Division of Immunology, Faculty of Chemistry, Biochemistry and Pharmacy, National University of San Luis, San Luis, Argentina
Laboratory of Immunopathology, Multidisciplinary Institute of Biological Investigations-San Luis (IMIBIO-SL), National Council of Scientific and Technical Investigations (CONICET), San Luis, Argentina

Tapas Kumar Sabui
Department of Pediatrics & Neonatology, Institute of Post Graduate Medical Education & Research, Kolkata, India

Syamal Sardar
Department of Neonatology, Institute of Post Graduate Medical Education & Research, Kolkata, India

Sumanta Laha
Department of Pediatrics, Burdwan Medical College & Hospital, Burdwan, India

Abhishek Roy
Department of Pediatrics, North Bengal Medical College & Hospital, Darjeeling, India

Maria J. H. de Hair, Marleen G. H. van de Sande , Danielle M. Gerlag and Paul P. Tak
Department of Clinical Immunology and Rheumatology, Academic Medical Center, University of Amsterdam, Amsterdam, The Netherlands

Mario Maas
Department of Radiology, Academic Medical Center, University of Amsterdam, Amsterdam, The Netherlands

Işıl Eser Şimşek, Müferet Ergüven and Olcay Bilgiç Dağcı
Göztepe Teaching and Research Hospital, Istanbul, Turkey

Andrew J. Sarkin , Rachel S. Lale and Kyle J. Choi
Health Services Research Center, University of California, San Diego, USA

Ari Gnanasakthy
Novartis Pharmaceuticals Corporation, East Hanover, USA

Jan D. Hirsch
Skaggs School of Pharmacy and Pharmaceutical Sciences, University of California, San Diego, USA

Daniel Jaramillo-Arroyave, Gerardo Quintana, Federico Rondon-Herrera and Antonio Iglesias-Gamarra
Internal Medicine, Rheumatology, Department of Internal Medicine, Rheumatology Unit, Universidad Nacional de Colombia, Bo- gotá, Colombia

Maria Giovanna Colella, Giuseppe Buttaro, Lucia Masi, Elena Palma and Raffaele Amelio
Pediatric Unit, "Dono Svizzero" Hospital, Formia, Italy

Alexander Vallone
Faculty of Medicine and Surgery, Università Cattolica, Rome, Italy

SaharAbou El-Fetou
Department of Clinical Pathology, Faculty of Medicine, Sohag University, Sohag, Egypt

Hanan S. Abozaid
Department of Rheumatology and Reha- bilitation, Faculty of Medicine, Sohag University, Sohag, Egypt

Mario Pérez , Ruben Asencio, Adolfo Camargo, Heladia Garcia, Miguel Angel Vazquez and Leonor Barile-Fabris
UMAE Specialty Hospital "Bernardo Sepulveda" CMNSXXI, IMSS, Mexico City, Mexico

Raul Ariza
Hospital Angeles del Pedregal, Mexico City, Mexico

Ikpeme A. Ikpeme and Ngim E. Ngim
Department of Surgery, University of Calabar Teaching Hospital, Calabar, Nigeria

Anthonia A. Ikpeme
Department of Radiology, University of Cala-bar Teaching Hospital, Calabar, Nigeria

Afiong O. Oku
Department of Community Medicine, University of Calabar Teaching Hospital, Calabar, Nigeria

Muhammad Ayaz Alam Qureshi and Jian Li
Department of Molecular Medicine and Surgery, Karolinska University Hospital, Karolinska Institutet, Stockholm, Sweden

Aisha Siddiqah Ahmed
Department of Clinical Neurosciences, Karolinska Institutet, Stockholm, Sweden

André Stark
Department of Clinical Sciences, Danderyd Hospital, Karolinska Institutet, Stockholm, Sweden;

Per Eriksson
Department of Medicine, Karolinska University Hospital, Karolinska Institutet, Stockholm, Sweden;

Mahmood Ahmed
Department of Neurobiology, Care Sciences and Society, Karolinska Institutet, Stockholm, Sweden

Eric L. Matteson
Division of Rheumatology, Rochester, USA
Department of Health Sciences Research, Rochester, USA

Tim Bongartz
Division of Rheumatology, Rochester, USA

Cynthia S. Crowson
Department of Health Sciences Research, Rochester, USA

Jay H. Ryu
Division of Pulmonary and Critical Care Medicine, Rochester, USA

Thomas E. Hartman
Department of Radiology, Mayo Clinic College of Medicine, Rochester, USA

Paul F. Dellaripa
Division of Rheumatology, Brigham and Womens Hospital, Boston, USA

Bernard Ng
Houston Veterans Affairs HSR&D Center of Excellence, Michael E. DeBakey Veterans Affairs Medical Center, Houston, USA
Department of Medicine, Baylor College of Medicine, Houston, USA

Antigone Delantoni
Department of Dentoalveolar Surgery, Implant Surgery and Radiology, Faculty of Dentistry, Aristotle University of Thessaloniki, Thessaloniki, Greece

Marta Olivieri, Maria Chiara Gerardi, Francesca Romana Spinelli and Manuela Di Franco
Rheumatology Unit, Department of Internal Medicine and Medical Specialities, Sapienza University of Rome, Rome, Italy

Christine Beyeler
Institute of Medical Education, Department of Rheumatology, Clinical Immunology and Allergology, University Hospital of Berne, Berne, Switzerland

Bernhard Dick and Brigitte M. Frey
Departments of Nephrology and Hypertension and Clinical Research, University Hospital of Berne, Berne, Switzerland

Howard A. Bird
Academic Department of Musculoskeletal Medicine, University of Leeds, Leeds, UK

Helena Lööf and Unn-Britt Johansson
Sophiahemmet University, Stockholm, Sweden
Karolinska Institutet, Department of Clinical Sciences, Danderyd Hospital, Division of Medicine, Stockholm, Sweden

Elisabet Welin Henriksson
Karolinska Institutet, Division of Nursing, Department of Neurobiology and Rheumatology Unit, Karolinska Hospital, Stockholm, Sweden

Staffan Lindblad
Karolinska Institutet, Department of Learning Informatics, Management and Ethics, Stockholm, Sweden

Fredrik Saboonchi
Karolinska Institutet, Department of Clinical Sciences, Danderyd Hospital, Division of Medicine, Stockholm, Sweden
Karolinska Institutet, Department of Neuroscience, Division of Insurance Medicine, Stockholm, Sweden
University of Stockholm, Stress Research Institute, Stockholm, Sweden
Red Cross University College, Stockholm, Sweden

Janet Pope
Schulich School of Medicine & Dentistry, University of Western Ontario, London, Canada
St. Joseph's Health Care, London, Canada

Bernard Combe
Department of Rheumatology, Lapeyronie Hospital, CHU Montpellier, Montpellier 1 University, Montpellier, France

Kanako Watanabe, Hiromi Sato, Ayano Ito, Tomomi Sato, Hana Sugai and Koichi Ueno
Department of Geriatric Pharmacology and Therapeutics, Graduate School of Pharmaceutical Sciences, Chiba University, Chiba, Japan

Aránzazu González-Canga
Assessment Area, Medicines for Veterinary Use Department, Agencia Española de Medicamentosy Productos Sanitarios (AEMPS), Madrid, Spain

Masahiko Suzuki
Research Center for Frontier Medical Engineering, Chiba University, Chiba, Japan

Takao Namiki
Department of Frontier Japanese-Oriental (Kampo) Medicine, Graduate School of Medicine, Chiba University, Chiba, Japan

Mariana Trivilin Mendes
Laboratory of Pharmacology, Unit of Translational Endocrine Physiology and Pharmacology, Instituto Butantan, São Paulo, Brazil
Department of Physiology, Instituto de Biociências, Universidade de São Paulo, São Paulo, Brazil

Paulo Flavio Silveira
Laboratory of Pharmacology, Unit of Translational Endocrine Physiology and Pharmacology, Instituto Butantan, São Paulo, Brazil

Mark Kosinski and Jakob B. Bjorner
Quality Metric Incorporated, Lincoln, Rhode Island

Ari Gnanasakthy and Usha Mallya
Novartis Pharmaceuticals Corporation, East Hanover, USA

Shephard Mpofu
Novartis Pharma AG, Basel, Switzerland

Owonayo Oniankitan, Prénam Houzou, Komi C. Tagbor, Eryam Fianyo, Viwalé E. S. Koffi-Tessio, Kodjo Kakpovi and Moustafa Mijiyawa
Department of Rheumatology, CHU Sylvanus Olympio, Lomé, Togo

Tatiana Reitblat, Lea Djin and Galina Reifman
Rheumatology, Barsilai Medical Center, Ashkelon, Israel

Zeev Weiler and Nelly Polyakov
Pulmonology, Barsilai Medical Center, Ashkelon, Israel

Alexander Reitblat
Medical Physics, Barsilai Medical Center, Ashkelon, Israel

Julia F. Simard
Department of Epidemiology, Harvard School of Public Health, Boston, USA
Clinical Epidemiology Unit, Karolinska Institutet, Stockholm, Sweden

Murray A. Mittleman
Department of Epidemiology, Harvard School of Public Health, Boston, USA

Nancy A. Shadick and Elizabeth W. Karlson
Department of Medicine, Division of Rheumatology, Immunology, and Allergy, Brigham and Women's Hospital, Boston, USA

Berit Grandaunet
KG Jebsen Center for Myeloma Research and Department of Cancer Research and Molecular Medicine, Norwegian University of Science and Technology, Trondheim, Norway

Silje Watterdal Syversen and Tore K. Kvien
Department of Rheumatology, Diakonhjemmet Hospital, Oslo, Norway

Mari Hoff
Depart- ment of Neuroscience, Norwegian University of Science and Technology, Trondheim, Norway
Department of Rheumatology, St. Olavs Hospital, Trondheim, Norway

Glenn Haugeberg
Depart- ment of Neuroscience, Norwegian University of Science and Technology, Trondheim, Norway
Department of Rheumatology, Sørlandet Hospital, Kristiansand, Norway

Désirée van der Heijde
Department of Rhe- umatology, Leiden University Medical Centre, Leiden, The Netherlands

Therese Standal
KG Jebsen Center for Myeloma Research and Department of Cancer Research and Molecular Medicine, Norwegian University of Science and Technology, Trondheim, Norway
Centre of Excellence for Molecular Inflammation Resear

Jason J. Lee
Schulich School of Medicine, Western University, London, Canada

Janet E. Pope
Schulich School of Medicine, Western University, St. Joseph's Health Care, London, Canada

Atsushi Kawase, Syoko Wada and Masahiro Iwaki
Department of Pharmacy, School of Pharmacy, Kinki University, Osaka, Japan

Hajime Yamanaka, Kenichiro Goto and Munetaka Suzuki
Department of Orthopaedic Surgery, National Hospital Organization Shimoshizu Hospital, Yotsukaido City, Japan

Tamborenea Maria Natalia, Silvia Moyano Caturelli, Jackeline Spengler and Grisel Olivera Roulet
Servicio Nacional de Rehabilitación (SNR), Buenos Aires, Argentina

Alison Cartwright and Oksana Kehoe
Keele University at Robert Jones and Agnes Hunt Orthopaedic Hospital, Oswestry, UK

Sophie King
Faculty of Medicine and Dentistry, School of Oral and Dental Sciences, University of Bristol, Bristol, UK

Jim Middleton
Keele University at Robert Jones and Agnes Hunt Orthopaedic Hospital, Oswestry, UK
Faculty of Medicine and Dentistry, School of Oral and Dental Sciences, University of Bristol, Bristol, UK

A. Hassani, S. Rostom, D. El Badri, I. Bouaadi, R. Bahiri, B. Amine and N. Hajjaj-Hassouni
Department of Rheumatology, El Eyachi Hospital, University Hospital of Rabat-Sale, Sale, Morocco

A. Barakat and B. Chkirat
Department of Pediatrics, Hospital of Children, University Hospital of Rabat-Sale, Rabat, Morocco

K. Elkari
Department of Nutrition, Faculty of Science of Kenitra, University Ibn Tofaïl, Kenitra, Morocco

Printed in the USA
CPSIA information can be obtained
at www.ICGtesting.com
JSHW052021301024
72690JS00004B/124

9 781632 39772